CASSELL DICTIONARY OF SEX QUOTATIONS

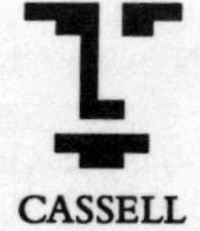

Compiled and Typeset by Market House Books

Commentary and Selection by Alan Isaacs

Assisted by an editorial team consisting of:

Jonathan Law
Elizabeth Martin
Anne Stibbs
Fran Alexander
Mark Salad
Amanda Isaacs

and a research team consisting of:

Mark Salad
Rupert Ward
David Parkinson
Ruth Salomon

Cassell
Wellington House
125 Strand
London
WC2R 0BB

First published as *Sex and Sexuality*, 1993; published under the title *Cassell Dictionary of Sex Quotations*, 1997

British Library Cataloguing-in-Publication Data
A catalogue entry for this book is available
from the British Library

ISBN 0 304 34939 9

Printed and bound in Great Britain by
MacKays of Chatham Ltd, Chatham, Kent

Contents

Preface

It is a pity that sex is such an ugly little word
D.H. Lawrence 'Sex versus Loveliness' (1930)

Ugly little word or not, it stands for something that almost everyone likes to do, think back on, and look forward to.

Sometimes the things people write or say on this subject are sharp or funny, sometimes they are quite silly; they always provide an interest and very occasionally titillate or even amaze.

The period covered by this book is roughly the whole of human history. Many writers, thinkers, moralists, and people in public life have commented quotably at one time or another on some aspect of love, sex, or marriage. And in these mass-media days men and women in the streets have often found their comments recorded too. A selection of what the famous and infamous, as well as the unknown, have said on the subject is presented here.

The quotations are arranged under some 50 headings and linked by a commentary. This was originally intended to provide a modest framework for other people's *bon mots.* From time to time, however, the commentary has emerged from the shadows to make a point or decry an injustice. Perhaps this is inevitable with a subject on which so many of us regard ourselves as world experts!

AI 1993

Abortion

The problem can be stated simply: 'Which is worse, an unwanted child or an abortion?' The antecedent events leading to the situation in which this decision has to be made are irrelevant. Only the future of the child and its parents are important. Perhaps the unwanted child will come to be loved by its parents and given a chance to build a useful life. Perhaps it will be denied love; perhaps a decision not to abort the fetus will result in a childhood and subsequent life of misery, pain, and deprivation. The problem is not new.

Abortion...this insoluble problem. I say insoluble because it has bothered mankind for at least 2500 years.

Aleck Bourne 'The Abortion Act' (a symposium held in 1966)

The number of children allowed to each marriage shall be regulated by the state, and...if any woman be pregnant after she has produced the prescribed number, an abortion shall be procured before the fetus has life.

Aristotle *Politics* (4th century BC)

Abortion does not seem the kind of moral issue which is just 'solved' once and for all; it can only be coped with.

D. Callahan *Abortion: Law, Choice and Morality* (1972)

The central question in the abortion issue is not whether fetuses are human, but whether all human beings, including fetuses, have the same moral status.

L. W. Sumner *Times Literary Supplement* (1981)

Historically, the law and the Church have seen fit to make their judgments, not on the effects on the child or its parents, but on abstract principles of one sort or another:

[The Law] *orders all the offspring to be brought up and forbids women either to cause abortion or to make away with the fetus; a woman convicted of this is regarded as an infanticide because she destroys a soul and diminishes the race.*

Flavius Josephus *Contra Apionem* (1st century AD)

It was as part of its comprehensive attempt to make the sexual act as difficult as possible that the Church devised laws against the practice of abortion. Neither Romans, Jews nor Greeks had opposed abortion, but Tertullian, following an inaccurate translation of Exodus XXI.22, which refers to punishing a man who injures a pregnant woman, but which appeared to prescribe punishment for injuring the fetus, gave currency to the idea that the Bible held abortion to be a crime.

Gordon Rattray Taylor *Sex in History* (1953)

But to us [Christians], *to whom murder has once and for all been forbidden, it is unlawful even to destroy the fetus in the womb whilst the blood is still forming into a human being. Prevention of birth is premature murder...That also is a human being, which is about to become one, just as every fruit exists already in the seed.*

Tertullian *Apology* (198)

A woman who deliberately destroys a fetus is answerable for murder. And any fine distinction as to its being completely formed or unformed is not admissible amongst us.

St Basil *Canonical Epistles* (374)

The advent of the Norman Conquest had consequences for the law relating to abortion...Abortion was regarded primarily as an ecclesiastical offence, the crime consisting in denying the prospect of eternal life to the soul of the unborn, and so unbaptized child...The ecclesiastical courts became more severe in their treatment of abortion and throughout the Middle Ages in Western Europe, guilty women were condemned on a capital charge, as the Sixth Ecumenical Council had ordained.

B. M. Dickens *Abortion and the Law* (1966)

Women who have illicit intercourse and destroy their unborn children, and those who help them to expel the fetus from the womb, are expelled from the Church for their lives by an old ruling, but now it is more leniently laid down that they should do penance for ten years. If a woman deliberately got rid of her fetus within forty days, she must do penance for four years; if it was done after it was alive, because it amounts to homicide, she must do penance for seven years.

Leges Henrici Primi (collection of English laws compiled in the reign of Henry I; 1100–35)

The infliction of death, whether upon mother or upon child, is against the commandment of God and the voice of nature: 'Thou shalt not kill!' The lives of both are equally sacred.

Pope Pius XI 'Casti Connubii' (1930)

If human life can be taken before birth, there is no logical reason why human life cannot be taken after birth.

Francis Schaeffer, speech at a rally of the Society for the Protection of the Unborn Child (June 1983)

The fetus is a human being (and is so in the fullest sense). Except (perhaps) as a judicial execution (and then only of someone whose crime merits the death penalty) or, in certain extreme cases, as a defensive measure against an aggressor, the deliberate killing of another human being is a grave violation of natural justice. Such killing is, to put it bluntly, murder. This abortion, the deliberate killing of the human fetus, is morally wrong, and to be legally prohibited, because it is a form of murder.

J. Foster *Personhood and the Ethics of Abortion* (1985)

Babies are not like bad teeth, to be jerked out just because they cause suffering.

Jill Knight MP *Hansard* (22 June 1966)

Abortion, however, was an abomination. In addition to being a violation of the precept against killing a living being, it was destruction of a potential Buddha and a crime against the maintenance of the human race. Mitigating factors such as impregnation by rape or incest may have been considered, but the Buddhist position against abortion was clear cut and has only been questioned in modern times.

John Stevens *Lust for Enlightenment* (1990)

The child, by reason of his physical and mental immaturity, needs special safeguards and care, including appropriate legal protection, before as well as after birth.

United Nations Declaration of the Rights of the Child (1959)

Indeed, in denigrating the fruit of the womb, abortionism automatically carries with it a sub-conscious denigration of women, because it diminishes the feeling and the experience of woman in her act of creativity...It is hardly surprising that high-abortion societies are societies in which women have on the whole poor status and hard lives – Japan and the USSR being prime examples.

Mary Kenny *The Tablet* (2 July 1983)

While popular opinion suggests that there exists a clear-cut opposition to abortion on the part of some religious bodies and a categorical support by others, it appears, in fact, that representatives of a variety of positions can be found in each of the major religions.

E. C. Moore-Cavar International Inventory of Information on Induced Abortion (1974)

While there are many people who believe that abortion is unacceptable under any circumstance, there are no advocates *for* abortion; there are, however, many who believe that the parents have a right to the choice of a termination in certain circumstances:

Historically the opposition to abortion and birth control...stemmed from the urgency of the need to decrease the mortality and morbidity rates and to increase the population...in the matter of abortion the human rights of the mother with her family must take precedence over the survival of a few weeks' old fetus without sense or sensibility.

Edith Summerskill *A Woman's World* (1967)

Abortion, it can be said, is contraception practised late. So the ethical rules that support contraception also support the abortion of a non-viable fetus, that is one not yet capable of living indefinitely outside the mother's body. Abortion is always sad, and depressing for the aborting woman. It negates her nature, and for that we should have pity. Yet it is her choice.

Francis Bennion *The Sex Code* (1991)

Most women decide to have abortions reluctantly, and with trepidation, as the lesser of two evils. No woman has an abortion for fun. They do not see why they should take on the responsibility of an unwanted child after their method of contraception has let them down...their circumstances – bad housing, lack of money, ill health – are such that they cannot cope with a new baby.

Joan Smith *Misogynies* (1989)

The abortion question is one of the most sickening, hypocritical symptoms of the illness of humanity. There is hardly a judge, parson, doctor, teacher, or any so-called pillar of society who would not prefer an abortion for his daughter than have his family face the disgrace of bastardy.

A. S. Neill *Summerhill: A Radical Approach to Education* (1962)

The 'immorality' of women, favourite theme of misogynists, is not to be wondered at; how could they fail to feel an inner mistrust of the presumptuous principles that men publicly proclaim and secretly disregard? They learn to believe no longer in what men say when they exalt woman or exalt man: the one thing they are sure of is this rifled and bleeding womb, the shreds of crimson life, this child that is not there. It is at her first abortion that woman begins to 'know'.

Simone de Beauvoir *The Second Sex* (1949)

Principles are all very well, especially if they apply to others. However, think of the plight of a 16-year-old schoolgirl who has been over-enthusiastic with her boyfriend. She knows that her devout parents will turn her out onto the streets if she tells them she is pregnant – it is possible, even, that her father will beat her up. She knows that this is inevitable because it has already happened to her sister. Suicide, if she had the courage, could be a solution. 'Principles' seem hardly relevant. A night away staying with a 'friend' with the help of a caring agency can solve her problem. The frightened guilt-ridden child-mother-to-be will have changed back overnight into the carefree schoolgirl.

The real question is not 'How can we justify abortion?' but 'How can we justify compulsory childbearing.'

Lana Phelan in *Birth Control and Women's Liberation* (1969)

Contrary to the folklore of abortion as lifelong trauma, it is not necessarily a profoundly scarring one either.

Helen Dudar 'Abortion for the Asking' *Saturday Review of the Society* (Apr. 1973)

The view that abortion is a lesser evil than the creation of an unwanted life rests on the assumption that such an operation can be quickly, safely, and effectively accomplished. In the civilized world this is now the case, although it has not always been so:

Methods used to procure abortions included traditional herbal remedies, savin, ergot of rye, penny royal, slippery elm, squills and hierpicra, compounds of aloes and iron; and compounds of iron and purgative extracts. Sometimes self-discovered methods were used: for example, after an epidemic of lead poisoning in Sheffield in the early 1890s it was noted that those who were poisoned had aborted.

Jeffrey Weeks *Sex, Politics and Society* (1981)

She should use diuretic decoctions which also have the power to bring on menstruation...If this is without effect, one must also treat locally by having her sit in a bath of a decoction of linseed, fenugreek, mallow, marsh mallow, and wormwood.

Soranus of Ephesus *Gynaecology* (2nd century)

If the woman suspects she is pregnant, she should indulge in violent movements and vigorous sexual intercourse. Joking too is useful.

Rhazes *The Spiritual Physick of Rhazes* (10th century)

She let me in and I was crying and I was feverish. There was a little table there and she put me on it. She started working on me and I was crying and she came and I will remember this till the day I die, she came and put her arms around me on the table and she said "Honey, did you think it was so easy to be a woman?"

Anon. account of a 1950s abortion, quoted in Joyce Johnson *Minor Characters* (1983)

A steel forceps mangles and extracts a murky mass of bloody tissue. There it lies now, soft and quivering. But in it are hands and feet, even eyes and a nose well formed. That tiny bleeding object dyed in red is a human being, no doubt about it. It whimpers now with a voice like a little kitten. It is tossed into a dark corner by itself. The cries become faint; now it is dead. Its life was short, but a few moments. Another artificial termination of pregnancy has been completed.

Anon. *Josei Jishin* (Japanese magazine; 1962)

Don't use your Hoover, ladies: it won't fit.

Lana Phelan in *Birth Control and Women's Liberation* (1969)

Some final words of wisdom:

Every induced abortion whether legal or criminal, is an expression of failure of one form or another – failed contraceptive technique, irresponsibility by one or both partners, ignorance, betrayal of trust or denial of human dignity.

John Stallworthy, in a letter to *The Times* (3 Jan. 1969)

Until that day when women, and only women, shall determine which American males must, by law, have vasectomies, then – and only then – will you or any man have the right to determine which American women can have abortions.

Betty Beale *Ms* (1982)

An Irish ban on information about the availability of abortions in Britain was ruled in breach of human rights by judges in Strasbourg today. The European Court of Human Rights dismissed Irish government claims that the ban was necessary to uphold the nation's constitution...the Norwegian president of the court, Rolv Ryssdal, said the restraint imposed on imparting information was disproportionate to the aim of protecting the right to life of the unborn, safeguarded in Article 40.3.3 of the constitution.

Oxford Mail (29 Oct. 1992)

Abortion is a universally practised but by no means universally approved procedure.

Barbara Brookes *Abortion in England* (1988)

In this generation we have removed the risks from abortion, but we have failed to create a society in which women no longer have to resort to it.

Jean Malcolm *Abortion in Debate* (1987)

Adultery

You know, of course, that the Tasmanians, who never committed adultery, are now extinct.

W. Somerset Maugham *The Bread-Winner* (1930)

There are those who argue that the sexual drive in men is so powerful that monogamy is unable to contain it:

Most societies recognise the necessity for accepting some extramarital coitus as an escape valve for the male, to relieve him from the pressures put on him by society's insistence on stable marital relationships. These same societies, however, less often permit it for the female.

Alfred Kinsey et al. *Sexual Behaviour in the Human Female* (1953)

See also MONOGAMY AND POLYGAMY

No man worth having is true to his wife, or can be true to his wife, or ever was, or ever will be so.

Sir John Vanbrugh *The Relapse* (1696)

Various antidotes and deterrents have been suggested:

Beneath the surge of elemental emotion which sex lets loose, nothing will suffice to hold us steady save the stabilising emotional power of a spiritual ideal which commands our wholehearted allegiance. The centrifugal forces of animal impulse can be balanced only by the centripetal power of religious faith.

David R. Mace *Facts About V.D.* (1948)

All this hocus-pocus, such as…magic herbs, formulae of exorcism, and love potions have no effect, as the example of Medea and Circe shows; both were famous enchantresses, and yet their black art did not avail to prevent the unfaithfulness of their husbands, Jason and Odysseus.

Ovid *Ars Amatoria* (1st century AD)

Geradas, one of the old Spartans, being asked by a guest, how the Spartans punished adulterers, replied: "There are no adulterers in Sparta." "But if there should be?" insisted the guest. "Then, as a punishment, he will have to give a bull large enough to stretch out his head over mount Taygetus and to drink from the river Eurotas." When the guest in amazement asked: "Wherever in the world could so big a bull be found?" Geradas laughed and said: "How could there be an adulterer in Sparta?"

Plutarch *Comparatio Lycurgi cum Numa* (2nd century)

The woman and the man
Guilty of adultery or fornication
Flog each of them
With a hundred stripes.

Koran

Moses comes down from the mountain after getting the ten commandments from God. At the bottom he sees the Children of Israel waiting. He says, "Look. I've got some good news and some bad news. First the good news. There's only ten. And now the bad news. Adultery's in."

Carol Clewlow *A Woman's Guide to Adultery* (1984)

If a man be found lying with a woman married to an husband, then they shall both of them die, both the man that lay with the woman, and the woman: so shalt thou put away evil from Israel.

Deuteronomy 22:22

And the scribes and Pharisees brought unto him a woman taken in adultery; and when they had set her in the midst, they say unto him, Master, this woman was taken in adultery, in the very act. Now Moses in the law commanded us, that such should be stoned.

John 8:3–5

For as much as Thomas Bray, of Yarmouth, a single person, and Anne, the Wyfe of Francis Linceford, have committed the act of Adultery, the court doth censure them as follows: that they be both severely whipt & that they shall weare two letters, viz. an AD for Adulterer, daily, upon the outeside of their uppermost garment, in a most emenent place thereof.

Ecclesiastical Court Records, Plymouth, New England (1641)

...in 1800 and again in 1856 and 1857, attempts were made to have Parliament impose the death penalty for adultery, but the motions were defeated.

Gordon Rattray Taylor *Sex in History* (1953)

Because, historically, men have paid the bills, they have assumed the right to make the rules:

The penalty inflicted on an adulterous wife is invariably greater than that inflicted on an adulterous husband.

Judith Armstrong *The Novel of Adultery* (1976)

Both cross-cultural and historical reviews of adultery laws reveal a remarkable consistency of concept: sexual intercourse between a married woman and a man other than her husband is an offence. It is often viewed as a property violation. The victim is the husband, who is commonly entitled to damages, violent revenge, or to divorce with refund of bride price.

M. Daly, M. Wilson, and S. J. Weghorst *Male Sexual Jealousy* (1982)

It is not immorality which is punished but theft. As the act of the wife, adultery is a revolt against the husband's property rights.

B. Crozier *Marital Support* (1935)

The woman who deceives her husband is the destruction of her house.

William the Conqueror (11th century)

If a husband has brought home some strumpet, unbeknown to his wife, and she finds it out, the husband goes scot free. But once a wife steps out of the house unbeknown to her husband, he has his ground and she's divorced. Oh I wish there was the same rule for the husband as for the wife!

Mercy me, if husbands too were taken to task for wenching on the sly, the same way as wanton wives are divorced, I warrant there'd be more lone men about than there are now women!

Plautus *Mercator* (3rd century BC)

I argued that the chastity of women was of much more consequence than that of men, as the property and rights of families depend upon it. "Surely" said she, "that is easily answered, for the objection is removed if a woman does not intrigue but when she is with child." I really could not answer her. Yet I thought she was wrong, and I was uneasy...

James Boswell, diary entry published in *Boswell: The Ominous Years 1774–1776* (ed. Charles Ryskamp and Frederick A. Pottle; 1963)

It had ever been the feeling of the House, indeed it was a feeling common to mankind in general that, although the sin in both cases was the same, the effect of adultery on the part of the husband was very different from that on the part of the wife. It was possible for a wife to pardon a husband who had committed adultery, but it was hardly possible for a husband ever really to pardon the adultery of a wife.

Lord Chamberlain, House of Lords debate (1857)

See also FEMINISM

This special insistence on female chastity may be largely a consequence of men's wish to know who sired the children produced by their wives:

As everyone since dim antiquity has known, or at least suspected, some wives conceive by men other than their husbands.

Paul Gebhard et al. *Pregnancy, Birth and Abortion* (1958)

Confusion of progeny constitutes the essence of the crime of adultery.

Samuel Johnson quoted by James Boswell in *The Life of Samuel Johnson* (1791)

Adultery by a wife not only subverts domestic tranquility, but has a tendency, by contaminating the blood of illustrious families, to affect the welfare of the nation in its newest interests.

Lord Thurlow, British Lord Chancellor (1779)

There have been, however, a few societies in which even this poses no problem:

In Sparta a husband could transfer his conjugal rights temporarily to one sexually stronger, from which he could expect beautiful and vigorous children, without the marriage being thereby upset.

Plutarch *Comparatio Lycurgi cum Numa* (2nd century)

Adultery is almost always regarded as a grave offence, even though there are a few communities which permit extra-marital intercourse in circumstances regulated by tribal law…

Judith Armstrong *The Novel of Adultery* (1976)

The Tyrrhenians bring up the children who are born, often without knowing who the father is. When they are grown up, they live in the same manner as those who reared them, often arrange drinking bouts and have connections with all the women they meet.

Theopompus of Chios (4th century BC)

Not religion, not flogging or threats of death, nor fear of discovery or social disapproval has ever held back the relentless tide of adultery –

Thys is now a common synne
For almost hyt is every-where
A gentyle man hath a wife and a hore,
And wyves have now comunly
Here husbands and a ludby [a lover]

John of Salisbury (12th century)

– for the obvious reason:

There can be no doubt that the lives of a very large proportion of married men and women are being enriched and made more meaningful by secret sexual relationships.

Tony Lake and Ann Hills *Affairs* (1979)

The crops are more abundant in fields belonging to others. The neighbour's herd has richer udders.

Ovid *Ars Amatoria* (1st century AD)

Unlike coitus itself, in which only two participants are involved:

Adultery needs three players. If one of these players refuses to play the role that is cast for them, the triangle cannot possibly continue.

Caroline Buchanan *Caught in the Act* (1990)

At least one of the players has to be a woman – and women, too, have voracious sexual appetities:

It's a question of taking married men, but not taking them seriously. Use them in a perfectly nice way, just as they use you.

Helen Gurley Brown *Sex and the Single Girl* (1962)

[Marriage] *is merely a mutual contract which if one party breaks, the other is free. Now, my husband I know has been unfaithful to me a thousand times. I should therefore have no scruple of conscience, I do declare, to have an intrigue.*

Anon. lady quoted in *Boswell: The Ominous Years 1774–1776* (ed. Charles Ryskamp and Frederick A. Pottle; 1963)

Let husbands know
Their wives have sense like them: they see and smell
And have their palates both for sweet and sour,
As husbands have. What is it that they do
When they change us for others? Is it sport?
I think it is: and doth affection breed it?
I think it doth: is't frailty that thus errs?
It is so too: and have not we affections,
Desires for sport, and frailty, as men have?
Then let them use us well: else let them know,
The ills we do, their ills instruct us so.

William Shakespeare *Othello* (1604)

As the extravagant woman
was minding the house on her own
she saw the lad she loved most
coming in to join her,
and he threw her upon the bed,
he did better than the man of the house.

Dafydd ap Gwilym 'The Man Under the Tub' (14th century)

Translations (like wives) are seldom faithful if they are in the least attractive.

Roy Campbell *Poetry Review* (1949)

It is as foolish to make experiments upon the constancy of a friend, as upon the chastity of a wife.

Samuel Johnson, letter to James Boswell (9 Sept. 1779)

Madame, you must really be more careful. Suppose it had been someone else who found you like this.

Duc de Richelieu, on discovering his wife with her lover (18th century)

Tis the established custom in Vienna for every lady to have two husbands, one that bears the name, and another that performs the duties.

Lady Mary Wortley Montague, letter to a friend (1716)

Promiscuous girls, you've had your fun:
Now marry and 'cleave unto one'
Lawfully. What a hope!

Martial *Epigrams* (1st century AD)

You mean apart from my own?

Zsa Zsa Gabor, when asked how many husbands she'd had (20th century)

There's beauty in a boy. But to a woman, no one's a true mate. She always loves the one who's there.

Theognis of Megara (6th century BC)

Men, according to Aphra Behn, suffer from the opposite weakness:

Since Man with that inconstancy was born,
To love the absent, and the present scorn...

'To Alexis' (1687)

Not all women, however, can commit adultery with a clear conscience. Some have scruples:

I say I don't sleep with married men, but what I mean is that I don't sleep with happily married men.

Britt Ekland (1970s)

and some cannot help feeling guilty:

Sara could commit adultery at one end and weep for her sins at the other, and enjoy both operations at once.

Joyce Cary *The Horse's Mouth* (1944)

Suffering...most often accompanies the notion of adultery in the female mind.

Carol Clewlow *A Woman's Guide to Adultery* (1989)

Although a few men have excused women's infidelity:

Women are not more to blame than men for unchastity, since the latter besiege them with solicitations and exert all their vaunted intelligence to bring about their capitulation.

Robert Vaughan *A Dyalogue defensyve for Women* (1542)

and some have given them ironic advice on how best to enjoy it:

Sometimes your lover to incite the more,
Pretend your husband's spies beset the door:
Tho' free as Thais, still affect a fright;
For seeming danger heightens the delight.

Ovid *Ars Amatoria* (1st century AD)

most men have reacted furiously to the unfaithfulness of their own wives:

When I had thrust open the door of the bedroom, those who entered first saw a man still lying beside my wife; those who came afterward saw him standing naked on the bed. I, gentlemen, knocked him down, bound both his arms behind him, and asked him why he had insulted the honour of my house. He admitted that he had done wrong, but begged and prayed me not to kill him, but to take from him a sum of money. To this I answered, 'I will not kill you, but the Law of the State will.'

Lysias *De Caede Eratosthenis* (4th century BC)

He bethought him that he had forgotten in his palace somewhat which he should have brought with him, so he returned privily and entered his apartments, where he found the Queen, his wife, asleep on his own carpet-bed, embracing with both arms a cook of loathsome aspect and foul with kitchen grease and grime. When he saw this he said, "If such case happens while I am yet within sight of the city, what will be the doings of this damned whore during my long absence at my brother's court?" So he drew his scimitar and, cutting the two into four pieces with a single blow, left them on the carpet and returned presently to his camp.

The Thousand and One Nights (trans. by Sir Richard Burton)

The records would probably show that women throughout the ages have been as ready to commit adultery as men, when the opportunity to do so undetected has arisen; modern sociologists have suggested that if, towards the end of the 20th century, there are more unfaithful wives, this is because there are more opportunities:

More women than ever are now having affairs...at least 40 per cent of women are cheating on their partners...Contraception has given women more freedom; and with more equality and more women working, the opportunities to be unfaithful are greatly increased.

Zelda West-Meads quoted by Caroline Buchanan in *Caught in the Act* (1990)

For men, opportunity has been much less of a problem – except perhaps for the working class:

Traditionally the only working-class sexual opportunists who actually succeed are travelling salesmen, soldiers living away from home, and sailors with a girl in every port.

Tony Lake and Ann Hills *Affairs* (1979)

The main difficulty for men lies in persuading themselves that what they are about to do, are doing, or have done, can be justified. Some have claimed patriotic motives:

Not even his friends could deny that he often committed adultery, though of course they said, in justification, that he did so for reasons of state, not simple passion – he wanted to discover what his enemies were at by getting intimate with their wives or daughters.

Suetonius *The Twelve Caesars*, 'Augustus' (2nd century)

Even if he did not feel drawn to any lady but his wife, a ruler was in honour bound to satisfy etiquette by taking a mistress, if only a nominal one.

Max von Boehn *Modes and Manners in the 19th Century* (1927)

For others, geography provides an excuse:

FRIAR BARNARDINE *Thou hast*
committed –

BARABAS *Fornication: but that was in another country;*
And beside the wench is dead.

Christopher Marlowe *The Jew of Malta* (c. 1590)

What men call gallantry, and gods adultery,
Is much more common where the climate's sultry.

Lord Byron *Don Juan* (1819–24)

My robust health disposed me to some follies which I afterwards repented and still do repent of. But as my wife refused to come over, and my temptations were great, I hope the faults I committed are the more pardonable.

Lord Herbert of Cherbury referring, in his autobiography (1619), to his years as English ambassador in Paris

Some men blame their marriages:

A true marriage may be what the laws call adultery, while the real adultery is an unloving marriage.

Thomas Nichols and Mary Nichols *Esoteric Anthropology* (1853)

While others put their trust in God's forgiveness – even in cases where the 'adultery' was purely mental:

I have looked on a lot of women with lust. I've committed adultery in my heart many times. God recognises I will do this and forgives me.

Jimmy Carter *Playboy* (Nov. 1976)

which, according to Jesus, is as bad as the real thing:

As a Jew, Jesus took seriously the Ten Commandments. But He totally confused the whole business of adultery by saying that even to entertain so much as a Carter-like lust for a woman is the equivalent of actually committing adultery.

Gore Vidal 'The Second American Revolution' *New York Review of Books* (1981)

Many other men are content to enjoy the fun, without seeking elaborate justifications:

If you think you love your mistress for her own sake you are quite mistaken.

François de La Rochefoucauld *Maximes* (1665)

The peculiar importance attached, at present, to adultery is quite irrational. It is obvious that many forms of misconduct are more fatal to married happiness than an occasional infidelity…

Bertrand Russell *Why I am Not a Christian* (1957)

See also JEALOUSY

A mistress should be like a little country retreat near the town, not to dwell in constantly, but only for a night and away.

William Wycherley *The Country Wife* (1675)

With all my heart. Whose wife shall it be?

John Horne Tooke, replying to the suggestion that he take a wife (18th century)

A joke upon which Thomas Moore elaborated:

"Come, Come" said Tom's father "at your time of life,
There's no longer excuse for this playing the rake –
It is time you should think, boy, of taking a wife" –
"Why so it is, father – whose wife shall I take?"

'A Joke Versified' (19th century)

Sometimes the unfortunate adulterer can find the whole thing somewhat bewildering:

Reading someone else's newspaper is like sleeping with someone else's wife. Nothing seems to be precisely in the right place, and when you find what you are looking for, it is not clear then how to respond to it.

Malcolm Bradbury *Stepping Westward* (1975)

Aphrodisiacs

If you don't know the way of intercourse, partaking of herbs is of no benefit.

P'eng Tsu, quoted by Li Tung Hsuan in *The Art of Love* (7th century)

Since earliest times people have claimed that certain substances, potions, and magical charms have the power to inspire love or lust and to enhance sexual performance as well as the pleasures derived from it:

Lust-provoking philtres were concocted by the ancients of Assyria, Persia, and China, with the earliest recorded recipes coming from undated Egyptian medical papyri from the Middle Kingdom, between 2200–1700 BC. *The greatest adepts were the Greek women of Thessaly, which was the home of magic and the cult of the arch sorceress Medea.*

Pamela Allardice *Aphrodisiacs and Love Magic* (1989)

People eager to find aphrodisiacs have experimented over the millenia with various plants and plant products. Anglo-Saxon manuals recommend St. John's wort, valerian, vervain...A fifteenth century manuscript prescribed French lavender for arousing venereal desire. Also taken from a plant was a gum known as 'dragon's blood' although according to a legend reported in Pliny it was extracted from a dragon or serpent crushed by a dying elephant; this gum is said to have been used for love into at least the tenth century...

From the works of Paulinus, medieval Europeans learned of various animals whose magical virtues could make amorous feeling; not only the testes of a hare or stag, a donkey's penis, the semen of a stag and the vaginal secretions of a sow were recommended, but also the urine of a bull, and the droppings of a hen, and the blood and brains of a sparrow.

Richard Kieckhefer quoted by Joyce E. Salisbury in *Sex in the Middle Ages* (1991)

The semen of virile young men should be mixed with the excrement of hawks or eagles and taken in pellet form.

Li-Shi-Chen *Medical Treatise* (14th century)

See also SEXUAL NONSENSE

Some aphrodisiacs were said to provoke or prolong an erection:

Erection is chiefly caused by parsnips, artichokes, turnips, asparagus, candied ginger, acorns bruised to powder and drunk in muscadel, scallion, sea shellfish, etc.

Aristotle *The Nicomachean Ethics* (4th century BC)

others were intended to inspire love:

When a mandrake root that has grown into male genital form is found, it will unquestionably secure feminine love.

Pliny the Elder *Natural History* (1st century AD)

The notion of the efficacy of love powders was so prevalent in the 15th century in our own country [England] *that in the Parliament summoned by King Richard III, on his usurping the throne, it was publicly urged as a charge against Lady Grey, that she had bewitched King Ed-*

ward IV by strange potions and amorous charms.

John Davenport *Aphrodisiacs and Antiaphrodisiacs* (1869)

Strait to the 'pothecary's shop I went,
And in love powder all my money spent;
Behap what will, next Sunday after prayers,
When to the alehouse Lubberkin repairs,
These golden flies into his mug I'll throw,
And soon the swain with fervent love shall glow.

John Gay 'Shepherd's Week' (18th century)

OBERON *Having once this juice,*
I'll watch Titania when she is asleep,
And drop the liquor of it in her eyes.
The next thing that she, waking, looks upon
(Be it on lion, bear, or wolf, or bull,
On meddling monkey, or on busy ape)
She shall pursue it with the soul of love.

William Shakespeare *A Midsummer Night's Dream* (c. 1595)

English country folk still say that a drop of blood from a man's little finger put in a woman's wine will make her fall passionately in love with him. This belief has its origins in fetishism, or sympathetic magic, which specified nail parings, bones and pieces of clothing as ingredients in love charms.

Pamela Allardice *Aphrodisiacs and Love Magic* (1989)

Many items thought of as aphrodisiacs have a noticeable resemblance to either the male or the female genitals. It has been suggested that objects originally used to represent the sexual organs in magical rituals may subsequently have been credited with aphrodisiac properties when taken internally:

Many lucky charms are strongly suggestive of the male member...From a historic point of view the mandrake root and the rhinoceros horn have provided the most potent sexual symbols and have thereby gained reputations as powerful aphrodisiacs.

Peter V. Taberner *Aphrodisiacs: The Science and the Myth* (1985)

The reputation of the oyster is probably due to sympathetic magic; they look (and even taste) like the female genitals.

Robert Anton Wilson *Sex and Drugs: A Journey Beyond Limits* (1988)

There have been many tales about the effectiveness of aphrodisiacs:

She took one pill herself, leaving three. Then she made the terrible mistake of giving him all three. She was afraid anything else would have no effect. Hsi-men shut his eyes and swallowed them. Before he could have drunk a cup of tea, the medicine began to take effect. Golden Lotus tied the silk ribbon for him and his staff stood up. He was still asleep. She mounted upon his body, put some powder on the top of his penis, and put that into her queynt; immediately it penetrated right to the heart of her...Hsi-men Ch'ing let her do everything she wished, but himself was perfectly inert.

Wang Shih-Chen *Chin P'ing Mei, or The Golden Lotus*

In 1917 Dr Brinkley, in the back-room of a country store, transplanted goat testicles into the scrotum of a farmer who complained of having 'no pep'. The following year the farmer's wife had a son.

G. L. Simons *Sex and Superstition* (1976)

One man supplies magical spells; another sells Thessalian charms by which a wife may upset her husband's mind, and lather his buttocks with a slipper; thence came loss of reason, and darkness of soul, and blank forgetfulness of all that you did but yesterday.

Juvenal *Satire VI* (2nd century)

The news from Marseilles is that M. Le Comte de Sade has just provided in this town a spectacle, pleasant at first but appalling in its consequences. He gave a ball, to which a large number of guests were invited. Into the pudding he inserted some chocolates so delicious that several people ate them. There were plenty of these and no-one went short, but in them he had inserted 'Spanish Fly'. The virtue of this preparation is well known; and all those who had eaten it, burning with unchaste desire, gave themselves up to all the excesses to which the most lascivious frenzy can carry one. The ball degenerated into one of those licentious parties renowned among the Romans. The most modest women could not do enough to give expression to the itch which had seized them. Several persons are dead from the excesses to which they gave themselves up in their priapic fury and others are still severely indisposed.

Louis de Bachaumont *Mémoirs historiques* (1808)

Despite this anecdotal testimony, most supposed aphrodisiacs are at best useless and at worst positively dangerous:

Dr John R Brinkley collected over twelve million dollars in twenty years for transplanting goat glands into sixteen thousand men, and for selling by mail his special Gland Emulsion. Readers who had doubts about their manliness could have an injection of coloured distilled water into hip or arm for only twenty-five dollars.

G. L. Simons *Sex and Superstition* (1976)

In human males, the drug does cause erection, but the erection is painful and it is a reflex action caused by inflammation of the urinary tract. In fact a dosage strong enough to have an effect on male or female genitalia may also be strong enough to cause acute, or even fatal kidney damage. Spanish Fly is therefore a dangerous substance and it is doubtful whether advertisers in pornographic magazines ever actually mail the 'real thing' to their customers.

Roy Eskapa *Bizarre Sex* (1987)

Mandragora, or mandrake, is a member of the potato family and contains the alkaloids atropine and scopolmine, and in large doses can cause mental confusion and death.

G. L. Simons *Sex and Superstition* (1976)

Methaqualone (Mandrax, Quaaludes or Ludes as the pills are called) is a hypnotic drug believed by some to produce incredible ultimate orgasms. They claim it has the effect of producing subjective euphoria – a form of excited hypnosis. Though particularly popular in the United States, the drug is also extremely dangerous because the user can overdose on a few tablets. For good reason, it is banned in both Britain and North America. It seems surprising that the drug should be thought of as a sex-drug. Users can seldom remember what happened when they were stoned on it.

Roy Eskapa *Bizarre Sex* (1987)

Drugs not considered to be aphrodisiacs as such may increase sexual desire, but not without accompanying risks. Cocaine may provoke violence and loss of control:

With the excitement of the brain, sexual desires loom up to the fore. In men there is increased sexual desire with erotic ideas developing into perversions which are carried even to the extent of violence. With women the same sexual stimulation occurs, but erotic manifestations are more marked, with a tendency to produce complete loss of moral sense and nymphomania.

Bernard Finch, on the effects of cocaine, in *Passport to Paradise?* (1959)

Although opium appears to have aphrodisiac properties, its continual use can have the opposite effect:

Of opium, it is well known that at first it increases sexual activity. Voluptuous phantasies and visions are also characteristic of these stages. Continued indulgence in opium, however, produces impotence.

Iwan Bloch *Strange Sexual Practices* (1924)

The use of aphrodisiacs was condemned by the early Christian Church:

As early as the sixth century, the penitential of Finnian prescribed six years of penance for anyone who administered a potion for the sake of wanton love...The seventh century penitential of Theodore condemns any woman who mixes her husband's semen into his food so that he will love her more fervently...Louis the Pious issued a capitulary in 829 condemning the use of love potions, enchanted foods, and charms worn on people's bodies to influence the minds of others.

Richard Kieckhefer quoted by Joyce E. Salisbury in *Sex in the Middle Ages* (1991)

In the modern Western world few people are prepared to set any store by magical charms and potions – although miracle cures for impotence and marvellous enhancers of sexual performance are still advertised.

Pheromone Technology is acknowledged by World Scientific Authorities and has been well proven in controlled tests by many leading journals as well as enjoying extensive testing on TV. PHEROMUSK will enhance your body chemistry making you irresistable to responsive females!

Advertisement in *Viz* (1 Dec. 1992)

The rules of the British Code of Advertising Practice state:

Advertisements should not suggest or imply that any product, medicine or treatment offered therein will promote sexual virility or be effective in treating sexual weakness, or habits associated with sexual excess or indulgence or any ailment, illness or disease associated with such habits.

Today, hormone treatment is often recommended to those who complain of a lack of sexual interest:

Sex hormones are the scientifically respectable aphrodisiacs of the modern world. Many doctors readily prescribe testosterone or oestrogen for impotent men or menopausal women worried about their libidos, and are convinced it helps. Yet there is growing evidence that these drugs, like all aphrodisiacs, work far more through the power of suggestion than anything else.

Guardian (11 Dec. 1992)

Aphrodisiacs do not necessarily have to be drugs, plants, or animal extracts:

Thus, although in theory an aphrodisiac is strictly an exciter of lust, in practice anything which, by any means, increases the capacity for sexual enjoyment will tend to increase the appetite and can be termed an aphrodisiac.

Peter V. Taberner *Aphrodisiacs: The Science and the Myth* (1985)

and the non-physical ones may be not only the safest but also the most effective:

Sexologists have long concluded rather vaguely that feelings of 'well being' enhance sexual desire. Could it be that a supportive social environment is the ultimate aphrodisiac? ...If so, the answer may lie, not in pharmaceutical potions, but in social engineering. The message from today's science? For an active sex life, choose supportive friends, workmates and lovers!

Guardian (11 Dec. 1992)

Power is the great aphrodisiac.

Henry Kissinger *New York Times* (19 Jan. 1971)

I will show you a love potion without drug or herb or any witch's spell; if you wish to be loved, love.

Hecato quoted by Seneca in *Epistles* (2nd century BC)

Bestiality

A man accused of having sex with a chicken told Nottingham Crown Court in October 1990 that he was checking to see if an egg was on the way. The prosecutor observed: "That fails quite markedly to explain why he should have his trousers down around his buttocks."

Observer (4 Oct. 1992)

All the evidence suggests that bestiality is found in both primitive and sophisticated cultures and amongst both sexes:

Apparently among all *primitive peoples bestiality is in some degree exhibited. It is eradicated only after a considerable intellectual and moral development.*

Professor George Barton *Encyclopaedia of Religion and Ethics* (1909)

Clearly, however, it has not yet been 'eradicated':

The precise incidence of zoophilia is not known, but, in America, according to Kinsey et al (1948 and 1953) about 8% of men and 3% of women admitted to sexual behaviour with an animal. Most prosecutions occur in rural areas. Kinsey estimated that about 17% of boys raised on farms experience orgasm as a result of direct contact with animals.

Roy Eskapa *Bizarre Sex* (1987)

In some ancient religions bestiality, whether real or simulated, formed part of the worship of sacred animals:

An ancient Vedic ceremony was the 'horse-sacrifice' which was the greatest animal sacrifice of those times. After the King had let the horse roam at will for a year, to enlarge his territory, it would be sacrificed and his wife lay by the horse and imitated copulation with it.

Geoffrey Parrinder *Sex in the World's Religions* (1980)

The god Anubis was represented by a priest clothed in the skin of a jackal, who in that animal form had ritual connection with a woman. A notorious scandal was caused in Rome...when a priest was bribed to allow a gentleman to take his place while a Roman matron was participating in the ritual...

The Iroquois tribes of New Netherlands regarded themselves as derived from the intercourse of women with bears, deer, or wolves.

Robert Briffault *The Mothers: a Study of the Origins of Sentiments and Institutions* (1927)

In Egypt the bull Apis, who represented Osiris, was treated with honours. During the first forty days after his installation in his temple at Memphis, the women stood before him and, raising their clothes, exposed their persons.

Diodorus Siculus (4th century BC)

The Islamic world provides a number of curious beliefs on the subject:

...according to many reports the dugong (sea-cow), when dragged up on land, is to be mounted by none but fishermen. This is such a general occurrence that the people who buy the meat of the sea-cow make the Islamic fisherman swear by the

Koran that he has had no sexual intercourse with the sea-cow he is offering for sale. They do not want the flesh of a creature that has served man as a beast of pleasure. That is cannibalism.

Robert E. L. Masters, *The Hidden World of Erotica* (1973)

The pilgrimage to Mecca is not complete without copulating with the camel.

Arab saying

Many Arabs also seem to have believed that bestiality was an effective cure for sexually transmitted diseases:

If, then, O men! you are sick and without medical aid, or if this latter has been powerless, you may fornicate with animals; but this fornication should cease, under penalty of the infraction of the law of Islam, from the time that you will have regained your health.

Omar Haleby *El Ktab* (8th century)

Commonly, bestiality was regarded as a cure for venereal diseases; so widespread has been this belief that there are few places in the world where the remedy has not been regarded as sure-fire at one time or another.

Robert E. L. Masters *The Hidden World of Erotica* (1973)

In the Judaeo-Christian tradition, bestiality has been seen as blurring the all-important distinction between animals as irrational beings without souls and humans as rational beings with souls. Because this demarcation was believed to have been created by God, breaking it incurred the harshest penalties:

If a man lie with a beast, he shall surely be put to death; and ye shall slay the beast. And if a woman approach unto any beast, and lie down thereto thou shalt kill the woman and the beast; they shall surely be put to death; their blood shall be upon them.

Leviticus 20:15–16

If a man and man, woman and woman, people and animals, are found to have sexual intercourse, they will be punished by death.

Article 116 of the Carolingian Law (1532)

The early Christian Church was firm in its condemnation:

Among its sexual regulations, the Council of Ancyra in 314 AD prescribed strict penalties against bestiality: fifteen years of penance for youths under twenty, twenty five years for married people over twenty, and for a married person over fifty, he or she must wait until the end of life to receive communion.

Joyce E. Salisbury *Sex in the Middle Ages* (1991)

The height of lechery is that one raves even over animals and over inanimate things.

John Climacus (7th century)

Medieval theologians and moralists became increasingly preoccupied with defining and maintaining the distinction between man and the animals:

In the 11th century bestiality joined homosexuality and masturbation as 'unnatural' offences carrying 'sanction of infamia' depriving the practitioners of respectable status in society. However in the 11th and 12th centuries outside the classroom of the canon lawyers, people's views on the relationship between humans and animals was changing in a way that would cause the scholastics of the 13th century to rank bestiality as the worst of the sexual sins…

None of the early Germanic secular law codes prohibited bestiality. These codes also suggest that for the early Germans animals were important as property and food, and it was in these areas that they legislated…

Alexander of Hales (d.1245) identified bestiality as the greatest sin against nature, for to sin with 'another species' and with 'things irrational' represents the furthest departure from human nature, and thus the most unnatural sin. The penalty for Alexander was simple and extreme: kill the human and the animal, and thus erase the memory of the act with the participants.

Joyce E. Salisbury *Sex in the Middle Ages* (1991)

Animals polluted by coitus with men are to be killed, the flesh thrown to dogs. But what they give birth to may be used and the hides taken.

Theodore of Canterbury *The Canons* (c. 741)

The animal participant was to be killed, burned and buried to prevent any memory of the crime to be renewed.

Thomas of Chobham (c. 1200)

In Renaissance Venice, too, the law made a distinction between bestiality and lesser sexual offences:

The Signori were not the least interested in masturbation except as it related to intercourse with a goat.

Guido Ruggiero *The Boundaries of Eros: Sex Crime in Renaissance Venice* (1989)

although it seems that mitigating circumstances could be taken into account:

As part of his defense the artisan named Simon claimed that he "had not been able to have sexual relations with a woman or masturbate for more than three years because of an accident" and so...had given in to the temptations of a goat.

Archivo di Stato, Venice (1357)

In the 17th century there were a number of executions of both humans and animals for the crime:

We executed two farmers, one of whom had fallen in love with his she-ass, and the other who had lain with his sow. Yet all the while there are women around at three for a farthing.

Jerónimo de Barrineuve *Aviscos* (1659)

One reason for this severity was the fear of monstrous offspring:

Sometimes when the movements of the active virtue are weak and do not manage to vanquish matter, their general character remains and an animal is formed; but this may have the head of a boar or bull, or else in a similar way a calf with the head of a man is engendered, or a lamb with the head of a bull. This type of monstrosity sometimes occurs in this way, that is, by means of coitus between different species, or by an unnatural type of copulation.

Vincent of Beauvais *Speculum Naturale* (1591)

Sexual relations with animals required harsh punishment, for colonists believed that these unions could have reproductive consequences. The mating of humans and animals, they feared, would produce monstrous offspring. For this reason colonists insisted in punishing not only the man but the beast, who might bear such monsters...

Sixteen year old Thomas Grazer of Plymouth confessed to buggery 'with a mare, a cow, two goats, five sheep, two calves, and a turkey.' The court ordered a line-up of sheep at which Grazer identified his sexual partners, who were 'killed before his face' before he himself was executed.

L. T. Ulrich *Goodwives: Image and Reality in the Lives of Women in Northern New England 1650–1750* (1983)

There was also a widespread association between bestiality and devil worship:

Sexual congress constituted an essential part of the magic ritual of European witches, who were united to the devil in the form of a he-goat.

Robert Briffault *The Mothers: a Study of the Origins of Sentiments and Institutions* (1927)

Numbers of the ancient writers have explained that for the purpose of depraving mankind, the demon assumed human flesh...and sometimes he preferred to be in animal or bird form.

C. L. 'Estrange Ewen *Witchcraft and Demonianism* (1970)

Even today bestiality remains a crime in Britain – one that carried a life sentence as recently as 1956:

It is felony for a person to commit buggery with another person or with an animal.

Sexual Offences Act (1956)

On 16 August 1983 at Manchester Crown Court before Judge Jelland accompanied by two Justices, the appellant pleaded guilty to an offence of attempted buggery and was sentenced to two years imprisonment. In view of the sentence one might have supposed that a woman or a young person, if not a child, was involved. In fact, the object of the appellant's attentions was a Pyrenean Mountain bitch.

Mr Justice Leggatt, Appeal Court Hearing (Jan. 1984)

In this country we now live in a society which is permissive and decadent, but that does not mean that the courts which act on behalf of the ordinary decent people in this area will countenance the maligned depravity which causes a man to attempt to satisfy his sexual lust by having intercourse with a dog.

When all is said and done, it is the appellant and indeed his wife, and not the dog, who need help.

Judge Jelland Manchester Crown Court (1983)

The chief interest which attaches to bestiality is not the practice of the act but the savage penalty which the law attaches.

Dr Anthony Storr *Sexual Deviation* (1964)

Even the mere allegation of bestiality has been enough to provoke legal action:

In the case of Edgar vs McCutcheon [Missouri Supreme Court Report 9:768] *the plaintiff complained that the defendant had slandered him in alleging that he had carnal knowledge of a mare. The word 'fuck' was used to convey the imputation. The defence claimed that since the word is not found in the dictionaries, it cannot be held to be comprehensible, and to utter an incomprehensibility cannot be a slander. The court upheld the judgment of a lower court; it* is *an English word, and it does not follow because it is not found in the dictionaries that it is not understood by those that hear it.*

Wayland Young *Eros Denied* (1964)

Others have taken a more nonchalant attitude:

Fool – don't put him in irons; put him in the infantry.

Frederick the Great, on being told that a cavalryman had been arrested for buggering his horse

The enormous variety of the animal kingdom provides a wide choice of partners and this – together with man's natural inventiveness – can result in some bizarre couplings:

In their book Prostitution and Morality *Harry Benjamin and Robert E. L. Masters report that animals trained to copulate or have other sexual relations with humans have been provided as a facility in brothels throughout history. Dogs, donkeys, goats, baboons and monkeys have commonly been used for this purpose, and also for stage performances. These authors mention avisodomy as a service provided in some French brothels. The client sodomizes the bird, cutting its throat as his climax approaches. This act raises the bird's body temperature, while provoking it to violently convulsive movements triggering the patron's orgasm.*

Francis Bennion *The Sex Code* (1991)

There is no accounting for tastes in superstition. Frederick Hanley would like to have a Bible bound with bits of skin stripped off live from the cunts of a hundred little girls and yet he could not be persuaded to try the sensation of fucking a Muscovy Duck while its head was cut off.

Sir Richard Burton, quoted by R. M. Milne in his *Commonplace Book* (1860)

He fucks a turkey whose head is gripped between the legs of a girl lying on her belly – while in action he looks quite as if

he were embuggering the girl. While he is at work he is being sodomized and the moment he discharges, the girl cuts the turkey's throat.

Marquis de Sade *120 Days of Sodom* (1785: early draft)

She would lie down on a sofa and separating her thighs would smear honey on and in the vulva. The flies thus attracted by the honey would tickle her until her sexual appetite was appeased...

A case is related where a number of congenial souls amused themselves with fishes, by inserting the tail ends of the live fish into the vulva and then by pressing the head of the fish, would start it to squirming, thus tickling the vulva.

G. Herzog *Medical Jurisprudence* (1894)

A most strange and unusual sexual behaviour has recently (1985) surfaced in the United States. The bizarre practice, labelled Gerbillophilia, involves the insertion of a living gerbil into the rectum...An abuser inserts a large funnel into his rectum and allows one of the little animals to creep inside. The funnel is then removed, and as the gerbil crawls and struggles against suffocating, toxic gases in the bowels, it provides, practitioners claim, sexual 'pleasure'.

Roy Eskapa *Bizarre Sex* (1987)

According to one German lawyer who made a special study of the subject:

Bestiality in women is a great deal more prevalent than it is in men.

G. Herzog *Medical Jurisprudence* (1894)

There is a common male slur that women are aroused by the sexual prowess of animals:

She [Mary, Countess of Pembroke] *was very salacious, and she had a contrivance that, in the spring of the years, when the stallions were to leap the mares, they were brought before such a part of the house, where she had a vidette to look on them, and please herself with their sport; and then she would act the like sport herself with* her *stallions.*

John Aubrey *Brief Lives* (written 17th century; published 1898)

BUGGERANTHOS *Dildoes and dogs with women do prevail,*
I caught one frigging with a cur's bob-tail:
My lord, said she, I do it with remorse,
For once I had a passion for a horse.

John Wilmot, Earl of Rochester 'Sodom' (17th century)

A different kind of allegation was made against female owners of lapdogs in the 18th century:

Stroak'd as thou slumberst, 'twixt thy Lady's knees.
As if thou hadst some secret Power to please,
Fondled all day, and then at Night prefer'd
To sleep in Holland, and be Honour's Guard,
That none without thy notice should approach
The Seat of Joy, which thou hast leave to touch,
And with thy icy Nose presum'st to kiss,
Without Offence, the very Gates of Bliss.

Edward Ward 'The Secret History of Clubs' (1709)

Perhaps because of the opportunity it gives for grotesque fantasy, authors of many different periods and cultures have relished writing about the subject:

And therewithall she eftsoons imbraced my body round about, and had her pleasures with me, whereby I thought the mother of Minotaurus did not causeless quench her inordinate desire with a Bull. When night was passed, with much joy and small sleepe, the Matron went before day to my keeper to bargaine with him another night, which he willingly granted, partly for gaine of money, and partly to find new pastime for my master.

Lucius Apuleius *The Golden Ass* (2nd century)

A Cossack whose hands were cold was warming them in his mare's cunt. The beast was neighing softly. Suddenly, the randy Cossack leapt on a chair behind his animal and, pulling out a prick as long as a wooden lance, slipped it joyfully into the creature's vagina, which must have dripped a very aphrodisiac hippomaniac juice, for the human brute discharged three times, his arse convulsing violently, before he finally withdrew.

The dog's penis, once it had penetrated refused to come out again. For half an hour both the woman and the beast had been making fruitless efforts to separate. A nodule on the Great Dane's prick held it firmly in my wife's clenched vagina. I threw cold water over them and this soon restored them to liberty. Since that day, my wife has shown no desire to make love with dogs.

Guillaume Apollinaire *Les Onze Mille Verges* (c. 1900)

The long prelude of exploration, she counting my teeth with her ballpoint pen, I searching in vain for nits in her copious hair. Her playful observations on the length, colour, texture of my member, my fascination with her endearingly useless toes and her coyly concealed anus. Our first 'time' (Moira Sillito's word) was a little dogged by misunderstanding largely due to my assumption that we were to proceed a posteriori. *That matter was soon resolved and we adopted Sally Klee's unique 'face to face', an arrangement I found at first, as I tried to convey to my lover, too fraught with communication, a little too 'intellectual'.*

Ian McEwan *In Between the Sheets*, 'Reflections of a Kept Ape' (1978)

Freddie smiled and went on tickling and whispering to her, caressing and tickling her tits with his large gentle fingers with their grubby nails...Every now and then she would give a little muted whinny, a sighing noise, a whimper, which she found she could not control, and which dissolved into a short bout of hysterical barking, not very loud, and an access of playfulness.

My Sister and Myself: The Diaries of J. R. Ackerley (1982)

When Deadeye Dick and Mexico Pete
Went down to Deadman's Creek,
They'd had no luck, in the way of fuck,
For well nigh half a week.
Bar a moose or two or a caribou
And a bison cow or so,
But Deadeye Dick was the king of pricks
And he found such fucking slow.

Anon. 'Eskimo Nell'

I have a particular lady friend at the moment who practises zoophilia with her dog, a large mongrel. Often she strips naked while doing her housework and allows him to excite her from any position she happens to be in, sometimes making a paste of chocolate powder, sugar and milk and spreading it on her breasts for him to lick off.

Greenwald and Greenwald *The Sex-Life Letters* (1974)

Curiosity and experimentation in childhood and adolescence may be one origin of such behaviour in later life:

Kinsey found that out of the 5,940 females in his sample, twenty-three had had dogs put their mouths to the genitalia, six had experienced the same things with cats, and only two had actually had coitus with animals (both dogs). A further interesting datum supplied by Kinsey is that of 659 females in his sample who had experienced orgasm before adolescence, in 1·7% this first full sexual experience had been with an animal.

Paul Ableman *The Mouth* (1969)

Dr Frank Caprio quotes a patient:

I was thirteen years old when I had my first animal contact. I had seen cows of ours on heat, chasing each other around the pasture and jumping on their backs. It excited me. So one time I decided to try and put my penis in the cow's privates. I stood on a stool and did this, hav-

ing intercourse with the cow. I remember the cow's privates were all wet and hot and I got an ejaculation real quick.
I did this for about three or four months and then I stopped. I think the reason was my stepmother nearly caught me...Another time I put my penis in a calf's mouth and it sucked at my penis exciting me so that I got an ejaculation. I did this several times and one time the calf started to butt me, which discouraged my doing it any more.

Variations in Sexual Behaviour (1957)

Often arousal is accidental:

A relatively common way in which children discover the possibility of pleasurable contact between mouth and genitalia, is through accidental contacts with animals. This form of initiation is much more common to girls than boys, the obvious reasons being that a dog or cat may perform cunnilingus spontaneously but not fellatio.

Paul Ableman *The Mouth* (1969)

Such accidental contact can have profound psychological effects:

A little girl of four, of nervous temperament and liable to fits of anger in which she would roll on the ground and tear her clothes, once ran out into the garden in such a fit of temper and threw herself on the lawn in a half-naked condition. As she lay there two dogs with whom she was accustomed to play came up and began to lick the uncovered parts of her body. It so happened that as one dog licked her mouth the other licked her sexual parts. She experienced a shock of intense sensation which she could never forget and never describe, accompanied by a delicious tension of the sexual organ. She rose and ran away with a feeling of shame, though she could not comprehend what had happened. The impression thus made was so profound that it persisted throughout life and served as the point of departure of sexual perversion, while the contact of a dog's tongue with her mouth alone afterward sufficed to evoke sexual pleasure.

Feré *Archives de neurologie* (1903)

According to one 19th-century researcher:

In most cases where four-footed animals are used, the man plays the active part, but there are instances where the animal is the active agent, the human male taking the part of the pathic; thus there is the case recorded where a farmer's rectum was seriously injured because he used a bull as the active agent...
Where the dog is used as the active agent, if the act is interrupted before the dog has ejaculated, owing to the swelling of the glans of the penis, which occurs during coitus and which disappears only after ejaculation, the sudden withdrawal of the penis will often cause a laceration of the anus...
In male animals the rectum is generally used, although in one reported case a man used the nostrils of a horse.

G. Herzog *Medical Jurisprudence* (1894)

The opinions of 20th-century 'experts' are, as usual, conflicting:

In cases of bestiality an animal becomes the symbol of the human being.

H. Havelock Ellis *Erotic Symbolism* (1926)

Man's sexual experience with the lower animals represents a diversion rather than a perversion.

Dr D. O. Cauldwell *Animal Contacts* (1948)

Sexual contacts with other animal species are much rarer...because, of course, they provide far fewer of the appropriate sexual stimuli.

Desmond Morris *The Naked Ape* (1967)

The elements that are involved in sexual contacts between the human and animals of other species are at no point basically different from those that are involved in erotic responses to human situations.

Alfred Kinsey et al. *Sexual Behaviour in the Human Male* (1948)

Perhaps the last word should go to an unnamed 19th-century English serving girl, who is recorded as having said in court:

> *When a woman has tasted a dog, she will never want a man again.*

Bisexuality

The assertion that we are all to a greater or lesser degree bisexual has become commonplace:

My feeling is that we are all bisexual. I don't believe there is anyone who could honestly say at some point in their lives they have not been attracted to a member of the same sex.

Ken Livingstone, in a speech during the general election campaign of 1987

Indeed, it is often argued that active bisexuality is an ideal to which we would all aspire were it not for the ill effects of social conditioning:

If one can speak of a 'normal' state, it is bisexuality. I am quite convinced that if you could bring up a child without any gender conditioning, that child would be bisexual.

Dr Charlotte Wolff *Love between Women* (1971)

Man is bisexual all his life long, and keeps his bisexuality. At the most he consents at one or another period of his life, as a concession to the moral code in fashion, to repress a portion – and it is a very small portion – of his homosexuality and in doing so, he does not destroy it, but merely narrows its range. And just as no-one is purely heterosexual, so no-one is purely homosexual.

Georg Groddek *The Book of the Id* (1923)

To the advocates of universal bisexuality, declaring oneself exclusively hetero- or homo- makes as little sense as (for example) resolving on principle to drink only tea or only coffee:

Each person experiences their sexuality differently and we feel it is right to fully acknowledge this. It is quite usual for the balance of a person's sexual preferences to change and evolve continuously for many reasons. Relationships may be emotional and/or physical, contemporaneous or consecutive. The emphasis should be on a fluid sexuality rather than a fixed one. Bisexuals are people who are not or have not been exclusively gay, lesbian or heterosexual. To be bisexual is to have the potential to be open emotionally and sexually to people as people, regardless of their gender.

Bisexual Lives (1988)

Recent decades have seen a reaction against the late 19th-century view of 'homosexual' and 'heterosexual' as fixed and mutually incompatible categories (see MALE HOMOSEXUALITY). This trend was anticipated by Kinsey's innovative study:

Males do not represent two discrete populations, heterosexual and homosexual. The world is not to be divided into sheep and goats. Not all things are black nor all things white, for nature rarely deals with discrete categories. Only the human mind invents categories and tries to force facts into separated pigeon-holes. The living world is a continuum in each and every one of its aspects. The sooner we learn this concerning human sexual behaviour, the sooner we shall reach a sound understanding of the realities of sex.

Alfred Kinsey et al. *Sexual Behaviour in the Human Male* (1948)

One recent view is that we should think less in terms of a preference for one gender over another, and more in terms of a predeliction for specific sexual acts:

It seems quite likely that there are some cases of male and female homosexuality, and some others of male and female bisexuality, or rather, cases that are so regarded, that would be much more profitably explained in terms of anal and oral sexuality, or of desire for anal or oral intercourse.

Robert E. L. Masters *The Hidden World of Erotica* (1973)

Earlier in the century, psychoanalysis did much to break down rigid ideas of sexual identity:

Since I have become acquainted with the notion of bisexuality I regarded it as the decisive factor, and without taking bisexuality into account, I think it would scarcely be possible to arrive at an understanding of the sexual manifestations that are actually to be observed in men and women.

Sigmund Freud *Three Essays on the Theory of Sexuality* (1905)

The idea that we are all (potentially) bisexual draws much of its plausibility from the fact that nobody is psychologically wholly 'male' or 'female':

Science draws your attention to the fact that portions of the male sexual apparatus also appear in women's bodies, though in an atrophied state, and vice versa in the alternative case. It regards their occurrence as indicators of 'bisexuality', as though an individual is not a man or a woman but always both – merely a certain amount more the one than the other.

Sigmund Freud *New Introductory Lectures* (pub. 1973)

There is no such thing as an absolute male or female. Every man has something of the woman in him, and every woman something of the man.

William Fielding *Sacrifice to Attis: a Study of Sex and Civilization* (1953)

In other cultures, most notably classical Greece, male bisexuality has been widely practised and accepted:

The Greeks...had no nouns corresponding to the English nouns 'a homosexual' and 'a heterosexual' since they assumed that (a) virtually everyone responds at different times both to homosexual and to heterosexual stimuli; and (b) virtually no male both penetrates other males and submits to penetration...at the same stage of his life.

K. J. Dover *Greek Homosexuality* (1978)

In years when the body is still strong and can perform the normal functions of love, the sexual desire assumes a dual aspect, sometimes playing a passive role and sometimes an active role. But for the old men who have lost their virile powers, all their sexual desire is turned in the opposite direction and consequently exerts a stronger desire for the feminine role in love. This is the reason why boys are also victims of this affliction, for like old men they do not possess virile powers.

Caelius Aurelianus *De Morbis et acutis chronicis* (mid 5th century, largely adapted from the work of the 2nd-century Greek physician Soranus of Ephesus)

They are men to women, and women to men.

Anon. Greek epigram (c. 300–100 BC) quoted in *Anthologia Palatina*

It is Cypris, a woman, who casts at us the fire of passion for women, but Eros himself rules the desire for males. Whither shall I incline, to the boy or to his mother? I tell you for sure that even Cypris herself will say, 'The bold brat wins'.

Meleager of Gadara (c. 60 BC)

Less is heard of female bisexuality in the ancient world, although this has also been recorded:

The women called tribades, because they practise both kinds of sex, are more eager to have sexual intercourse with women than with men, and pursue women with almost masculine jealousy.

Caelius Aurelianus *De Morbis et acutis chronicis* (mid 5th century)

Much Roman literature similarly seems to take it for granted that men will be attracted to both women and boys:

Postumus, are you really
Taking a wife?...
Isn't it better to sleep with a pretty boy?
Boys don't quarrel all night, or nag you for little presents
While they're on the job, or complain that you don't come
Up to their expectations, or demand more gasping passion.

Juvenal *Satire VI* (2nd century)

When you're feeling randy
If a girl or boy is handy,
Attack at once!
Or would you rather suffer in silence?
Not me!
I like love fast and easy.

Horace *Satires* (c. 30 BC)

According to one source, Julius Caesar himself was known as

Every woman's man and every man's woman.

Curio the Elder, quoted by Suetonius in *The Twelve Caesars* (1st century AD)

Elsewhere, too, male bisexuality has been accepted within certain social contexts and conventions:

Shamans in eastern Asia put on female clothing and keep it all their lives. Bisexuality in the priests is acceptable because they are mediators between female Earth and male Heaven.

Jean Rhys Brain *Sex Reversal in the Ancient World* (1979)

The attitude of the Japanese towards homosexuality was at this period [1927] *considerably more tolerant than that of (say) the English. It was semi-respectable, in part at least because of the* samurai *tradition, which, like that of Plato's Athens, did not discourage a warrior from keeping both a wife and a catamite. Indeed, a man who had been through a frenetically active homosexual phase in youth might (and apparently often did) settle down to a lifelong marriage, his friends not thinking this out of the ordinary.*

Peter F. Alexander *William Plomer: A Biography* (1989)

Although it is quite common for bisexuals to marry, the demands of monogamy often prove frustrating:

It appears that very few bisexual men get divorced because of an unsuccessful marriage. Generally they make good, responsible caring fathers. That they cannot be faithful to their wives is due to the fact that without male sexual companionship, a very important part of their nature remains frustrated and unfulfilled.

Anon. woman quoted in *Bisexual Lives* (1988)

The most serious effect of the bi-sexual tendency is that it unfits many women for happy, married life.

William Fielding *Sacrifice to Attis: a Study of Sex and Civilization* (1953)

In Western societies, open bisexuality has until recently been restricted mainly to the artistic and literary elite:

Bloomsbury's sexual relationships crossed lines Carrington in her youth assumed to be firm. Maynard Keynes had relationships with men before marrying in middle age; Duncan Grant, despite fathering a child with Vanessa Bell was primarily homosexual and had an affair with David Garnett who later married Duncan and Vanessa's daughter Angelica; Virginia and Leonard Woolf had a celibate marriage; Lytton [Strachey] *was, of course homosexual, and continued to have affairs with men despite his relationship with Carrington.*

Gretchen Gerzina *Carrington: A Life of Dora Carrington 1893–1932* (1989)

Oh, you mean I'm homosexual! Of course I am, and heterosexual too. But what's that got to do with my headache?

Edna St Vincent Millay (20th century), in response to a doctor who hinted that her severe recurring headaches might be due to repressed lesbian impulses

Some have always taken a highly pragmatic view of the whole business:

Well, I might have loved boys too; but girls are what I prefer. If I tire of one as a girl, I can still use her as a boy.

J. W. von Goethe *Venetian Epigrams* (c. 1786)

Hetero-sex is best for the man of a serious turn of mind,
But here's a hint, if you should fancy the other:
Turn Menophila round in bed, address her peachy behind,
And it's easy to pretend you're screwing her brother.

Marcus Argentarius 'Hetero-Sex is Best'

Nor shall our love-fits, Chloris be forgot,
When each the well-looked linkboy strove t'enjoy,
And the best kiss was the deciding lot
Whether the boy fucked you, or I the boy.

John Wilmot, Earl of Rochester 'The Disabled Debauchee' (17th century)

Certainly, bisexuality can greatly widen one's opportunities:

I'm a practising heterosexual...but bisexuality immediately doubles your chances for a date on Saturday night.

Woody Allen (20th century)

We had heard through Dr. Dickinson of a man who had kept an accurate record of a lifetime's sexual behaviour. When we got the record after a long drive to take his history, it astounded even us, who had heard everything. This man had had homosexual relations with 600 pre-adolescent males, heterosexual relations with 200 pre-adolescent females, intercourse with countless adults of both sexes, with animals of many species and besides had employed elaborate techniques of masturbation. He had set down a family tree going back to his grandparents, and of thirty-three family members he had sexual contacts with seventeen. His grandmother introduced him to heterosexual intercourse and his first homosexual experience was with his father.

W. B. Pomeroy *Dr. Kinsey and the Institute for Sex Research* (1972). Pomeroy assisted Kinsey in his research

By the same token, however, most human beings find attraction to one sex quite troublesome and time-consuming enough without choosing to complicate the problem. For many heterosexuals, the absence of any sexual element is one of the chief attractions of single-sex friendships. (The same is presumably true of friendships between gays and members of the opposite sex.) Ultimately this, rather than social conditioning, may be why the number of people who choose to define themselves as bisexual and to pursue an actively bisexual lifestyle remains statistically small.

In the 1990s there are also prudential reasons for abstaining from any casual flirtation with bisexuality:

Many bisexual spokespeople advocated bisexuality as superior (for various reasons) to either form of 'exclusivism' (heterosexual or homosexual); they also held it to be much more threatening to the prevailing sexual norms, precisely because it potentially involved everyone rather than a small minority which could be ghettoized.

With the AIDS crisis in the 1980s, bisexuals were targeted as the most serious source of infection for the heterosexual majority, and 'bisexual chic' passed as quickly as it had arisen. With it, for the most part, went the bisexual liberation movement. Its self-description as threaten-

ing had been realized all too quickly, but in a way none of its leaders had foreseen.

Wayne R. Dynes (ed.) *Encyclopedia of Homosexuality* (1990)

See also SEXUALLY TRANSMITTED DISEASES

Castration

He that is wounded in the stones, or hath his privy member cut off, shall not enter into the congregation of the Lord.

Deuteronomy 23:1

While the Old Testament writers clearly regarded a eunuch as ungodly, the Gospel According to St Matthew records Jesus as apparently advocating self-castration as a way of entering the kingdom of heaven:

For there are some eunuchs which were so born from their mother's womb; there are eunuchs...which made themselves eunuchs for the kingdom of heaven's sake.

Matthew 19:12

The idea of making oneself into a eunuch for religious reasons has a long history. In ancient Phrygia the Greek goddess Cybele had only castrated priests, known as Corybantes. She also had a lover, Attis, who became so demented by her jealousy that he castrated himself:

Attis borne in speedy vessel
on the crest of seas profound,
when eagerly with restless foot
he reached the Phrygian woodland
and entered the dark tree-crowned
demesne of the goddess,
driven on by raging madness
and wandering in his mind
he there cut off the weights
of his groin with a sharp flint.

Catullus (1st century BC)

The origins of ritual castration go back even earlier:

Castration in the mother-cults may have imitated the reaping of crops. Only stone tools could be used for ritual castration; bronze or iron was forbidden, indicating the custom's prehistoric origins. Edith Weigert-Vowinhel endorses the view that the Phrygians borrowed castration from the Semites, who altered it over time to circumcision, and that the celibacy of Catholic priests is a substitute for castration.

Camille Paglia *Sexual Personae* (1990)

The association between castration, mythology, and the 'mother complex' clearly fascinated Freud:

I am delighted with your mythological studies. Much of what you write is quite new to me, e.g. the mother-lust, the idea that priests emasculated themselves to punish themselves for it. These things cry out for understanding, and as long as the specialists won't help us, we shall have to do it ourselves.

Sigmund Freud, in a letter to Carl Jung (21 Nov. 1909)

The subject has continued to intrigue psychiatrists:

The themes of self-castration and castration have re-emerged in modern psychiatry: if a man cuts off his own penis, psychiatrists call him schizophrenic, but if he can persuade a surgeon to cut it off for him they call him a transsexual... Although doctors now seem eager to enable persons to perform sexually, regardless of how or with whom – until recently they were just as eager to disable persons with 'perverse' erotic interests from satisfying their sexual appetites.

Such sexually disabling operations [castration] *– for homosexuals as well as for men who like to wear feminine clothing – were popular both before and after the second world war (especially in the Scandinavian countries).*

Thomas Szasz *Sex; Facts, Frauds and Follies* (1981)

In the case of the 3rd-century Church father, Origen, a literal interpretation of Christ's words about eunuchs is reputed to have led to self-castration in a fit of religious fervour (see CHASTITY AND CELIBACY). For Peter Abelard, however, the castration preceded the religious fervour:

In 1116 or 1117, the reader will recall, the great scholar and teacher Peter Abelard married his mistress Héloïse, niece of a canon of the cathedral of Notre-Dame in Paris. It was the briefest of unions. Her uncle had Abelard castrated, which Abelard took for a divine judgement: he insisted on their marriage being dissolved by the only legal means – by both entering religious orders.

Christopher Brooke *The Medieval Idea of Marriage* (1989)

Abelard wrote to Héloïse in about 1130:

So intense were the fires of lust which bound me to you that I set those wretched, obscene pleasures, which we blush even to name, above God as above myself; nor would it seem that divine mercy could have taken action except by forbidding me these pleasures altogether, without future hope. And so it was wholly just and merciful...that this member should justly be punished for all its wrongdoing in us, expiate in suffering the sins committed for its amusement, and cut me off from the slough of filth in which I had been wholly immersed in mind as in body. Only thus could I become more fit to approach the holy altars, now that no contagion of carnal impurity would ever again call me from them...

When divine grace cleansed rather than deprived me of those vile members which from their practice of utmost indecency are called 'the parts of shame' and have no proper name of their own, what else did it do but remove a foul imperfection in order to preserve perfect purity?

The 4th-century theologian Cassianus tells a story about a prurient old man who wanted to be pious:

Cassianus writeth, that St Syren being of body very lecherous, and of mind wonderfull religious, fasted and prayed to the end his body might be reduced miraculously to chastity. At length came an angel unto him by night, and cut out of his flesh certain kernels, which were the sparkes of concupiscence; so as afterwards he never had any more motions of the flesh.

Reginald Scott *The Discovery of Witchcraft* (1584)

But a mother complex or a religious obsession with the impurity of sex are not the only reasons for wanting to be castrated:

Love causes more pain than pleasure. Pleasure is only illusory. Reason would command us to avoid love, if it were not for the fatal sexual impulse – therefore it would be best to be castrated.

Karl von Hartmann *Philosophie des Unbewursten* (1869)

There seems, too, to be some kind of wild and perverse sexual gratification involved in the idea of immolating the member that is responsible for the gratification:

They went into a back room, where several acts of the grossest indecency passed; in particular he pressed her to cut off the means of generation, and expressly wished to have it cut in two. But this she refused.

Anon. *An Essay on the art of Strangling etc., ...with Memoirs of Susannah Hill...* (1791)

If Henry had cut off his thingy with a scythe he knew why. "If thy right hand scandalise thee cut it off and cast it from thee. For it is better for one member to die than that the whole body be consumed in the everlasting fire." How often he had thought of those words as he had held his own recalcitrant member out in front of him.

Michael Carson *Sucking Sherbet Lemons* (1988)

As the Galli sing and celebrate their orgies, frenzy falls on some of them, and many who have come as mere spectators afterwards are found to have committed the great act...Any young man who has resolved to this action, strips off his clothes and with a loud shout bursts into the middle of the crowd and picks up a sword from a number of swords which I suppose have been kept ready for many years for this purpose. He takes it and castrates himself, and runs wild through the city bearing in his hands what he has cut off.

Lucian *Erato* (2nd century)

The door opened, and Lucy and Pauline carried in a small, low table. Through his fear O'Bryne felt excitement once more, horrified excitement. They arranged the table close to the bed. Lucy bent low over his erection. 'Oh dear...oh dear,' she murmured. With tongs Pauline lifted instruments from the boiling water and laid them out in neat silver rows on the starched white tablecloth she had spread across the table. The leather noose slipped forwards fractionally. Lucy sat on the edge of the bed and took the large hyperdermic from the bowl. 'This will make you a little sleepy,' she promised. She held it upright and expelled a small jet of liquid. And as she reached for the cotton wool O'Bryne's arm pulled clear. Lucy smiled. She set aside the hyperdermic. She leaned forwards once more...warm, scented...she was fixing him with wild red eyes...her fingers played over his tip...she held him still between her fingers. 'Lie back, Michael, my sweet.' She nodded briskly at Pauline. 'If you'll secure that strap, Nurse Shepherd, then I think we can begin.'

Ian McEwan *In Between the Sheets*, 'Pornography' (1978)

However, the effects of castration are not always clear-cut:

The basic fact is that the results of surgical castration are unpredictable.

Anthony Storr *Sexual Deviation* (1964)

Although academic commentators taught that a castrated man could not marry, an Augsburg judge thought otherwise, for he held in a case on 9 March 1350 that a eunuch (spado) had successfully consummated his marriage.

James A. Brundage *Law, Sex and Christian Society in Medieval Europe* (1987)

It is said that those who, having attained the age when the genital member is capable of copulation, have cut off their testicles, burn with greater desire for sexual union, and that...they think they can defile any women they meet.

Basil of Ancyra *De Virginitate* (c. 365)

They say castrated eunuchs, when abortive lust challenges them to female embraces and encounters beyond their power, are consumed with unsatisfied ecstasies on the tumbled bed: until their passion, tickled for an instant, blazes in a last fling and completes the sportive act with a bite of the mouth.

Ausonius *Ephemeris* (4th century)

There are girls who adore unmanly eunuchs, so smooth, so beardless to kiss, and no worry about abortions!

Juvenal *Satire VI* (2nd century)

Eunuchs often develop a distinct physical appearance, characterized by hairlessness, a flaccid physique, and signs of premature ageing:

This would be the answer for those who wished to abstain from sexual contact, if vigour and virility were not removed along with the testicles.

Galen (2nd century)

Look at that specimen – you could spot him a mile off,
Everyone knows him, displaying his well endowed person.
At the baths: Priapus might well be

jealous. And yet
He's a eunuch. His mistress arranged it.
So,
Let them sleep together.

Juvenal *Satire VI* (2nd century)

Geoffrey Chaucer gave a very clear portrait of a suspected eunuch:

This Pardoner hadde heer as yelow as
wex,
But smothe it heeng as dooth a strike of
flex;
By ounces henge his lokkes that he hadde,
And therwith he his shuldres overspradde...
A voys he hadde as smal as hath a goot.
No berd hadde he, ne nevere sholde have;
As smothe it was as it were late shave.
I trowe he were geldying or a mare.

The Canterbury Tales, 'Prologue' (late 14th century)

The effect of the testicles and the hormones they produce on the growth of both facial and head hair has long been known:

...Let the testicles ripen
And drop, fill out till they hang like
two-pound weights:
Then what the surgeon chops will hurt
no-one's
trade but the barber's.

Juvenal *Satire VI* (2nd century)

It is an infallible sign of this, if a man is bald and not old; but if old and not bald, you may conclude he hath lost one of his stones or both.

Giovanni Sinibaldi *Rare Verities* (1657)

They also have a profound effect on the voice. In the 16th century, when women were not allowed to sing in church choirs, another reason for castration was discovered. If young singers were castrated before puberty they turned into adult sopranos and contraltos of great power:

The unique tone quality of the voice, coupled with the ability of the intensively trained singers to execute extremely difficult florid vocal passages, made the castrati the rage of opera audiences and contributed to the spread of Italian opera. In 18th-century opera the majority of male singers were castrati.

Encyclopaedia Britannica

This inhumane practice was brought to an end in 1878 by Pope Leo XIII.

Many other cultures have found specialized uses for the emasculated male. In the polygamous societies of the Muslim world, eunuchs were traditionally employed in the harems of potentates. In this way the ruler could ensure the chastity of his wives and the legitimacy of his succession. Eunuchs were also for many centuries employed at the court of imperial China, where they often acquired considerable wealth and influence:

Traditionally the emperor had three thousand eunuchs, the princes thirty each, the emperor's children and nephews twenty each, his cousins and the descendants of the Tartar princes who helped Nurhachi found the dynasty ten each. They had been recruited into the palace through the princes who provided five fully trained eunuchs every five years...but this method had never furnished enough, and by the reign of Hsien-feng a register had been opened in which the names of candidates were inscribed. That the state had any charms at all seems incomprehensible, but the squalor, misery and abject poverty in which many Chinese lived, combined with their reverence for the emperor, made the lure of his service extremely powerful. Within there were riches, luxury, food in the belly and money in the palm – it was an overwhelming bribe...For although a palace eunuch was only given ten taels a month and daily rice, he was entitled to a cut on all money that passed through his hands, and jewels, jade, fur, silk, antiques, paintings, vases were sent as gifts and tribute to the emperor in such quantities that a little pilfering, or even a great deal, went by quite unnoticed...The family who performed the castrations jealously guarded their hereditary rôle because, while the operation was cheap, they hired out the testicles or sold them back at an exorbitant rate to their client...for at the annual inspections which were carried out in the Imperial City by the Chief Eunuch each one was required to prove himself by producing his remains, bottled and labelled. Also, according to Confucian doctrine, mutilation of the body reflected the imperfection of the spirit. All eunuchs desired to be buried whole, so that their spirit could enter eternal life intact.

Marina Warner *The Dragon Empress* (1972)

In China the eunuchs were widely despised for their corruption and insidious politicial influence:

These two can be neither taught nor led: wives and eunuchs.

Chan-Yang *Book of Odes* (c. 4th century)

Elsewhere, castration of a man against his will was not infrequently used as a form of punishment:

But if Church authorities in the seventh, eighth and ninth centuries were sometimes reluctant to deal with deviant sexual practices, secular authorities were not so restrained. In Spain the Visigothic laws prescribed castration for homosexual offences.

James A. Brundage *Sex, Law and Christian Society in Medieval Europe* (1987)

While I was lying senseless they called in a barber, who cut off my testicles and cauterized the wound: so that when I recovered my senses I found myself a eunuch with nothing left. My master wagged his finger at me with evident satisfaction, saying "You have taken away from me things that I valued dearly: I have taken away from you things which you held most precious."

Tales from the Thousand and One Nights, 'The Tale of Kafur the Black Eunuch'

In 1983, a South Carolina judge sentenced three rapists guilty of a particularly horrific incident to choose between either thirty years in prison or castration. Castration or testalectomy is a radical and irreversible surgical removal of the testes. The practice was first recorded by Farel in 1892. Once the testes are removed, there is a dramatic reduction in the male sex hormone, testosterone, libido or sexual desire decreases in response to this absence of male hormone.

Roy Eskapa *Bizarre Sex* (1987)

In the 20th century castration was also practised in German slave camps as part of the Nazis' evil and insane plan to create a German *Herrenvolk*:

Himmler wanted all non-Aryans to be a slave force for the Reich, he felt that the vast majority of them would have to be sterilized. This would prevent race-mixing and control the slave population. By 1942...it was decided to use long, high doses of X-rays, which were known to cause sterility...This time Jewish men were chosen for the experimentation...The strongest and brightest among the men were selected to be exposed to high doses of radiation. These were men who would make excellent workers in a slave society. Unfortunately, no one knew the exact level of dosage that was important, so variations were used...approximately four weeks later, those who had survived and done well were brought back and castrated so that their testicles could be dissected and studied. In that manner, the perfect dosage for sterilization was determined.

The initial action was to be applied to the European Jews at first. There were two to three million such individuals in captivity who were deemed healthy enough to be of use in a work program.

Testing took place at Auschwitz and Ravensbruck, the results being a disappointment for Dr. Schuhmann. The concept was a good one, but it was expensive and not 100 percent effective for men. Castration by operation was a better approach, the doctor explained, since the operation took approximately six minutes to complete. Unfortunately, the added time factor made such large-scale castration impractical.

Ted Schwarz *Walking with the Damned* (1992)

It is ironic that the leader of these diabolical people should himself have been, as the Hebrew Bible has it, 'wounded in the stones':

> *In the scrotum, which is singed but preserved, only the right testicle was found. The left testicle could not be found in the inguinal canal.*
>
> Soviet autopsy report on Adolf Hitler (1945)

Rumours of this deficiency were gleefully embroidered by marching British and American soldiers (to the tune of Colonel Bogey):

> *Hitler has only got one ball*
> *Goering has two – but very small*
> *Himmler has something similar,*
> *But poor old Goebbels has got no balls at all.*

Chastity and Celibacy

Although the words chastity and celibacy are often used interchangeably, they are not synonyms:

Chastity, a 13th-century word from the Latin *castitās*, means abstention from illicit sexual intercourse.

> *The first degree of chastity is pure virginity, and the second faithfulness in matrimony.*
>
> William Bauldwin *Moral Philosophy* (1547–64)

Celibacy, a 17th-century word from the Latin *caelibatus*, means the state of being unmarried, especially as a result of taking a religious vow.

A faithfully married man or woman can therefore be described as chaste but not celibate, while a Roman Catholic priest takes a vow of celibacy but not of chastity. Inevitably, attitudes to sexual abstinence will depend on attitudes to the sexual act itself. In an age characterized (in the West at least) by the weakening of traditional religious sanctions and the availability of safe and effective contraception, few people see sexual abstinence as a virtue:

> *The omnipresent process of sex, as it is woven into the whole texture of our man's or woman's body, is the pattern of all the process of our life.*
>
> H. Havelock Ellis *The New Spirit* (1890)

> *We might as well make up our minds that chastity is no more a virtue than malnutrition.*
>
> Dr Alex Comfort *The Joy of Sex* (1986)

> *I will find you twenty lascivious turtles 'ere one chaste man.*
>
> William Shakespeare *The Merry Wives of Windsor* (1599)

Marriage has many pains, but celibacy has no pleasures.

Samuel Johnson *Rasselas* (1759)

Those who restrain Desire, do so because theirs is weak enough to be restrained.

William Blake *The Marriage of Heaven and Hell* (1793)

Chastity is a monkish and evangelical superstition, a greater foe to natural temperance even than unintellectual sensuality; it strikes at the roots of all domestic happiness, and consigns more than half the human race to misery…A system could not well have been devised more studiously hostile to human happiness…

Percy Bysshe Shelley *Queen Mab* (1813)

Marriage may often be a stormy lake, but celibacy is almost always a muddy horse-pond.

Thomas Love Peacock *Melincourt* (1817)

Chastity is the most unnatural of all the sexual perversions.

Remy de Gourmont (late 19th century)

Mr Mercaptan went on to preach a brilliant sermon on that melancholy sexual perversion known as continence.

Aldous Huxley *Antic Hay* (1923)

If you resolve to give up smoking, drinking and loving, you don't actually live longer; it just seems longer.

Clement Freud *Observer* (27 Dec. 1964)

More than 100 million acts of sexual intercourse take place every day, the

World Health Organisation has calculated.

Nigel Hawkes *The Times* (25 June 1992)

The view that sexual intercourse is a normal, universally practised, human activity is sometimes taken further by its enthusiasts:

'Bed,' as the Italian proverb succinctly puts it, 'is the poor man's opera.'

Aldous Huxley *Heaven and Hell* (1956)

Life can little more supply
Than just a few good fucks and then we die.

John Wilkes *Essay on Woman* (1763)

The dangers of abstinence have also been stressed by many writers:

If one should resolve to abstain from sexual intercourse, one's spirit will not develop since the interchange of Yin and Yang will then come to a halt. How could one thus supplement one's vital essence?

Su-nü-Ching *Fang Nei Chi (Secrets of the Bedchamber)* (7th century)

If a man abstains too long from emitting semen he will develop boils and ulcers.

Sun-szu-mo *Priceless Recipes* (7th century; printed 1066)

Sexual abstinence in a normally constituted person is always pathogenic. We have been given sex organs to use them. If we don't use them, they decay and cause irreparable damage to body and mind. This is blunt, firm, indisputable, and true.

Dr Barbara Bross 'How to Love like a Real Woman' *Cosmopolitan* (June 1969)

On the other hand, reverence for virginity and an insistence on abstinence outside marriage have featured in many religions, most notably Christianity. The Church's idealization of celibacy probably derived originally from the virginity of both Christ and (according to orthodox doctrine) his mother. Christ himself is reported to have spoken approvingly of

...eunuchs, which have made themselves eunuchs for the kingdom of heaven's sake.

Matthew 19:12

– a puzzling remark, traditionally taken as a metaphorical reference to those who choose celibacy for religious reasons. Few Christians now take this text literally – although there have been suggestions that it inspired the 3rd-century theologian Origen to castrate himself in his youth,

so as to work freely in instructing female catechumens.

Encyclopaedia Britannica

See also CASTRATION

For most early Christians, including St Paul, marriage was regarded as a second option for those who found celibacy too difficult:

He that giveth his virgin in marriage doeth well; but he that giveth her not in marriage doeth better.

I Corinthians 7:38

He that is unmarried careth for the things that belong to the Lord, how he may please the Lord.
But he that is married careth for the things that are of the world, how he may please his wife.

I Corinthians 7:32–33

This downgrading of the married state was largely based on the fanatical assumption that the end of the world was imminent:

...the time is short: it remaineth, that...they that have wives be as though they had none...for the fashion of this world passeth away.

I Corinthians 7:29–31

Another factor in the promotion of celibacy as a Christian ideal was undoubtedly a primitive fear of sexuality:

The Church's profound loathing for sex was proclaimed by Odon of Cluny, for the Church saw sexuality as the principal means by which the Devil secured his hold on the creation.

Georges Duby, writing about the 11th century in *Medieval Marriage* (1938)

In Christendom this attitude appears as early as St Paul, but is at its most virulent in writers of the later Roman empire, such as St Jerome and St Augustine:

All sexual intercourse is impure.

St Jerome (4th century)

But I was an unhappy young man, wretched as at the beginning of my adolescence when I prayed to you for chastity and said: 'Grant me chastity and continence, but not yet.' I was afraid you might hear my prayer quickly, and that you might too rapidly heal me of the disease of lust which I preferred to satisfy rather than suppress.

St Augustine *Confessions* (397–400)

If you do not *think about it you have no hope...he who does not fight against the sin and resist it in his spirit will commit the sin physically.*

Abba Cyrus of Alexandria (3rd century)

There are six degrees of chastity. The first consists of not succumbing to the assaults of the flesh while conscious. In the second, the monk rejects voluptuous thoughts. In the third, the sight of a woman does not move him. In the fourth, he no longer has erections while awake. In the fifth, no reference to the sexual act in the holy texts affects him any more than if he was in the process of making bricks, and in the sixth the seduction of female fantasies does not delude him while he sleeps. (Even though we do not believe this to be a sin, it is nevertheless an indication that lust is still hiding in the marrow.)

John Cassian *Collationes* (c. 420)

When one wants to take a town, one cuts off the supply of water and food. The same applies to the passions of the flesh. If a man lives a life of fasting and hunger, the enemies of his soul are weakened.

John the Dwarf (3rd century)

Although the practice of clerical celibacy had grown steadily since the emergence of a distinction between clergy and laity in the 2nd century, there were no attempts to enforce it until the 4th century. The Council of Nicaea (325) ruled that celibacy was required of bishops but not of the lower clergy, a position that is still held by the Eastern Church. However:

Celibacy became mandatory for priests at the Second Lateran Council in 1139. Pope Innocent II decreed that ordination was an impediment to marriage. Up to then, married priests had been the norm. Afterwards canon law stated (and continues to state) that matrimony and celibacy were mutually exclusive.

Kate Saunders and Peter Stanford *Catholics and Sex* (1992)

Before this, clerical marriages were permitted on the condition that the partners abstained from intercourse, a manifestly unenforceable prohibition that declined into a formality in most parts of Western Christendom. The insistence on celibacy was not seriously challenged until the rise of Protestantism in the 16th century and the abolition of clerical celibacy in the Reformed Churches (in 1549 in the Church of England). The Council of Trent (1563) reacted to the Protestant encouragement of married priests with an uncompromising restatement of the traditional view. Anathema was pronounced on those who denied

that it is more blessed to remain in virginity or in celibacy than to be joined in marriage.

Council of Trent, XXIV session (11 Nov. 1563)

Despite the incomprehension of the secular world and rising unrest among its own ranks the Catholic Church continues to maintain its traditional position:

[Celibacy] *is a singular source of spiritual fertility in the world.*

Pope John Paul II in the apostolic exhortation *Pastores dabo vobis (I Will Give You Shepherds)* (Apr. 1992)

Modern apologists for clerical celibacy offer two main arguments. One is that by forsaking worldly ties the priest frees himself to live a life of self-sacrificing love that would be impossible if he had to consider the welfare of a wife and children. Another is that by renouncing sexual love the priest affirms that even the highest natural goods are transcended by a greater supernatural good:

To live in the midst of the world, with no desire for its pleasures; to be a member of every family, yet belonging to none; to share all sufferings, to penetrate all secrets, to heal all wounds; to go daily from men to God, to offer Him their homage and petitions, to return from God to men, to bring them His pardon and His hope; to have a heart of iron for chastity and a heart of flesh for charity; to teach and to pardon, console and bless and to be blessed for ever. O God, what a life is this, and it is thine, O priest of Jesus Christ.

Henri Lacordaire (19th-century French Dominican)

What a priest has to offer his people, that no one else has to offer, is the unique relationship he can have with them as their priest. Just as a couple's activity takes on a deeper significance and even a new meaning to the degree that there is genuine commitment and bonding between them, so priestly activity becomes truly 'priestly' to the degree that it reflects a genuine commitment and bonding between himself and his people.
Enter celibacy. As a catalyst speeds up and enhances the chemical reaction of two elements without being essential to that reaction, the charism of celibacy deepens and enhances the relationship of the priest with his people, without being essential to that relationship.

Charles A. Gallagher and Thomas L. Vandenberg *The Celibacy Myth; Loving for Life* (1987)

On the other hand there are a number of commonsense objections to compulsory priestly celibacy. The first, of course, is that a vow of celibacy cannot ensure chastity; secret liaisons have always been commonplace in spite of the various decrees since the Council of Nicaea forbidding them:

A survey by Richard Sipe, a psychiatrist at Johns Hopkins University, Baltimore, revealed that 20 per cent of US priests were having sex at any one time. Only 2 per cent were truly chaste.

Kate Saunders and Peter Stanford *Catholics and Sex* (1992)

As it is certain that there have always and everywhere been priests who lived exemplarily, so a noticeable proportion, especially among the parish clergy, kept able-bodied women in their prime, when they had no blood relations, in order to look after the housekeeping and agriculture...
They lived together with them and by them had children who often grew up in the vicarage... We know of many cases where these 'keepers of concubines' possessed the sympathies of their parishioners and were looked on as good and virtuous pastors...
The keepers of concubines were in many dioceses punished by fines and then tolerated; what is much worse is that these fines (commonly known as the 'whore tax') formed a not inconsiderable source of income for the Bishop and Archdeacon.

H. Jedin 'The Celibacy of Priests in the 16th Century', an unpublished document prepared for the Second Vatican Council (1963)

A real Catholic doesn't expect that his priest is a saint. They are sinners like everybody else. I asked Graham Greene once whether he was in favour of celibacy, and he said he was in favour of priests having cooks. Lady cooks, you know – this was the traditional way; all these cooks were of course mistresses.

Josef Skvorecky, interviewed in the *Independent* (27 June 1992)

In fact there is a Catholic story (no doubt apocryphal) about an elderly priest in a rural parish being visited by his bishop:

"Are you ever lonely?" asked the bishop.
"I have my Rosary," replied the old man.
"But what about spending the long winter nights all alone?"
"I have my Rosary."
When the bishop asked for a cup of

> *coffee, the elderly priest called into the kitchen: "Rosary, bring his Eminence a cup of coffee, please."*

It has also been said that everyone calls a Catholic priest 'father', except his children – who call him 'uncle'.

> *Every time I did a marriage, every time I see people married I say: 'That could have been me.' So I think a successful celibate has to regret that he wasn't married.*

Cardinal Hume, in an interview on BBC Radio (12 July 1992)

Not all priestly diversions have been heterosexual however:

> *So there is the chastity of the Romish Priests, who forsooth may not marry and yet may miscarry themselves in all abominations, especially in sodomy, which is their continual pleasure and practice.*

William Lithgow *Rare Adventures* (1620)

> *Inevitably, one asks today whether a commitment to celibacy is not a way of hiding from one's self or others a psychological disinclination to marriage that stems from instincts having little to do with religion.*

Robert Bernard Martin *Gerard Manley Hopkins: A Very Private Life* (1991)

> *It has been estimated that at least 33 per cent of all priests and religious in the Catholic Church are homosexual.*

Dr Elizabeth Stuart, convener of the Catholic Caucus of the Lesbian and Gay Christian Movement, in the Channel 4 television programme 'Roman Catholics and Homosexuality' (1990)

Recently a great scandal ensued over the discovery that Dr Eamonn Casey, Bishop of Galway, was the father of a 17-year old boy. More scandalous still, that Dr Casey had supported his lover and his son from misappropriated church funds. Not exactly the kind of bishop that Raymond Chandler had in mind:

> *It was a blonde, a blonde to make a bishop kick a hole in a stained-glass window.*

Farewell My Lovely (1940)

A second objection to a celibate priesthood, put forward by the president of the American Psychiatric Association (himself a Catholic), is that it produces emotionally immature ministers:

> *We take promising young men from thirteen to twenty years of age, feed them well, educate them diligently, and eight to twelve years later we ordain them, healthy, bright, emotional thirteen-year-olds.*

Leo Bartmeyer, quoted by Richard Sipe in an address (1988)

Their ignorance of sexual matters may verge on the ludicrous:

> *...at Oxford the select preacher, one evening service, speaking of venery, said "And let me implore you, my young friends, not to imperil your immortal souls upon a pleasure which,* so I am credibly informed, *lasts less than one and three-quarter minutes."*

T. E. Lawrence *The Mint* (1955)

Unsurprisingly, ex-priests do not always make very good family men:

> *Priests aren't very practical husbands. All their training is intellectual, and idealism can be rather cloying...*
> *They say the Pope gets letters saying, "please take him back, and I'll rear the kids on my own." Some people say that's why he's not giving dispensations, but I don't believe it...*
> *Financially they are hopeless. They haven't a bull's notion about money.*

Comments by anonymous wives of laicized priests, quoted by David Rice in *Shattered Vows* (1990)

However, the former priest David Rice recalls being told by the wife of another former priest that her husband in mid-passion called out:

> *Thank you God, thank you – I never thought it could be like this.*

Shattered Vows (1990)

A third, and to the Roman Catholic Church most important, objection to compulsory celibacy is that it is now creating a shortage of priests:

42 percent of all American priests leave [the priesthood] *within twenty-five years of ordination.*

Richard Schoenherr *Corpus Reports* Vol. 1 (1987)

As many as 100,000 priests worldwide (a quarter of the total) have left the Church in the last 20 years.

Movement for the Ordination of Married Men

...Christian communities have a right to leaders and to the Eucharist, and if compulsory celibacy is depriving them of such leaders, then it must be questioned. In such a situation Church legislation, which can in any case be changed, must give way to the more urgent right to the apostolic and Eucharistic building up of the community.

Edward Schillebeeckx *Ministry* (1981)

I do not believe it [compulsory celibacy] *to be a just law or a good law, or a law which the Church had the right to make, and I am convinced that it does not express God's will for the Church today, if it ever did... Wherever one turns, the clericalism which puts celibacy above ministry is strangling the Church.*

Andrew Hastings *Commonweal* (1978)

...the requirement of celibacy must help shape the type of entrant [to the Roman Catholic priesthood]. *Some good men must be lost...*

Editorial, *Independent* (9 May 1992)

Not all religions take the same view of these matters as Christianity. This advice is given by a Buddhist elder:

Most young men who keep themselves strictly chaste find themselves visited by sexual fantasies and tortured longings which are worse for them than occasional visits to flower-houses, while marriage is far better still...Perfect chastity is dangerous, unless you have really mastered such longings. Buddhism does not enjoin enforced chastity, which is the road to madness, but the gradual mastery of desire.

J. Blofeld *The Wheel of Life* (1988)

In Judaism, celibacy is frowned upon; the first commandment in the Old Testament is

Be fruitful and multiply, and fill the waters in the seas, and let fowl multiply in the earth.

Genesis 1:22

Judaism is opposed to it [asceticism], *regarding all things in life as good when enjoyed within limits and under discipline.*

The New Standard Jewish Encyclopedia (1970)

The Jews scorn the beauty of virginity, and this is hardly surprising since they treated Christ himself with contempt, and he was born of a virgin. The Greeks admire and revere this beauty, but the Church of God is unique in directing toward its devotion.

St John Chrysostom *De virginitate* (4th century)

In Islam

The Quran *regards celibacy definitely as something exceptional – to be resorted to only under economic stringency...however, many Sufis preferred celibacy, and some even regarded women as an evil distraction from piety...*

Encyclopaedia Britannica

Many Christians regard celibacy as a charism (a gift from God for the benefit of others). For the Hindu, however:

...the world-renouncing ascetic is the type universally admired, and his renunciation is in no sense altruistic or philanthropic, but is purely self-regarding, since it is every man's business and licence to look after his eternal welfare; and to be concerned with delivering oneself from the generally accepted chain of rebirth, and from the cycle of biological existence; is not considered to be a blemish upon one's character. Gandhiji was nobly inconsistent when he made unselfish service of his fellow-men part of the discipline to which he subjected himself in order to free his

soul from the bonds of the flesh, since self-forgetful service of others is a Christian, not a Hindu idea.

A. C. Bouquet *The Religion of Man* (1931)

Gandhi was 36 when he took his vow of celibacy:

It has not been proved to my satisfaction that sexual union in marriage is itself good and beneficial...momentary excitement and satisfaction there certainly was. But it was invariably followed by exhaustion. And the desire for union returned immediately the effect of exhaustion wore out. Although I have always been a conscientious worker, I can clearly recall that this indulgence interfered with my work. It was the consciousness of this limitation that put me back on the track of self-restraint and I have no manner of doubt that the self-restraint is responsible for the comparative freedom from illness that I have enjoyed...and for my output of energy and work both physical and mental.

Mahatma Gandhi *Collected Works* Vol. 1 (1975)

The intensity of his desire led him to the source of power itself. Deep in meditation Gandhi began to see how much of his vital energy was locked up in the sexual drive. In a flood of insight he realised that sex is not just a physical instinct, but an expression of the tremendous spiritual force behind all love and creativity which the Hindu scriptures call kundalini, *the life force of evolution.*

E. Easwaran *Gandhi the Man* (1983)

In many non-Western cultures women are still subjected to a rigid code of chastity:

Japanese women often became nuns upon the death of their husbands and lovers, vowing to remain chaste until they joined their partners again in the next world.

John Stevens *Lust for Enlightenment* (1990)

In Africa

Tribal societies still use extreme methods to ensure chastity. Some modern Nubian women willingly submit to a surgical operation when their husbands have to be away for any length of time. It involves infibulation (sewing up) as a shield against penetration: the operation can be reversed when the husband returns.

Reay Tannahill *Sex in History* (1980)

See CIRCUMCISION (FEMALE)

This practice is reminiscent of the chastity belts imposed on some European women in earlier centuries:

...made of iron, and consisting of a belt and a piece which came up under and was locked in position, so neatly made that once a woman was bridled it was out of the question for her to indulge in the gentle pleasure, as there were only a few little holes for her to piss through.

Pierre de Bourdeille, Seigneur de Brantôme (16th century)

Such devices were still being manufactured in the 19th century:

The advantages are manifold. Not only will the purity of the virgin be maintained, but the fidelity of the wife exacted. The husband will leave the wife without fear that his honour will be outraged and his affections estranged.

An advertisement for a French chastity belt, quoted by Eric Dingwall in *The Circle of Chastity* (1880)

The allegation that he locked a steel chastity belt of mediaeval design on his wife formed the basis of a charge of 'atrocious assault and battery' brought against a 39-year-old wood worker. His wife...was quoted by Police-Captain Webb as having declared that he padlocked the belt about her before he left for work. She was brought to police headquarters, where a locksmith removed the belt by cutting one of the one-inch steel links in the chain. The police stated that when arrested...he said he manufactured the belt during his spare time, and applied it to his wife to 'keep her from running around'.

News of the World (US) (16 June 1946)

Child Abuse

Paedophilia, incest, and the sexual abuse of children have occurred throughout history and in almost every culture. However, what constitutes an abuse and who should be treated as a child are questions largely determined by social and cultural attitudes.

In ancient Greece the assault of a child was illegal:

> *The Law of Outrage stipulates that the assailant of a child, whether the victim be free or a slave, shall be charged and the due penalty applied or else he shall pay a fine determined by the court.*

Aeschines *Against Timarchus* (4th century BC)

However, it was not considered an abuse for men to have intercourse with prepubescent boys; prepubescence ended when the boys began to grow beards – after which they were no longer regarded as desirable:

> *Boys in the flower of their youth are loved, the smoothness of their thighs and soft lips is adored.*

Solon (594 BC)

> *Plato declares that men who have proven their worth should be permitted to caress any fair lad they please. Lovers who lust only for physical beauty, then, it is right to drive away; but free access should be granted to lovers of the soul.*

Plutarch *Education* (1st century AD)

See also MALE HOMOSEXUALITY

Although pederasty was not thought of as child abuse in ancient Greece – indeed the boy was often materially and socially rewarded for his cooperation by the older man – the boy was not expected to enjoy the act of sodomy:

> *The Athenian vases clearly show that only the adults were considered to derive satisfaction from pederastic intercourse; the boy usually looks as if he is solving some academic problem.*

Professor Jan Bremmer *Greek Pederasty and Modern Homosexuality* (1989)

> *Schoolboys are hardly so well-educated in kissing, their embraces are awkward, their love-making is lazy and devoid of pleasure.*

Achilles Tatius *Leucippe and Cleitophon* (5th century BC)

The difference in social status between freeborn boys and slaves considerably affected what the ancient Greeks judged to be abuse:

> *Freeborn boys wore a gold ball around their necks when very young, so that men could tell which boys it was not proper to use sexually, when they found a group in the nude.*

Plutarch *Lives* (1st century AD)

There were also certain rules concerning the running of a school or gymnasium:

> *Consider the case of teachers – it is plain that the lawgiver distrusts them. He forbids the teacher to open the schoolroom, or the gymnastics trainer the wrestling school, before sunrise, and he commands them to close the doors before sunset; for he is exceeding suspicious of their being alone with a boy, or in the dark with him.*

Aeschines *Speeches* (4th century BC)

This suspicion of teachers was shared by many ancient Romans:

If inadequate care is taken in the choices of respectable governors and instructors, I blush to mention the shameful abuse which scoundrels sometimes make of their right to administer corporal punishment or the opportunity not infrequently offered to others by the fear thus caused in the victims. I will not linger on this subject; it is more than enough if I have made my meaning clear.

Quintilian *Instituto Oratorio* (1st century AD)

Although the Roman moral tradition put greater emphasis on sexual restraint than that of the ancient Greeks, paedophilia still occurred:

While buggering a boy, refrain from stirring the groin with poking hand. Nature has separated the male: one part has been produced for girls, one for men. Use your own part.

Martial *Epigrams* (1st century AD)

It was, however, disapproved of:

So, shun damnable deeds.
For this there's at least one good reason –
Lest our children repeat
The crimes we have taught them.

Juvenal *Satire XIV* (2nd century AD)

Apart from the classical world, pederasty was also customary in some other cultures. In Papua, for example:

Bachelors remained truly celibate until they entered upon sexual relations with their own wives. They had recourse to sodomy, which was actually a custom of the country. It is actually regarded as essential to the growing boy to be sodomized...

The Father bids his son stoop to drink and as he does so catches him at a disadvantage.

F. E. Williams *Papuans of the Trans-Fly* (1969)

In Britain, child abuse was legislated against in the 16th century but was still widespread in the 19th century:

It wasn't until 1548 that any legal protection from sexual abuse was offered to children. In that year England passed a law protecting boys from forced sodomy. In 1576 another law was enacted which prohibited the forcible rape of girls under the age of ten. In the 1700s some educators warned parents to protect their children from abuse by supervising them at all times and by ensuring that they were never nude in front of adults, and in general suggested enforced modesty. This warning was one of the earliest indications that the larger society recognized children could be sexually exploited...

Pornography and child prostitution also increased during the Victorian period. Men, who dared not 'prevail upon their wives to perform their duty too often' and who shielded their children from explanations of sexuality, thought nothing of frequenting child prostitutes in city slums. In the early nineteenth century, American slave owners had delighted in 'breaking in' their young slaves or using them for breeding. Eleven-, twelve-, and thirteen-year old girls were often impregnated.

Cynthia Crosson Tower *Understanding Child Abuse and Neglect* (1989)

The reluctance of adults to admit that children have any sexual knowledge or feelings has often made it easier for child abuse to continue undetected:

Unfortunately, the idea that children are innocent and cannot be corrupted is a common defense by child molesters against admitting that their abuse is harming the child, so the mediaeval fiction that the child is innocent only makes our sources less revealing, and proves nothing about what really went on.

Lloyd Demause *The Evolution of Childhood* (1974)

The belief that children should not be told about sex in order to protect them is dangerous;

ignorance may, in fact, render them more vulnerable to abuse:

I look for the kid who looks vulnerable – you know – the one who doesn't have much confidence, who's probably been taught to obey adults no matter what. And I really know that I have it made if no one's explained anything about sex to the kid. Then I can tell him or her anything I want and he or she will believe me. When parents don't talk to kids about sex or abuse and when the kid knows he or she can't ask questions, that's when I have no trouble getting a child to go along with me. Maybe parents should know that. If they want to protect their kids against someone like me, they should talk to them – tell them honestly what could happen.

Convicted child abuser, quoted by Cynthia Crosson Tower in *Understanding Child Abuse and Neglect* (1989)

There was also a belief that to talk publicly about child abuse, even in parliament, would incite ordinary people to become abusers:

It is argued that to speak out on this subject is only to suggest the very evil you want to cure, and to do more harm than good...let us recognize once and for all that the modest silence has landed England in child harlotry.

Earl of Halsbury, debate on the Incest Bill, House of Lords (1903)

In many cases children are abused by members of their own family. Even now, many people refuse to accept that such abuse occurs or are reluctant to confront it in case they disrupt the family. This wall of silence can make children afraid to speak out, and can leave sympathetic adults feeling unable, or too ashamed, to offer help:

The fact remains that sexual offenses against children are barely noticed except in the most violent and sensational instances. Most offenses are never revealed, and when revealed, most are either ignored or not reported. If reported, a large percentage are dismissed for lack of proof, and even when proof can be established, many cases are dropped because of the pressure and humiliation forced on the victim and family.

Florence Rush *The Sexual Abuse of Children: a Feminist Point of View* (1971)

The sexual abuse of children is an outrage to which people universally react in uncontained horror when that rare manifestation, a mutilation murder, occurs. Yet the routine *occurrence of child molestation remains a subject from which people prefer to avert their eyes.*

Susan Brownmiller *Against Our Will* (1975)

Many children who ring childline refuse to identify themselves because they still deeply love and need the parents who cause them pain; the children know that calling for help may bring about the total destruction of their family. As one child told me, "I don't want to hurt my brothers or break up my family so I have to put up with it till he drops down dead. I will be happy then. Please help the other children who are suffering. I am a stupid coward, no one can help me, it's my job now".

Esther Rantzen, in a foreword to *Innocent Victims* by Dr Alan Gilmour (1988)

See also Incest

There is also the problem of what the authorities should do if they believe they have identified a case of child abuse within the family. In 1987 in Cleveland, in the UK, two doctors sent 200 children into care for alleged abuse. They were subsequently severely criticized by a public inquiry.

Unfortunately, one of the greatest worries about the Cleveland furore in 1987 was that the public reaction to what appeared to be excessive diagnosis and family disruption during an apparent epidemic of sexual abuse, would bring back an atmosphere of rejection, by professionals and public. This fear was borne out for me by a colleague, who received a series of telephone calls from a teenage girl, who told of well-established sexual abuse by her father. She felt that she could cope with this, but was worried for her younger sister, who was beginning to be a victim too. She refused to give any name or address, saying, "Even if you did get us taken into care, after this Cleveland business we'd only get sent back to him, wouldn't we?" She disappeared, a sad victim of loss of trust in society...

Anger, though understandable, though justifiable, is the most destructive emotion if we really want to protect children.

Dr Alan Gilmour *Innocent Victims* (1988)

Almost unbelievably, a repeat performance occurred in Orkney in 1991, in which nine children were snatched from their beds in a dawn raid. A government inquiry later accused social workers of making hasty decisions that:

...subordinated the interests of the children to the anxiety to find evidence of abuse.

and concluded:

It is not easy to find any individual among the principal actors...who is not open to some criticism.

Sunday Times (1 Nov. 1992), quoting from Lord Clyde's report.

The fact that children sometimes make false accusations of abuse has also hindered attempts to help those in genuine danger. In the Orkney case problems arose because some children were believed too readily:

The police and social workers failed to distinguish adequately between taking the children's allegations seriously and believing them.

The Times (28 Oct. 1992), quoting from Lord Clyde's report.

Many small girls reflect the public hysteria over the prospect of 'being touched' by a strange person; and many a child, who has no idea at all of the mechanics of intercourse, interprets affection and simple caressing from anyone except her own parents, as attempts at rape. In consequence, not a few older men serve time in penal institutions for attempting to engage in a sexual act which at their age would not interest most of them, and of which many of them are undoubtedly incapable.

Alfred Kinsey et al. *Sexual Behaviour in the Human Female* (1953)

I wrote to you several months ago about a male relative molesting my 3-year old girl. Your answer was to confront him with it and get him to a doctor, fast. We had already confronted him, and of course, he denied everything. 'She makes up stories,' he said. How can a 3-year old make up stories of this kind? I talked with the police department and was told you cannot accuse someone of molesting without proof. Will they take the word of a 3-year old against that of a grown man who is admired and respected by all? NO! I was made to look like an hysterical mother having hallucinations. Can you understand why each night I pray for God to take him?

Letter signed 'DAZED' *New York Post* (11 Feb. 1972)

Paradoxically, current social attitudes condemn acts of child abuse while apparently condoning a view of children as sexually desirable:

It is clear that our current society harbors a contradiction in its view of children and sexuality. On one hand we state children should not be exploited sexually, but child pornography thrives and the courts are often more likely to believe molesting adults than molested children. Television commercials use nubile girls posed seductively. Such practices can only give molesters and children a mixed message about what society believes about sexual abuse and the sexual exploitation of children.

Cynthia Crosson Tower *Understanding Child Abuse and Neglect* (1989)

Our culture teaches young girls, implicitly and explicitly, that seductive behaviour is a way to get what they want. Acting cute or sexy, even when they are quite young, garners compliments and attention. Furthermore, a girl's socialization teaches her at the same time to internalize guilt for such learned behaviour. Therefore the female incest victims in effect have been programmed to blame themselves – they feel they must have done something bad *to have caused the abuse to happen.*

S. Butter *Conspiracy to Silence* (1978)

It has not been unusual to hear clinicians claim that the daughters who are victims of incest with their fathers, in addition to being 'seductive' were also masochistic and thereby precipitated the incest.

Paula J. Caplan *The Myth of Women's Masochism* (1984)

One psychoanalyst has argued that Freud deliberately misrepresented the cases of women who came to him as patients claiming to have been abused as children:

Not one analyst has called or written to discuss my book or agreed to take part in debates... They are reacting not as analysts but as men, *because here we are touching on the last taboo, the most shameful secret of all, the* male *secret. All the favourable letters I have received came from women, hundreds, saying that their analysts refused to believe their stories of abuse, or that it was relevant.*

Dr Jeffrey Masson, interviewed in the *Guardian* (1985)

The children, themselves, can react in various ways:

The word 'incest' suggests consent, yet most young girls are not in a position to agree or oppose. Very often they do not know what 'sex' is, and are searching for love and affection, so can get this confused with other shows of affection.

Jane Dowdeswell *Women on Rape* (1986)

He never had a kind word to say to me. Just say You gonna do what your mammy wouldn't. First he put his thing up gainst my hip and sort of wiggle it around. Then he grab hold my titties. Then he push his thing inside my pussy. When that hurt, I cry. He start to choke me, saying You better shut up and git used to it.

Alice Walker *The Color Purple* (1983)

My father and I came to each other out of great neediness. I wanted emotional sustenance, an assurance of love, an obliteration of the fear of abandonment. He wanted sexual gratification, perhaps to ease the pain of his own emptiness, to deny the inexorable movement of time, to assuage his bruised ego. And in a sense, at that time we served each other very well.

Katherine Brady *Father's Days* (1979)

Sharing a bedroom with my two brothers, I took part in sex play with them from an early age. I was ten when I first experienced full intercourse with my eldest brother (then 13), and I subsequently became very active with my brothers and their friends, usually in group situations. At puberty I withdrew from this promiscuity, but continued and deepened my intimacy with my brothers.

Greenwald and Greenwald *The Sex-Life Letters* (1974)

It may not occur to children who have been taught by their parents never to take sweets from strangers that the bar of chocolate being offered by daddy ought to be refused for exactly the same reason.

Jean Renvoize *Incest* (1982)

And then there was the pain. A breaking and entering when even the senses are torn apart. The act of rape upon an eight-year-old body is a matter of the needle giving because the camel can't. The child gives, because the body can, and the mind of the violator cannot.

Maya Angelou *I Know Why the Caged Bird Sings* (1971)

Children are encouraged to model what they see in pornographic films and pictures. In turn they are compelled to become involved in the manufacture of pornographic materials. Often drugs are used as incentives or rewards or to ensure compliance. The fact that pornography and drugs are illegal is used by ringleaders as insurance against disclosure. The children realize that to tell means they, as well as others in the ring, will suffer censure or prosecution.

A. Burgess *Response Patterns in Children and Adolescents Exploited through Sex Rings and Pornography* (1984)

Most victims are female:

Kinsey and his co-workers found that twice as many girls as boys are paedophilia victims and published the alarming fact that, of American women interviewed, 24 per cent reported that they had as children been sexually approached by an adult male...A 1985 survey in Britain estimated that over a million children could expect to be sexually assaulted before the age of fifteen; but the results of polls vary, between 10 and 20 per cent of British adults claiming to have been sexually approached by an adult in childhood.

Roy Eskapa *Bizarre Sex* (1987)

There is no need for parents to fear homosexual teachers. Ninety-seven percent of child seduction is heterosexual.

Dr Benjamin Spock (1945)

Without an understanding of male supremacy and female oppression, it is impossible to explain why the vast majority of incest perpetrators (uncles, older brothers, and fathers) are male, and why the majority of victims (nieces, younger sisters, and daughters) are female.

Judith Lewis Herman *Father-Daughter Incest* (1981)

According to most authors, father-daughter and stepfather-stepdaughter incest are recognized as the two forms of incest most frequently recorded in Western civilization.

H. Maisch *Incest* (1972)

The law relating to incest most explicitly reveals the doctrine of female sexual passivity, since a woman can never actually 'commit' incest but only 'permit' it.

Susan Edwards *Female Sexuality and the Law* (1981)

In modern Western society boys who are seduced by older women are usually proud of the experience, while girls characteristically feel victimized or 'dirty':

Female victims outnumbered male victims by 10 to 1. Male victims were chiefly involved in homosexual activity. These statistics are suspect since women who sexually exploit young boys are rarely reported. In such situations, boys usually do not consider themselves to be victims. Due to the sexual socialization process in our society, young males are likely to view such contacts as sexual initiations while females view these encounters as sexual violations.

M. Tsai and N. Wagner *Incest and Molestation* (1979)

There are exceptions to the general pattern of males abusing females:

Boys and men do experience sexual abuse at the hands of men. The homophobes distorting concentration on this fact, which cannot and must not be denied, neatly eliminates from view the primary victims of male sexual abuse: women and girls. This is congruent with the fact that crimes against females are ultimately viewed as expressions of male normalcy, while crimes against men and boys are viewed as perversions of that same normalcy.

Andrea Dworkin *Pornography: Men Possessing Women* (1981)

It would seem to be the Victorian assumption that women are devoid of sexual desire which is responsible for the fact that several of these regulations, passed in the last century, apply only to men. Thus the law does not provide for the contingency, by no means impossible, that a woman should abduct a boy, or that she should seduce a male imbecile.

Gordon Rattray Taylor *Sex in History* (1953)

Indecent assault by an adult woman on a small boy is more common than is thought. In 1842 the Court of Assizes of the Seine convicted a girl of rape on two children. A case has been reported where several women seized a young man. Such cases are rare. The mores of the community...define sexual deviation as acts committed by males.

B. Karpman *The Sexual Offender and His Offences* (1954)

With women there are ways of being sexual without touching: men are far more overt. What's so agonizing about mother/daughter incest is that it's one oppressed woman doing it to another who is even more powerless than she is, a little kid.

Jean Renvoize *Incest* (1982)

Often girls who are abused as children fail to have normal and fulfilling sex lives in adulthood:

Women who were mistreated as children also experience confusion as to what they really wanted when the adult male expressed his sexual will on them, but must as a condition of forced femininity, accept the male as constant aggressor and forced sex as normative.

Andrea Dworkin *Pornography: Men Possessing Women* (1981)

Even though she derives no pleasure from sex, her need for self-punishment as a response to her guilt may lead her to have sex with a variety of men. She may be promiscuous as a means of self-degradation, while at the same time seeking through sex the affection she never quite found in incest. Because she confuses love, guilt and sex, she ends up too often being used as a sexual object. Through her continual self-punishment she tries to cleanse herself of guilt, but her feelings won't wash away.

Susan Forward and C. Buck *Betrayal of Innocence: Incest and its Devastation* (1981)

Sometimes abused girls react by running away from their homes. When they do so, they usually head for big cities, which are inevitably centres of prostitution, where the pimps will be watching out for them:

Typically the victims of sexual abuse at the hands of their father, stepfather, or uncle, girl hustlers see prostitution as an exit from an intolerable home life.

D. Campagna *Sexual Exploitation of Children: Resource Manual* (1985)

The majority of girls I've gotten so far got raped by their fathers or uncles or somebody.

New York pimp, quoted in 'New York: White Slavery', *Time* (5 June 1972)

Pimps, who are acknowledged experts in the field of female psychology, intuitively, or perhaps empirically, understand that rape is the fastest way to 'turn out' a likely teen-age candidate, and they have been known to set up intricate gang-rape situations when they have spotted a prospect, as a sort of good-business practice.

Susan Brownmiller *Against Our Will* (1975)

See also PROSTITUTION

As more effort is made to help victims of abuse, it is to be expected that more crimes will be reported:

As an expert in the field of sexuality, I can only condemn the sexual abuse of children. But as a historical expert, I also have to challenge the statements...that child sexual abuse is increasing. I know of no evidence that this is the case. I would agree, however, that today child sexual abuse is more likely to be reported than in the past. One has to remember that not too long ago 'respectable' newspapers like The Times *would not publish stories dealing with child sexual abuse. That there is publicity, a healthy thing, does not mean that the incidence has increased.*

Professor Vern Bullough, letter to the *New York Times* (17 Apr. 1984)

Prevention may depend on understanding the psychology of abusers:

Pedophilia implies an erotic craving for a child of the same or different sex on the part of an adult, which is distinctly asocial only when it attains overt proportions.

J. H. Cassity *Psychological Considerations of Pedophilia* (1927)

The typical incestuous father is not mentally retarded, psychotic, or pedophilic, but is characterized by some sort of personal disturbance that interferes with his ability to control his impulses in a situation where his temptation to commit incest exists.

K. Meiselman *Incest* (1978)

The data conclusively show that absence from the home or uninvolvement in the early socialization of the child dramatically increases the risk of sexual child abuse.

Seymour Parker *The Precultural Basis of the Incest Taboo* (1976)

Russell (1984) found that 17% of the women in her San Francisco sample with a stepfather had been sexually abused by him (8% very seriously) as against 2.3% abused by their natural father (0.5% very seriously).

Bill Gillham *The Facts about Child Sexual Abuse* (1991)

The pedophile collector of kiddie porn is the archetype of sexual exploitation; his is a world of sexual obsessions and, in a sense, moral consumption. The deeper he plunges into the market, buying, selling, and trading duplicate and triplicate films and photos of child pornography, the harder it is for him to recognize and accept legal and social bans. Like a stamp or coin collector, he devotes a sizeable portion of his discretionary income towards the purchase of pornography.

D. Campagna *Sexual Exploitation of Children: Resource Manual* (1985)

Some psychologists believe that the whole family becomes involved when abuse is occurring:

Incest is a relationship among at least three persons, the two participants and the nonparticipating parent.

A. Rosenfeld *The Clinical Management of Incest and Sexual Abuse of Children* (1979)

The secret of incest tightens bonds rather than loosens them; the family becomes even more cemented together as a result of sexual abuse…

An unexpected finding is that a number of incestuous families are extremely religious; and to some incest is thought to be preferable to adultery…

Another rationalization given is that they want their children to have a proper introduction to sexuality and that first experiences with a loving father will be beneficial.

Jean Renvoize *Incest* (1982)

The question of how to treat abusers is now being addressed more openly:

One of the modern treatments for child-molesters is by hormone drugs such as Androcur and Oestradiol. These reduce the sex drive. The hormone implant operates by swamping the male hormone testosterone with the female hormone oestrogen. The offender's male sex drive wilts, and often disappears, for as long as treatment is continued. There are side-effects. The men find their breasts swelling. Not infrequently this becomes so embarrassing as to require surgical treatment. This is a straightforward operation: the offending breasts are cut off. One should not be too distressed about this however, since a clever technique enables the nipples to be reattached. After healing the scar tissue is not too extensive.

Francis Bennion *The Sex Code* (1991)

One major problem in counselling abusers is getting them to accept that their behaviour is wrong. Paedophiles frequently justify their actions to themselves and others by claiming that their victims were willing participants:

Kids love sex and become joyous when they are sexually happy. I'm not just rationalizing when I say that ninety per cent of the trouble we have with teenagers is the result of sexual frustrations. When I see a really happy well-adjusted boy I say to myself: 'He's getting some good sex somewhere.'

Pederast quoted by Dr Parker Rossman in *Sexual Experience between Men and Boys* (1979)

Paedophilia has always been and shall always be as much a healthy part of our species as red hair or left-handedness.

Stephen Freeman *Guardian* (5 Dec. 1984)

It's a dangerous over-simplification to condemn any sexual activity involving a child on the ground that ipso facto it constitutes 'abuse'. Children have sexual needs of their own. A report in the Independent *(13 Oct. 1990) described a 'child abuse' ring in Australia involving 300 boys aged between seven and seventeen. The ring operated in a highly organized way, and kept computer records of the boys. No doubt the operation was highly reprehensible, but one item in the report strikes a redeeming note. The computer records included the sexual preferences of the boys.*

Francis Bennion *The Sex Code* (1991)

However, not all sexual behaviour involving children should be reacted to with hysteria:

Under certain specific circumstances sibling incest may not be a traumatic or even unpleasant experience. If the children are young and approximately the same age, if there is no betrayal of trust between them, if the sexual play is the result of their natural curiosity and exploration, and if the children are not traumatized by disapproving adults who stumble upon their sex play, sibling sexual contact can be just another part of growing up. In most such cases both partners are sexually naive. The game of show-me-yours-and-I'll-show-you-mine is older than civilization and between young siblings of approximately the same age it is usually harmless.

Susan Forward and C. Buck *Betrayal of Innocence: Incest and Its Devastation* (1978)

Circumcision (male)

Circumcision in males, the cutting away of the foreskin of the penis, is a procedure that is both widespread and of great antiquity. Who invented this bizarre form of mutilation in the first place, and why, is not clear:

> *Circumcision did not originate among the Jews: they took the custom from either the Babylonians or the Negroes, probably the latter. It has been practised in West Africa for over 5000 years.*
>
> *Baley and Love's Short Practice of Surgery*, revised by A. J. Harding Rains and H. David Ritchie (1984)

Whatever its origins, circumcision is still a part of the way of life of Jews, Muslims, Coptic Christians, and many African tribes, as well as primitive peoples throughout the world. For the Jews, it was introduced as a sign of the covenant established between God and Abraham:

> *And God said unto Abraham...this is my covenant, which ye shall keep between me and you and thy seed after thee. Every man child among you shall be circumcised. And ye shall circumcise the flesh of your foreskin; and it shall be a token of the covenant betwixt me and you...And the uncircumcised man child whose flesh of his foreskin is not circumcised, that soul shall be cut off from his people; he hath broken my covenant.*
>
> Genesis 17:9–14

As a first sign of His special favour towards Abraham, God arranged for his wife Sarah, previously childless, to bear him a son who would continue the covenant:

> *And God said, Sarah thy wife shall bear thee a son indeed; and thou shalt call his name Isaac: and I will establish my covenant with him for an everlasting covenant, and with his seed after him.*
>
> Genesis 17:19

Abraham, then 99, duly had himself circumcised, impregnated the 90-year-old Sarah, and became the father of Isaac. On the strength of this biblical legend succeeding generations of Jewish boys have been, and still are, ritually circumcised when they reach the age of 8 days:

> *The use of flint knives, in the stories of both Moses and Joshua, showed that the practice of circumcision was very ancient, in vogue before metal knives were known. What the purpose of circumcision was originally is hard to say and various theories have been put forward, of which the most likely may be that it was a preparation for sexual intercourse by removing any tightness of the foreskin.*
>
> Geoffrey Parrinder *Sex in the World's Religions* (1980)

An early Jewish philosopher from Alexandria thought almost entirely the opposite:

> *Circumcision is for the excision of passions, which bind the mind. For some among all passions that of intercourse between man and woman is greatest, the law givers have commanded that that instrument which serves this intercourse, be mutilated, pointing out, that these powerful passions must be bridled, and thinking not only this, but that all passions would be controlled through this one.*
>
> Philo Judaeus *Works* (1st century AD)

A view endorsed by a medieval Jewish philosopher:

I believe that one of the reasons for circumcision was the diminution of sexual intercourse and the weakening of the sexual organ; its purpose was to restrict the activities of this organ and to leave it at rest as much as possible. The true purpose of circumcision was to give the sexual organ that kind of physical pain as not to impair its natural function or the potency of the individual, but to lessen the power of passion and of too great desire.

Maimonides *Treatise on Poison, Haemorrhoids, Cohabitation* (12th century)

This opinion may be a reflection of the unsophisticated tools with which the operation was once performed. The usual modern view is that it makes no difference to either of the participants in the sexual act whether the man is circumcised or not:

Cutting off this structure [the foreskin] *is possibly the oldest human sexual ritual. It still persists – on the ground, now, either that cancer of the penis and cervix is rarer when it is done...or that it slows down orgasm (for which there is no evidence).*

It probably doesn't make very much difference either to masturbation or to intercourse...Normally one retracts it anyway for all these purposes... Women who have experienced both are divided – and over which looks sexier. Some find the circumcised glans 'neater' and are even turned off by an unretracted prepuce...while others love the sense of discovery which goes with retraction.

Dr Alex Comfort *The Joy of Sex* (1972)

However:

A few years ago a survey conducted among prostitutes, whose opinion on male sexual performance is unlikely to be influenced by emotion, showed that more than 90 per cent preferred intercourse with a circumcised man, both on the grounds of cleanliness and function.

Dr Thomas Stuttaford *The Times* (15 Oct. 1992)

In reality, circumcision as a means of either facilitating or restricting sexual intercourse has little credibility. The Jews and other habitual circumcisers are patently no more or less prolific than the uncircumcised, nor do they gain more or less pleasure from the act of procreation. There are, perhaps three reasons for the survival of the practice. First the hygienic:

Urologists and paediatricians generally favour circumcision on hygienic grounds, since smegma, an accumulation of dead skin and dirt, can build up under the foreskin with resultant infection.

Roy Eskapa *Bizarre Sex* (1987)

Research in Australia has shown that there is no sexually transmitted disease which is not more readily spread to the uncircumcised. Similar results have come from Africa, where it has been shown that men from uncircumcised tribes catch HIV up to eight times more readily than the circumcised...It has long been accepted that circumcision in early childhood saves the adult, of whatever race, from any risk of later developing penile cancer.

Dr Thomas Stuttaford *The Times* (15 Oct. 1992)

The second reason for its survival could be eugenic:

Some see in it a tribal badge. If this be the true origin of circumcision, it must go back to the time when men went around naked. Mutilations (tattooing, removal of teeth and so forth) were tribal marks, being partly sacrifices and partly means of recognition.

Encyclopaedia Britannica (11th ed.; 1910)

Here, perhaps, lies an unsuspected clue. Jewish girls have always been under great parental pressure to marry Jewish men – uncircumcised boys, however handsome, clever, and attractive, are regarded as unclean. The tribal badge, visible as it is to lovers, is a powerful custodian of the gene pool.

In addition to the hygienic and eugenic factors is a third more sinister force – the sadistic. The Old Testament, for example, relates the story of David's application for the hand of Michal,

Saul's daughter. David, a poor man, had no dowry to offer:

> *And Saul said, thus shall ye say to David, the king desireth not any dowry, but an hundred foreskins of the Philistines... Wherefore David arose and went...and slew of the Philistines two hundred men; and David brought their foreskins, and they gave them in full tale to the king, that he might be the king's son in law.*
>
> I Samuel 18:25–27

An ugly story, with continuing reverberations:

> *While the civilized world considers circumcision at puberty, with or without an anaesthetic, to be barbaric, it still accepts the surgical removal of a newborn's foreskin without an anaesthetic. Contrary to popular myth, newborn infants do feel pain, as is evidenced by their screams during the ritual.*
>
> Roy Eskapa *Bizarre Sex* (1987)

All Jewish men know that they were themselves subjected to this ritual mutilation as babies and they therefore, perhaps, experience some sadistic compulsion to expose their infant sons to it. Make him suffer – make a man of him – do to him what they did to me – and my father – and my father's father...The whole ritualistic procedure is an abandonment of reason in favour of an ethically compelling sophistry deriving ultimately from magic, superstition, and, above all, ignorance. Rituals have no need to be rational, they must only have been happening for a long time.

This, from the Talmud (two collections of early Jewish writings), emphasizes the departure from any semblance of reality:

> *In the hereafter Abraham will sit at the entrance of Gehinnom (Hell) and will not allow any circumcised Israelite to descend into it. As for those who sinned unduly, what does he do to them? He removes the foreskin from children who had died before circumcision, places it upon them and sends them down to Gehinnom.*
>
> Talmud

In spite of Abraham's covenant with God, the Jews have throughout their history found circumcision an embarrassment:

> *The penis was considered sacred, particularly the glans. An exposed glans penis was seen as shocking and awe-inspiring. The prepuce was kept over it, and the penis was often tied with a string or closed with a clasp. Even during the Olympic Games when men would compete in the nude, the prepuce would have to cover the glans. For that reason, a circumcised man would not be permitted to compete in the Olympic Games. Jews of Greece who wanted to be part of the Hellenic civilization would avoid circumcising their sons so that they could participate equally, even though this broke the Covenant of Abraham.*
>
> Sander J. Breiner MD *Slaughter of the Innocents* (1990)

So important was the covering of the glans to the ancient Greeks that they invented a surgical remedy for those born with short foreskins:

> *When the foreskin wasn't sufficiently long to cover the glans, an operation was sometimes performed whereby the skin was cut around the base of the penis and the skin drawn forward.*
>
> Lloyd Demause *The Evolution of Childhood* (1974)

> *Some Jews who wished to take part in public games and other activities which required nakedness underwent operations to lengthen their foreskins again, but such practices were strongly opposed by the orthodox.*
>
> Geoffrey Parrinder *Sex in the World's Religions* (1980)

> *Male circumcision has been the cause of social unrest and martyrdom in the past. Under the Greek Antiochus Epiphanes, the conquered Jews were forbidden to circumcise their male infants (164–168 BC). The* Encyclopaedia Judaica *reports the murder of two women for circumcising their sons...Later the Roman emperor Ha-*

drian, also forbade male circumcision by Jews, who, as slaves to the Romans, carried the practice to various parts of the empire. The outlawing of circumcision, among other sanctions, contributed to the successful Jewish rebellion Bar Kokhba against the Romans in AD 132.

Roy Eskapa *Bizarre Sex* (1987)

And more recently:

In the shower Steve noticed I'd been circumcised. "Why?" I didn't know. "To make it lighter? You know, Milligan, if Jerry took you prisoner, that could've got you into a concentration camp." It was really something, when your prick could get you sent to a concentration camp. "Believe me, Spike," says the Yew, "anyone that sends someone to a concentration camp is a prick." Amen.

Spike Milligan *Where Have All The Bullets Gone?* (1985)

Circumcision is still required of all Jews and all converts to orthodox Judaism:

In Jewish reform movements of the nineteenth century circumcision came under criticism, and especially the regulation which required it to be imposed upon proselytes converted to the Jewish faith. Since this necessitated operations on adults it was felt to be harsh, and in 1892 the American Reform Movement dropped the requirement of circumcision of converts, which was followed by reformed synagogues elsewhere.

Geoffrey Parrinder *Sex in the World's Religions* (1980)

For gentile converts to Christianity some 2000 years earlier, circumcision also presented a problem:

And certain men which came down from Judæa taught the brethren, and said, Except ye be circumcised after the manner of Moses, ye cannot be saved.
When therefore Paul and Barnabas had no small dissension and disputation with them, they determined that Paul and Barnabas...should go to Jerusalem unto the apostles and elders about this question.

Acts 15:1–2

The message they brought back was that members of the Church were not obliged to follow this 'law of Moses', in spite of the fact that Jesus himself had been circumcised:

The foreskins, still extant, of the Saviour, are reckoned to be twelve in number. One was still in the possession of the Monks of Loulombs; another at the Abbey of Charroux; a third at Hildesheim, in Germany; a fourth at Rome, in the Church of St Jean-de-Latran; a fifth at Antwerp; a sixth at Puy-en-Velay, in the Church of Notre Dame, etc.

John Davenport *Aphrodisiacs and Anti-Aphrodisiacs* (1869)

For Muslims following the example of the prophet Mohammed, circumcision is also required; nevertheless

...it is a civic and not a religious rite, and it is not prescribed by the Koran.

Robert Briffault *The Mothers: a Study of the Origins of Sentiments and Institutions* (1927)

Amongst modern gentiles, the pros and cons of infant circumcision have been much debated. The practice has gone in and out of fashion. There was a revival in late Victorian England:

Circumcision is like a substantial and well secured life annuity...parents cannot make a better saving investment for their little boys, as it ensures them better health, greater capacity for labour, longer life, less nervousness, sickness, loss of time, and less doctor bills, as well as it increases their chance for an euthanasian death.

P. C. Remondino *History of Circumcision* (1891)

That British circumcision is to be seen primarily as an imperial phenomenon is, finally, demonstrated statistically by its differential adoption among various social groups. It was chiefly characteristic of the upper and professional classes, pioneered by doctors and army officers.

Ronald Hyman *Empire and Sexuality* (1990)

Before the second world war circumcision was often a concealed status symbol in Britain, denoting that a boy had come from the affluent middle classes: this aspect of the procedure has remained, but to a lesser extent, in America: whereas sociologists have detected no class or economic differences between the circumcised and the uncircumcised in Australia.

Dr Thomas Stuttaford *The Times* (15 Oct. 1992)

Male circumcision is still generally popular in the United States, despite the fact that it reduces sexual sensitivity, hinders masturbation and deforms the unclothed male figure. The ostensible excuse is hygiene.

Francis Bennion *The Sex Code* (1991)

Although this now seems to be a minority view, the procedure is not without its risks:

In the United States, about 1,325,000 neo-natal circumcisions are performed each year. The practice gives cause for alarm, since it results in about 230 deaths each year as a result of accident or infection.

Roy Eskapa *Bizarre Sex* (1987)

It is this small but genuine risk that has persuaded paediatricians against the procedure:

Paediatricians sit in judgment on the future of the foreskin but as they only see the male when the sex organs have no sexual role their conclusions may be suspect. In these more promiscuous days, when society is haunted by HIV and herpes, perhaps the decision should be more influenced by doctors who look after the genitalia when they are fulfilling their adult purpose.

Dr Thomas Stuttaford *The Times* (15 Oct. 1992)

One recent development is the advent of bloodless circumcision:

Israeli doctors have performed their first circumcision by laser on a 14-year-old Jewish immigrant from Moscow because a rare blood disease made it risky to do the usual way. Dr Shlomo Wallfish said: "We consulted with the rabbis who agreed to the laser technique."

Oxford Mail (12 Oct. 1992)

Finally two quips relating to circumcision. The first is a remark that Lloyd George is said to have made about his Jewish Liberal colleague, Herbert Samuel, whose philosophical superiority he sometimes found irritating:

When they circumcised Herbert they threw away the wrong bit.

Which is reminiscent of the second – a staple of the feminist repertoire:

Q. *What do you call the useless piece of flesh at the end of a penis?*

A. *A man!*

Circumcision (female)

In one sense female circumcision is very much less controversial than the male variety, because it is so widely condemned. The operation can take various forms:

Female circumcision…entails different things in different cultures. The mildest form – known to Muslims as 'sunna' and the least common – involves the removal of the prepuce or hood of the clitoris. It is the only operation analogous to male circumcision. Excision involves the removal of the clitoris and the labia minora: while infibulation involves the removal of all the external genitalia and the stitching up of the two sides of the vulva to leave only a tiny opening for the passage of urine and menstrual blood…

There is no doubt that the practice is a means of suppressing and controlling the sexual behaviour of women. Female circumcision is a physiological chastity belt.

Sue Armstrong *New Scientist* (2 Feb. 1991)

In some communities, clitorectomy was and still sometimes is performed to reduce sexual sensation as a safeguard against premarital relations and loss of virginity, without regard to reduction of enjoyment in marriage subsequently.

Elizabeth Draper *Birth Control in the Modern World* (1972)

Female circumcision, or more properly, clitoridectomy, is practised in many parts of Africa, though not in all…with the apparent aim of making sexual penetration easier for the man and removing any opposition or rivalry in intercourse from the woman…Its purpose seems to aim at ensuring male pleasure and dominance, without considering the woman.

Geoffrey Parrinder *Sex in the World's Religions* (1980)

Female circumcision is practised in the name of religion, for improved sexual attractiveness and to curb the 'natural promiscuity' of women. The ritual is performed on every inhabited continent…and is endorsed by the Koran and consequently much of the Islamic world. President Jomo Kenyatta of Kenya defended female circumcision in a 1938 paper, when he wrote that no Kikuyu tribe member should even consider marriage to an uncircumcised woman.

Roy Eskapa *Bizarre Sex* (1987)

The almost unbelievable savagery of clitoridectomy and infibulation is described by two writers almost exactly a century apart:

After the operator has cut out the clitoris and the lips of the labia…she then sews up the parts with a pack needle and a thread of sheepskin, while a thin tube is inserted for the passage of urine. Before marriage the bridegroom trains himself for a month on beef, honey, and milk; for if he can open the bride with his natural weapon he is a mighty sworder. If he fails, he tries penetration with his fingers, and by way of last resort, whips out his knife and cuts the parts open. The sufferings of the bride must be severe.

Sir Richard Burton *Love, War, and Fancy; Notes to the Arabian Nights* (c. 1888)

Infibulation is practised primarily in Somalia. The ritual is typically performed on an eight- to ten-year-old child by her mother while female relatives stand guard outside the ceremonial circumcision hut. The child sits on a chair as her legs are prised apart by several women. The mother separates the labia and fastens them aside with acacia thorns, leaving the clitoris totally exposed. Typically a kitchen knife is used to remove the clitoris. Cutting goes down to the bone so that the surrounding parts of the labia can be taken out. The child comes close to biting off her tongue out of sheer pain. To prevent this, hot pepper is placed on the tongue every time it sticks out. The pepper ensures a rapid return of the tongue to the mouth. When the torturous operation is over, the mother closes both sides of the vulva with the acacia thorns...

One group in Sierra Leone performs mass clitoridectomy. The initiation rite, witnessed by the whole tribe, is carried out at full moon. The object here is to render the girl sexless and to prevent her from seducing men. After 'surgery', the girls are locked in huts until a man asks their fathers to permit marriage. All the clitorides are collected at the mass ritual and are buried in the river bank...

Among the Australian aborigines, female circumcision is performed in tandem with group rape. The operation is performed by clan brothers on a girl as soon as she reaches puberty. A stone knife is used to make an incision from the vagina to the clitoris, thereby cutting the perineum. The young girl is then forced to have sexual intercourse with all those who participate in the ritual. 'Clitoris-free women' are considered to be more sexually desirable and pure.

Roy Eskapa *Bizarre Sex* (1987)

It is not, therefore, surprising that:

By the Arabs, as well as by most peoples who practice female circumcision, the utmost secrecy is observed in regard to it, and nothing is ever said about it. So that our information is very far from representing the full extent of the distribution of the practice.

Robert Briffault *The Mothers: a Study of the Origins of Sentiments and Institutions* (1927)

The operation is sometimes carried out in the West, where the same secrecy is observed:

Female circumcision is performed in Western countries, it being reported as recently as 1983 that clitoridectomies were being carried out by surgeons in London's prestigious Harley Street (ITN News). These surgeons provided the service to wealthy Saudi Arabian businessmen who had brought wives, children and concubines with them to England. The extent of the procedure is unknown, since it is performed in total secrecy. Doctors at the London Hospital, a National Health Service hospital, claimed that they performed clitoridectomies on the daughters of immigrants because, if they refused, the mothers would perform the operation themselves in the absence of sterile conditions.

Roy Eskapa *Bizarre Sex* (1987)

Although in the UK, at least, the position changed in 1985 with the Prohibition of Female Circumcision Act which made it

...an offence, punishable with up to five years' imprisonment, to excise or otherwise mutilate the external genital organs of a woman, or to aid or abet a woman mutilating herself in this way.

Elizabeth Martin *A Concise Dictionary of Law* (1990 ed.)

Nevertheless in 1992 a case was reported of a Pakistani surgeon offering to perform a female circumcision in a London clinic by misdescribing it as 'repair to vulva':

As part of a Sunday Times *investigation, a female journalist* [Donu Kogbara] *posed as a Nigerian whose fiancé wanted her to have the operation...Kogbara met Siddique at the clinic...and paid him the*

money [£500] *in cash...Siddique told Kogbara: 'I have done the operation a number of times'...The operation was halted just minutes before Donu Kogbara was due to be anaesthetized...Siddique fled when confronted by* The Sunday Times.

Sunday Times (18 Oct. 1992)

Nearly everyone in the civilized world, who is not emotionally or financially involved with female circumcision in some way, has condemned the practice. Nearly everyone –

Of the two operations, that upon the female has infinitely more to recommend it from a sanitary point of view. Had the practice of female circumcision survived among the Jews or the Romans, we should no doubt have a large medical literature setting forth the sanitary advantages of the measure. Male circumcision on the other hand, apart from the status which the mutilation owes to Biblical sanction, can only be regarded as a savage, senseless, and disgusting practice.

Robert Briffault *The Mothers: a Study of the Origins of Sentiments and Institutions* (1927)

Feminists have seen clitoridectomy as an extreme version of the denial of female sexuality found in many other cultures:

...the ritual sexual mutilations imposed on African women since time immemorial constitute the exact physical counterpart of the psychical intimidations imposed in childhood on the sexuality of European little girls.

Marie Bonaparte *Female Sexuality* (1953)

In the past, Western women have occasionally been subjected to similar physical treatment for pseudo-medical reasons:

There was, for instance, some attempt to use clitoridectomy as a cure for dysuria or amenorrhoea, for epilepsy, hysteria, sterility or insanity, in the 1860s. It was believed that all of these were produced by sexual arousal so the surgical removal of the clitoris was a sure cure for the disease.

Jeffrey Weeks *Sex, Politics and Society* (1987)

The ultimate in male chauvinism is surely the man who mutilates his bride or concubine in order that his pleasure will be increased and hers will be eradicated entirely. What then are the arguments used by Muslims and others for allowing these cruel procedures to continue? Some believe that it enhances the chances of conception:

A newly married wife waits six months, and if not pregnant by then she gets herself circumcised, whereon pregnancy usually ensues.

H. A. Rose *A Glossary of the Tribes and Castes of the Punjab and NW Frontier Province* (1911)

Others have put forward a variety of suggestions, most of which owe more to mythology than to reason:

The Dogon, who inhabit the interior of Mali, West Africa, have a cosmological explanation for female circumcision. According to their mythology, the god Amma created the world by having sexual intercourse with his wife. Unfortunately, Amma bumped into his wife's clitoris, the 'termite mound in the earth.' Amma was very angry and tore out the 'termite mound', which resulted in his wife's circumcision. Thus the Dogon imitate their venerable god.

Roy Eskapa *Bizarre Sex* (1987)

The Dogon (of the Western Sudan) are said to believe that man, like the primordial beings, has two souls of opposite sexes. One lives in his body and the other lives in the sky or water. When a boy is circumcised he is freed from the element of femininity, which he had in his childhood. Similarly when a girl is circumcised or excised she is freed from the male element and her clitoris no longer prevents intercourse. At circumcision prayers are offered for the stabilization of the soul, of the boy or girl, and spiritual force is thought to be released.

Geoffrey Parrinder *Sex in the World's Religions* (1980)

As is usual in these quasi-religious circumstances, ignorance plays the dominant role; some African tribes believe that if the clitoris is not removed, it will grow long and masculine, making its unfortunate possessor unmarriageable; others believe that the sex drive of an uncircumcised woman cannot be controlled; some Nigerian tribes believe that if the baby's head touches the clitoris during childbirth, the baby will die.

Strangest of all is the fact that many African girls look forward to circumcision – even if it involves infibulation – because it symbolizes for them a rebirth as a mature woman, a rite of passage in which they pass from the ownership of their father to the ownership of their husband. Ultimately they accept it as part of their cultural heritage and because uncircumcised they would be unmarriageable.

In her recent book, the Black US writer Alice Walker has written about a young African American woman's desire to become a fully accepted member of her tribe by submitting to circumcision. The result is horrifying:

It now took a quarter of an hour for her to pee. Her menstrual periods lasted ten days. She was incapacitated by cramps lasting nearly half the month. There were premenstrual cramps: cramps caused by the near impossibility of flow passing through so tiny an aperture as M'Lissa had left after fastening together the raw sides of Tashi's vagina with a couple of thorns and inserting a straw so that in healing, the traumatized flesh might not grow together, shutting the opening completely: cramps caused by the residual flow that could not find its way out, was not reabsorbed into her body and had nowhere to go. There was the odour too, of soured blood, which no amount of scrubbing ever washed off.

Possessing the Secret of Joy (1992)

The World Health Organization estimates that there are some 90 million circumcised females alive today, mostly in Africa but also in Arab states in Asia:

The campaign against female genital mutilation began in earnest around 12 years ago. Originally much of the impetus came from Western feminists, but African women have become increasingly active and now predominate…The leading international organization in this context is the IAC [Inter-African Committee Against Harmful Traditional Practices] *which now has member groups in 23 African countries…Education, especially of women, is the single most important factor in persuading parents to abandon the practice. Not only can education impart health dangers, but it provides an alternative context in which precious notions about feminine sexuality and marital responsibility can be upheld.*

Janie Hampton *New Internationalist* (Feb. 1993)

Contraception

Contraceptives should be used on every conceivable occasion.

Spike Milligan *The Last Goon Show of All* (1972)

Birth control has been a preoccupation of the human race since the beginning of history. There have always been couples who do not wish a particular act of love to result in pregnancy or who wish to plan their families in an orderly way. The issue of population control first arose in the early 19th century:

Populations, when unchecked, increase in a geometrical ratio. Subsistence only increases in arithmetical ratio...the perpetual struggle for room and food.

Thomas Malthus *An Essay on the Principle of Population* (1798–1803)

Over the last 200 years the need to restrict the population of the planet has become increasingly obvious, providing a further argument for the responsible use of contraception:

The command 'Be fruitful and multiply' was promulgated according to our authorities, when the population of the world consisted of two people.

Dean Inge *More Lay Thoughts of a Dean* (1931)

See also REPRODUCTION

Abstinence, advocated by Malthus, is contrary to human nature (see CHASTITY AND CELIBACY): nevertheless, it was for centuries the only method permitted to couples by moralists and the medical establishment:

"Yes, yes – I know, Doctor," said the patient with trembling voice, "but," and she hesitated as if it took all of her courage to say it, "what can I do to prevent getting that way again?"

"Oh, ho!" laughed the doctor good naturedly. "You want your cake while you eat it too, do you? Well, it can't be done...I'll tell you the only sure thing to do. Tell Jake to sleep on the roof!"

Margaret Sanger *My Fight for Birth Control* (1931)

Coitus interruptus was presumably devised as soon as mankind had recognized the connection between coitus, the emission of sperm, and childbirth (no mean feat when the last event does not occur until nine months after the first two). However, this method has both physical and psychological drawbacks:

I fucked her once, but I minded my pullbacks. I sware I did not get it.

John Harrington, unsuccessfully denying paternity in a 1771 New England courtroom quoted by Wells in *Illegitimacy* (1980)

How a gentleman could make a practice, in the very moment of unutterable ecstasy of withdrawing from the arena, is more than I can conceive.

Anon. pamphlet 'On the Use of Night-Caps' (1830s)

Withdrawal has an evil effect upon the woman's nervous condition. She has not completed her desire, she is under a highly nervous tension, her whole being is perhaps on the verge of satisfaction. She is then left in this dissatisfied state, which is far from humane.

Margaret Sanger quoted in *Birth Control in America: the Career of Margaret Sanger* (1920s)

The sort of intercourse that takes place followed by withdrawal hardly ever produces any feeling in the wife except disgust and nerviness; once I happened to mention in a woman's paper the case of a young man who was worried because his wife always had an attack of hysterical weeping after he had made love to her. During the next few days I had about a hundred letters from husbands telling me the same thing; in each case the method of birth control they practised was withdrawing.

Leonara Eyles *The New Commonsense About Sex* (1956)

It has also come in for a good deal of moral censure – perhaps deriving ultimately from the Biblical story of Onan, who incurred God's wrath by 'spilling his seed on the ground' (see MASTURBATION):

A woman on whom her husband practises what is euphemistically called 'preventative copulation' is necessarily brought into the condition of mind of a prostitute. As regards the male, the practice, in its character and in its remote effects, is in no way distinguishable from masturbation.

The Lancet (1869)

First, let me state that I look upon conjugal onanism as a great moral crime...Masturbation is mean and bad enough, and much to be reprehended, because it is fostered by a filthy spirit which can no longer control the sexual impulses. But here, at least, there is no partner in the sin, and no pure woman is degraded thereby. Conjugal onanism places both the man and the woman below the instincts of the brute creation.

C. H. F. Routh *The Moral and Physical Evils likely to Follow Practices Intended to Act as Checks to Population* (1879)

Nevertheless, it was standard practice for many couples:

We were on the bus and Harold knew the conductor and he asked Harold if we were married. He said "Don't forget, always get off the bus at South Shore, don't go all the way to Blackpool." That was how they kept the family down. It was just that the men had to be careful.

Anon. Englishwoman (1920s) quoted in Elizabeth Roberts *A Woman's Place* (1984)

With abstinence not satisfying their needs at all and withdrawal doing so only partially, men and women set about devising more congenial means of contraception. Many early methods are based purely on superstition:

This girl had heard that when a woman is going to conceive, the seed remains inside her and does not fall out...One day she noticed that the seed had not come out again. When I heard it I told her to jump up and down, touching her buttocks with her heels at each leap. After she had done this no more than seven times there was a noise, the seed fell out on the ground, and the girl looked at it in great surprise.

Hippocrates *On the Seed* (5th century BC)

A woman forbids herself to conceive and fights against it, if in her delight she aids the man's action with her buttocks, making undulating movements with all her breast limp; for she turns the share clean away from the furrow and makes the seed fail of its place. Whores indulge in such motions for their own purposes, that they may not often conceive and lie pregnant, and at the same time that their intercourse may be more pleasing to men; which our wives evidently have no need for.

Lucretius *On the Nature of Things* (1st century BC)

Anticonceptional: wear cat liver in a tube on the left foot, or wear the testicles of a cat in a tube around the umbilicus.

Wear part of the womb of a lioness in a tube of ivory. This is very effective.

Aëtios of Amida *On Medicine* (6th century AD)

When during the sexual act, the man feels he is about to ejaculate, he should quickly and firmly, using the fore and middle fingers of the left hand, put pressure on the spot between scrotum and anus, simultaneously inhaling deeply and gnashing his teeth scores of times, without holding his breath. Then the semen will be activated but not yet emitted; it returns from the Jade Stalk and enters the brain.

Yü-fang-chih-yao *Important Matters of the Jade Chamber* (c. 600 AD)

Nor is superstition in these matters restricted to prescientific societies:

Some women have that flexibility and vigour of the whole muscular system that they can, by effort of will, prevent conception.

Russell Thacker Thrall *Sexual Physiology* (1868)

The chances of conception are greatest early in the night, for the air of beds before morning is well known to become so foul as to extinguish burning tapers...

A remedy of corrective or fruitful nature might be found by embracing only in vessels filled with carbonic acid or azotic gas. Coition will always be unfruitful unless it be done in the pure air, so that some oxygen may be protruded before the penis into the uterus.

Thomas Ewell MD, US naval surgeon, *Medical Matters* (1911)

...in a 1974 paternity suit in Sweden ...the Israeli psychic Uri Geller was sued for allegedly bending the metallic contraceptive IUD of an unsuspecting woman. The woman claimed that Geller was liable to child support because she became pregnant after he, using his telekinetic powers, bent her IUD and made it ineffective – even though he had never had any physical contact with it.

Roy Eskapa *Bizarre Sex* (1987)

There's the Greek method. Apparently one can temporarily sterilize oneself by heating one's organs in boiling water.

Anon. British teenager quoted in Michael Schofield *Sexual Behaviour of Young People* (1965)

See also SEXUAL NONSENSE

Other early methods may have had some medical basis (although they are not necessarily recommended):

...wherefore, since if the parts be smooth conception is prevented, some anoint that part of the womb on which the seed falls with oil of cedar, or with ointment of lead or with frankincense, comingled with olive oil.

Aristotle *History of Animals* (347–335 BC)

It also aids in preventing conception to smear the orifice of the uterus all over before with old olive oil or honey or cedar resin or juice of the balsam tree, alone or together with white lead; or with a moist cerate containing myrtle oil and white lead; or before the act with moist alum, or with galbanum together with wine; or to put a lock of fine wool into the orifice of the uterus; or, before sexual relations to use vaginal suppositories which have the power to contract and to condense...

The woman ought, in the moment during coitus when the man ejaculates his seminal fluid, to hold back a little, so that the semen cannot penetrate into the mouth of the uterus, then immediately get up and sit down with bent knees, and in this position provoke sneezes.

Soranus of Ephesus *On Midwifery and the Diseases of Women* (2nd century AD)

The ancient Greeks also used a type of enema, usually made from goatskin and ivory, both for douching the vagina as a contraceptive measure and for cleansing the bowel:

I, only, am allowed to fuck a wife,
Quite openly, at her own mate's request.
I mount young lads, those in the prime of life,
Old men, maids – at their grieving parents' behest.
I'm anti lust, loved by the healer's hand,
Performing Herculean tasks each time.
I'll even take on Pluto and demand
The lives of those whom I've lain with. For I'm
The offspring of an elephant and goat –

A white-tusked child with a good leather coat.

Anon. 'On a Clyster'. A clyster is an early name for an enema

While some of these methods may have worked sometimes, it was not until the introduction of a primitive condom that contraception became effective. Penile sheaths were sported by the ancient Egyptians, but not for contraceptive purposes:

More than 3000 years ago the Egyptians were wearing fine linen sheaths (with very little else), but mostly for decoration, doubling as a coloured bandage of rank and a defence against insects and tropical diseases.

Jeannette Parisot *Johnny Come Lately; A Short History of the Condom* (1987)

In modern Europe it seems that condoms first came into use as a protection against syphilis. The disease was apparently brought to Portugal from Haiti by Columbus's sailors in 1494 and thereafter spread rapidly throughout the civilized world (see SEXUALLY TRANSMITTED DISEASES). In 1594 the Italian Gabriello Fallopio recommended the use of a linen sheath, moistened with a lotion, for protection. These sheaths were not, however, used as contraceptives until the 18th century, when they were generally made of sheep's gut and tied on to the scrotum with a ribbon:

The New Machine as a sure defense shall prove
And guard the sex against the Harm of Love.

Joseph Gay 'The Petticoat' (1716)

The man, dear Friend, who wears a C....m,
May scour the Hundreds at random,
Whether it please him to disport
In Wild Street, or in Coulson's Court,
He fears no danger from the Doxies,
*Laughs at their F*****, and scorns their Poxes.*

Nicholas Rowe 'Horace's Interger Vitae' (1741)

Despite its obvious benefits, many rakes rejected the condom, finding it cumbersome and passion-quelling:

The Condum being the best, if not the only Preservative our Libertines have found out at present...yet, by reason of its blunting the Sensation, I have heard some of them acknowledge, that they had often to choose to risk a Clap, *rather than engage with spears thus sheathed.*

Anon. (1717) quoted by Richard Davenport-Hines in *Sex, Death and Punishment* (1990)

For the first time I did engage in armour, which I found but dull satisfaction.

James Boswell, diary entry (1763) published in *Boswell's London Journal* (ed. Frederick A. Pottle; 1950)

An armour against enjoyment and a spider's web against danger.

Madame de Sévigné (17th century) quoted by John Camp in *Magic, Myth and Medicine* (1973)

The vulcanization of rubber in 1843, by Goodyear and Hancock, led to a more effective sheath that was thinner, more sensitive, and easier to keep in place. Some men, however, persisted in their aversion to condom use, finding sex in a sheath

Like eating toffees with their wrappers on.

Anon.

Next we come in contact
with what's called a sheath.
Though it helps repulse VD
and Aids and sharp teeth,
I will stand up to state
that this method's the worst:
I'd strangle the geezer
who thought of it first
and each time I'm in one
I pray it will burst.

I'm sentenced to stop
in a cellophane bracket.
I squirm around like mad
in my plastic straight-jacket
attempting to put
matters into reverse,
but they pull me up quick

with a short breathless curse
and push it back harder
which makes me feel worse.

We all have our time
of endurance allotted,
but I really do wish
that the sheath would get knotted:
I get so restricted
when one is around,
I feel so uptight
and I can't hear a sound,
and then at the climax
I nearly get drowned.

Charles Tomlinson 'The Penis Poem' (20th century)

In the 19th century various simple barrier devices were also used by informed and resourceful women:

Before sexual intercourse, the female introduces into her vagina a piece of sponge as large as can be pleasantly introduced, having previously attached a bobbin or bit of narrow riband to withdraw it, it will be found a preventive to conception, while it neither lessens the pleasure of the female nor injures her health...

The English Duchess never goes out to dinner without being prepared with the sponge.

Richard Carlile *Every Woman's Book or What is Love?* (1838)

Contraceptive information remained largely confined to the educated classes until after World War I, when such campaigners as Marie Stopes in Britain and Margaret Sanger in America began to challenge the taboo on public discussion of such matters:

I read about what you were going to do and about the Mothers Clinic that you have opened what I would like to know is how I can save having any more children as I think that I have done my duty to my Country having had 13 children 9 boys and 4 girls.

Anon. letter to Marie Stopes (22 Mar. 1921)

We want far better reasons for having children than not knowing how to prevent them.

Dora Russell *Hypatia* (1925)

The early campaigners gradually made the subject respectable by treating it as an issue of public health rather than private gratification:

The protagonists of contraception...saw in a diminishing birth-rate the answer to poverty, residential overcrowding, maternal ill-health, the problems of the unmarried mother, the prevalence of prostitution, abortion and infanticide, and the desire to give fewer children a better education.

Judith Armstrong *The Novel of Adultery* (1976)

At times this led to a dubious flirtation with eugenics:

[Birth Control can be]...*nothing more or less than the facilitation of the process of weeding out the unfit, or preventing the birth of defectives.*

More children from the fit, less from the unfit.

Margaret Sanger, quoted in *Birth Control in America: the Career of Margaret Sanger* (1920s)

If instead of birth control every one would preach drink control, you would have little poverty, less crime, and fewer illegitimate children...I speak feelingly; for as my brother Harold John Tennant and I were the last of twelve children, it is more than probable we should never have existed had the fashion of birth control been prevalent in the eighties.

Margot Asquith *Places and Persons* (1925)

The most revolutionary development in the field of birth control was the appearance of oral contraceptives. Although the principle of controlling conception by the use of hormones was understood as early as the 1920s, it was not until the late 1950s that satisfactory formulations had been produced or the reluctance of medical practitioners and religious bodies to interfere with nature had been overcome. However, once the Pill became generally available it brought about two major social changes. First, it gave women a reliable method of contraception that enabled them to combine an active sexual life with the chance of a fulfilling career:

The contraceptive pill may reduce the importance of sex not only as a basis for the division of labor, but as a guideline in developing talents and interests.

Caroline Bird *Born Female* (1968)

I wonder anew whether and how the human female will ever transcend the lower, more dependent, less rights-ful station to which her reproductive nature has until the last-minute invention of The Pill confined her.

Shana Alexander *State-by-State Guide to Women's Legal Rights* (1975)

Secondly, with the fear of unwanted pregnancies removed there seemed to be no good reason why girls should not sleep with their boyfriends or, for that matter, anyone else – the swinging sixties had arrived:

The pill signified an important break with the past. It made contraception – and sex – a more accessible subject for public debate. Dealing with a drug taken in pill form removed embarrassing images of 'private parts' (which continued to inhibit public discussion of the sheath); talking about hormones rather than genitals turned contraception into an issue of medicine rather than morality. The pill shifted responsibility for contraception onto women. It gave them autonomous control over their reproductive choices. By releasing women to enjoy sex without fear of pregnancy, it challenged one of the central tenets of the social control of women, that their primary role and fulfilment in life was bound to motherhood. For they now had real choice.

Cate Haste *Rules of Desire* (1992)
See also PROMISCUITY

I want to tell you a terrific story about oral contraception. I asked this girl to sleep with me and she said 'no'.

Woody Allen quoted by Adler and Feinman in *Woody Allen: Clown Prince of American Humor* (20th century)

Not being an intrusive barrier method, the Pill is also much preferred on aesthetic grounds. Despite popular belief to the contrary, however, it is no more 100% effective than any other technique:

Because it is easy to accuse a woman of not taking it when she should, failures are explained away as the patient's fault ('you know these women; no good with numbers'). Oddly enough, most women seem to have one or two friends who can count but who somehow got pregnant on the pill anyway.

Lucina Cisler *Birth Control and Women's Liberation* (1969)

In recent years the possible links between cancer and the long-term use of the Pill by older women have also contributed to a swing back towards barrier methods.

While medical technology has given people the chance to plan their families, controversy still surrounds the subject on religious and ethical grounds. Traditional Christian teaching associated sexual intercourse with guilt (see CHASTITY AND CELIBACY) and argued that it could only be justified on the grounds of reproduction. Largely because of this heritage, contraceptive use has often been condemned as selfish and unnatural, or as a way of trivializing the sexual act:

Taking Physick before-hand to prevent your being with Child is wilful Murther, as essentially and as effectively, as your destroying the Child after it was formed in your womb.

Daniel Defoe *Conjugal Lewdness: or Matrimonial Whoredom* (1727)

Let the mothers do their duty by their children, and suckle them as they are bound to do, and so they shall not procreate more frequently than is consistent with health. Ameliorate, improve, raise her moral position. Use her as a helpmate worthy of an honourable man, not as a vessel for unbridled lust.

C. H. F. Routh *The Moral and Physical Evils likely to Follow Practices Intended to Act as Checks to Population* (1879)

It is therefore a real sin when a young married woman refuses to bear a family or neglects the nurture and the welfare of her children, in the pursuit of pleasure, or even in the performance of works which are indeed good, and which ought to be accomplished, but not by her.

Mary Scharlieb *The Seven Ages of Woman* (1915)

Nations which practise artificial prevention of conception, and who therefore have no restraint on their sexual passions, are likely to become effeminate and degenerate. The removal of the sanction of matrimony, and the unhindered and unbalanced sexual indulgence that would follow, would war against self-control, chivalry and self-respect.

Mary Scharlieb (1921)

No one will wish to propose that contraception in any form is an absolute good. The bond between love and life is so strong and so spontaneous that any arbitrary *separation of one from the other would surely seem to be 'unnatural'.*

It may be suggested that every sexual expression of marital love which is so planned or executed as to deliberately exclude the possibility of procreation will be experienced by the Christian married couple as a gesture of love which is less adequate than, ideally and in the abstract, they would wish it to be.

Stanley E. Kutz *Conscience and Contraception* (1964)

To accept the pleasures of sexual attitudes and practices without relating them to the purposes for which these pleasures were intended is a form of perversion and must be condemned as delinquent.

Lord Soper in *Does Pornography Matter?* (ed. C. H. Rolph; 1961)

Skullion had little use for contraceptives at the best of times. Unnatural, he called them, and placed them in the lower social category of things along with elastic-sided boots and made-up bow ties. Not the sort of attire for a gentleman.

Tom Sharpe *Porterhouse Blue* (1974)

Condom vending machines could stop Australia being a great nation.

Headline, *New Australian Express* (10 Sept. 1987)

The Roman Catholic Church's continuing ban on artificial methods of contraception has outraged those who see overpopulation as the world's primary problem:

Every conjugal act has to be open to the transmission of life.

Pope Paul VI *Humanae Vitae* (1968)

If the possibility of conceiving a child is artificially eliminated in the conjugal act, couples shut themselves off from God and oppose his will.

Pope John Paul II, sermon given in Chihuahua, Mexico (11 May 1990)

I would not give a baby from one of my homes for adoption to a couple who use contraception. People who use contraceptives do not understand love.

Mother Teresa, in a radio interview while on a visit to London (1983)

To the non-Catholic, the underlying objective of the ban on birth control is obvious: to make more Catholics.

Brenda Maddox *The Pope and Contraception* (1991)

Any Protestant woman in her senses would object to marrying a Roman Catholic... They prohibit the use of proper hygienic Birth Control methods preferring that a woman's health should be entirely ruined and that she should bring forth feeble, dying or imbecile infants rather than that proper hygienic methods should be used.

Marie Stopes, letter to an Irish Catholic (18 Oct. 1920)

To any man who says population control is a form of genocide, I say, ask any woman.

Judith Hart at a Food and Agricultural conference on birth control (1969)

Some are unhappy at using contraceptive techniques because these are 'unnatural'. Of course they are – but all of us are constantly manipulating and thwarting nature in everyday life. It is not 'natural' to drink purified water, to treat disease by medicines, to take even an aspirin, to shave or to visit a dentist.

R. F. R. Gardner *Abortion: the Personal Dilemma* (1972)

Birth control is thought wicked by people who tolerate celibacy, because the former is a new violation of nature and the latter an ancient one.

Bertrand Russell 'Why I am Not a Christian' (1957)

He no play-a da game. He no make-a da rules!

Earl Butz, referring to the Pope's strictures against contraception (1974)

Protestant women may take the Pill. Roman Catholic women must keep taking the Tablet.

Irene Thomas (1970s). The *Tablet* is a British Roman Catholic newspaper

The Pope does not know about American Catholics. He doesn't know how to gear down a Porsche, he can't work a cigarette machine, doesn't know about Bank Americard – doesn't know about any of your problems.
And the big issue, contraceptives – he never makes it with anybody! He lives in a state of celibacy, and I respect him for this, but he cannot relate to a problem about it, then, if he is that far removed from it, man.

Lenny Bruce (1960s)

The Church in its continuing campaign of sexual pessimism, stubbornly links the abortion question with sex. It believes in something it calls the 'contraceptive mentality'. Women who get used to taking the pill, goes the argument, have already decided that if the pill fails, they will automatically opt for an abortion. We believe this view insults women. We have never met anyone who had an abortion for fun. We maintain that women – particularly Catholic women – take contraceptive precautions in order to avoid facing this situation. The Church has a powerful and laudable reverence for human life. Its great mistake is attaching the same amount of sin-value to two entirely different acts – preventing conception and terminating a pregnancy. The logic here is deeply flawed. If abortion is so terrible, all the more reason to make contraceptives widely available and morally acceptable, so that fewer abortions will be necessary in the first place.

Kate Saunders and Peter Stanford *Catholics and Sex* (1992)

For Catholic women the only form of family planning permitted by the Church is the highly inefficient rhythm method:

It is now quite lawful for a Catholic woman to avoid pregnancy by a resort to mathematics, though she is still forbidden to resort to physics and chemistry.

H. L. Mencken *Notebooks*, 'Minority Report' (20th century)

Q. *What do you call people who use the rhythm method?*
A. *Parents.*

Anon.

In the past, ideas about the so-called 'safe period' during a woman's cycle have often been quite erroneous:

In order to avoid conception it is necessary to abstain from coitus during the days favourable to conception, for example, at the beginning or end of menstruation.

Aëtios of Amida (6th century)

Other religious traditions have been less absolute in their attitude to contraception:

Since birth control could be interpreted as an attempt to interfere with the workings of Karma, there was a tendency in Buddhism to discourage artificial contraception. In reality, however, the necessity of birth control was tacitly recognized.

John Stevens *Lust for Enlightenment: Buddhism and Sex* (1990)

Under certain circumstances, however, the rabbis permitted family limitation, preferably by contraception. "There are three classes of women who should employ an absorbent: a minor, lest pregnancy should prove fatal; a pregnant woman, lest abortion should result; and a nursing mother, lest she become pregnant and prematurely wean the child so that it dies."

N. E. Himes *Medical History of Contraception* (1970)

For its part, the Church of England declared that contraception was morally permissible in certain circumstances in 1930.

In recent years the Catholic Church's unrelenting attitude has been further called into question by the fact that condom use offers one of the few effective remedies against the spread of AIDS:

The Pope has swept through Africa, where 5 million people are already infected with the AIDS virus and which expects by the end of the century to have 10 million orphans whose parents have died of AIDS – and told them not to use condoms.

Brenda Maddox *The Pope and Contraception* (1991)

The history of the condom has, in a sense, come full circle, in that it is now once again regarded mainly as a preventive against disease rather than as a contraceptive measure. The last five or six years have seen a marked increase in the use of the sheath – formerly regarded by many younger people as inherently ludicrous and anti-erotic:

The condom is the third most popular method of contraception (16 per cent) after sterilisation (25 per cent) and the pill (23 per cent of women), and about two million British women used condoms as their main method of contraception in 1991.

Alice Thomson 'Is This the Age of the Condom?' *The Times* (27 Oct. 1992)

For those who are certain that they want no more children, sterilization or vasectomy may well be the best solution (although the latter can sometimes be reversed). At the same time many people are reluctant to commit themselves to something they believe to be irreversible: the desire to have children can unexpectedly reassert itself – especially in cases of remarriage. Until recently, men have been particularly reluctant to have vasectomies, despite the advantage noted by the US harmonica virtuoso Larry Adler:

Vasectomy means not ever having to say you're sorry.

Curiously, a primitive type of 'vasectomy' was popular amongst Australian aborigines as this letter, written in 1928 to Marie Stopes, makes clear:

Their method is to make an insertion in the male organ, underneath, near junction with the body. This cut is healed much the same as perforation with earring. They can fulfill all obligations except propagate; as the seed is passed out at the perforation. We call them whistle-cocks.

Sterilization has sometimes been abused by those intent on social engineering:

One staff member would lie to the patient if he felt she had too many kids and tell her her uterus needed to come out when it didn't.

Anon. quoted in *Workbook on Sterilization* (1978)

Even those forms of contraception that have no lasting effect on the user's fertility may provoke an occasional twinge of regret or feeling of 'what if?'

Where are the children I might have had? You may suppose I might have wanted them. Drowned to the accompaniment of the rattling of a thousand douche bags.

Malcolm Lowry *Under the Volcano* (1947)

When you take your Pill,
It's like a mine disaster
I think of all the people
Lost inside you.

Richard Brautigan 'The Pill versus the Springhill Mine Disaster' (1968)

It's funny how in spite of my reluctance to get pregnant, I seem to live inside my own cunt. I seem to be involved with all the changes of my body. They never pass unnoticed. I seem to know exactly when I ovulate. In the second week of the cycle I feel a tiny ping and then a sort of tingling ache in my lower belly. A few days later I'll often find a tiny spot of blood in the rubber yarmulke of the diaphragm. A bright red smear, the only visible trace of the egg that might have become a baby.

Erica Jong *Fear of Flying* (1973)

A final pertinent question from the poet Zygmunt Frankel:

WITH ALL THE
pills
IUDs,
condoms
diaphragms,
safe periods,
coitus interruptus,
abortions,
accidents,
wars,
and emigration,
why is the bus so crowded?

Obviously no one is taking the simple piece of advice offered by a wisely anonymous delegate at an International Planned Parenthood Conference:

The best contraceptive is a glass of cold water: not before or after, but instead.

Exhibitionism

What is exhibitionism? Two clinical definitions:

The act of exposure can range from a partial showing of the flaccid penis without a conscious experience of sexual satisfaction to a full exposure of the genitalia with erect penis, masturbation, and an intense experience of sexual satisfaction… Exposure is, however, not a determinant of clinical exhibitionism unless it represents the final sexual gratification without any intention of further sexual contact.

J. W. Mohr, R. E. Turner, and M. B. Jerry *Pedophilia and Exhibitionism* (1964)

An exhibitionist is a person, who has an irresistible, repetitive impulse to show his sexual organs, usually to strangers, in order to achieve a psychic discharge that other sexual practices do not give him.

Preben Hertoft *Psychosexual Problems* (1976)

Psychiatrists differ as to whether such behaviour is always evidence of deep-seated abnormality:

The exposure is an act of more or less normal individuals, and is in the nature of an anomalous form of the ordinary sexual advance.

D. T. Maclay *The Diagnosis and Treatment of Compensatory Types of Indecent Exposure* (1956)

Many normal males, regardless of age, may under temporary stress or temptation expose their genitals to females.

Clifton D. Bryant *Sexual Deviancy in Social Context* (1977)

Exhibitionism, as a sexual deviation, is included under disorders of character, behaviour, and intelligence in the International Statistical Classification of Diseases. Every exhibitionist is therefore prima facie psychiatrically ill and would be classified as such.

J. W. Mohr, R. E. Turner, and M. B. Jerry *Pedophilia and Exhibitionism* (1964)

Exhibitionism is not necessarily an indication of mental abnormality. In certain slum neighbourhoods this is an accepted form of courting, and only in respectable middle-class areas are passers-by likely to call the police.

Melitta Schmideberg *On Treating Exhibitionism* (1972)

Whether or not it should be classified as abnormal, male exhibitionism is a criminal offence in most countries. In the UK the Vagrancy Act of 1824 is still used for most prosecutions of this kind:

Every person wilfully, openly, lewdly and obscenely exposing his person with intent to insult any female is a rogue and a vagabond.

Vagrancy Act (1824)

Exhibitionism is the only deviated sexual offence which is punishable on summary conviction and not on indictment. The law therefore commonly recognizes that exhibitionism is more of a social nuisance than a danger.

J. W. Mohr, R. E. Turner, and M. B. Jerry *Pedophilia and Exhibitionism* (1964)

Female exhibitionism is not recognized as an offence in law:

> *A woman may take off her clothes in public but cannot be charged with indecent exposure…*
> *The exposure of the female genitalia was not regarded to be as threatening to social morals as the exposure of the penis.*

Susan Edwards *Female Sexuality and the Law* (1981)

Although rare, it undoubtedly occurs:

> *There's a woman lives near us who is not quite right in the head. You know there's been a full moon these last few days, well – this woman came up to Mrs. —, as she was standing talking to a friend in the street, and this woman whisked up her skirt and ripped down her knickers and said, 'How's that, then!'*

Anon. quoted by Iona Opie and Moira Tatem in *Dictionary of Superstitions* (1989)

> *Lesbia, why are your amours*
> *Always conducted behind open,*
> *unguarded doors?*
> *Why do you get more excitement out of a*
> *voyeur than a lover?*
> *Why is pleasure no pleasure when it's*
> *under cover?*

Martial *Epigrams* (1st century AD)

So who are exhibitionists? The stereotype of the 'dirty old man' in the 'flasher's mac' has little foundation in reality:

> *Exhibitionists as a group are young; offences occurring at an older age frequently indicate other factors, such as alcoholism, organic deterioration, or another sexual deviation, especially pedophilia.*

J. W. Mohr, R. E. Turner, and M. B. Jerry *Pedophilia and Exhibitionism* (1964)

Sometimes the offence is a momentary aberration, triggered by unusual circumstances or a sudden inexplicable impulse:

> *For some the act* [of exhibitionism] *is preceded by a profound state of anxiety, depression, or tension; others are unaware of any precipitating factors and the act is impulsive and spontaneous.*

Clifton D. Bryant *Sexual Deviancy in Social Context* (1977)

This is, however, rare: most flashers are trapped in a pattern of compulsive behaviour that can be traced back to childhood:

> *At the age of five a boy had his first sexual experience. An older playmate enticed him to a wood and induced him to undress completely and fondle his own penis. The experience was very pleasurable, especially the act of being naked out in the open and in broad daylight. The little boy was discovered and scolded by his mother. In the course of time he became an exhibitionist.*

Francis Bennion *The Sex Code* (1991)

Because exhibitionists do not form a homogenous group of people all suffering from the same deviation, psychiatrists have offered varying accounts of their motives. Interestingly, some have normal sex lives in which the exhibitionism is a supplementary activity, while for others it is the sole form of gratification. This diversity makes understanding of the problem extremely difficult. According to some psychiatrists, the exhibitionist craves recognition:

> *The exhibitionist shows off his body, or part of his body, or some highly prized function or skill trying to overcome that haunting isolation and loneliness of one who feels his 'real' or 'true' self has never been disclosed to and confirmed by others. The man who compulsively exhibits his penis substitutes disclosure through this 'thing' rather than through living.*

R. D. Laing *Self and Others* (1971)

Others argue that he seeks power over his victims:

> *The exhibitionist feels that he has effected a psychic defloration.*

H. Havelock Ellis *Erotic Symbolism* (1926)

or his own abasement:

> *The word 'exhibitionistic' is not adequate because it would presume that the demonstrator is proud of what he displays or*

considers it to be beautiful or commendable.

Theodor Reik *Masochism in Modern Man* (1957)

Many exhibitionists seem to derive excitement from the risk of being caught:

Exhibitionism always involves considerable risk taking and thus can be viewed from the point of adolescent excitement or daring and not from the perspective of a behavioral disorder.

Clifton D. Bryant *Sexual Deviancy in Social Context* (1977)

Some appear to invite arrest:

Arrest tends to alleviate the sense of guilt and shame and gives him a feeling of excitement and manliness for posing such a threat.

James L. Mathis *Medical Aspects of Human Sexuality* (1969)

In fact, although his activities may cause distress and embarrassment, especially to the young girls who are often his targets, the exhibitionist very rarely poses a serious threat:

The cases thus far recorded are exclusively those of men who ostentatiously expose their genitals to persons of the opposite sex, whom in some instances they even pursue, without, however, becoming aggressive.

Richard von Krafft-Ebing *Psychopathia Sexualis* (1886)

For this reason, and because of the compulsive nature of the offence, some modern commentators take a tolerant view:

Should you see an exhibitionist in action, do regard him as a fellow human being, not as a leper! Try to understand the touching and pathetic element in his behaviour. Above all, do not report him to the police – nothing but harm can come of that. We ought to allow our fellow human beings the beneficial magic of the exhibitionist rite.

Lars Ullerstam *The Erotic Minorities* (1967)

Exhibitionism is a clinical entity, but it does not appear to occur in cultures which tolerate nakedness, even if only to a degree which allows the growing child to satisfy his curiosity. Such harm as the persistent exhibitionist does results from the attitude of his audience rather than the emotional character of the offence. In another context of custom he might be an object of ridicule rather than of fear, and those individuals whose income and intelligence permit them to veil their abnormality under a guise of hygiene and nudism attract little attention.

Alex Comfort *Sexual Behaviour in Society* (1950)

Indeed, exhibitionists often expose not only their penises, but also their vulnerability:

In 1980, Julie Barlow, an anthropology student at the University of Chicago, was stepping out of a phone booth one evening when a man approached her displaying himself and asking, "What do you think of that then?" "It looks like a cock to me," she said, "only smaller."

Gyles Brandreth *The Bedside Book of Great Sexual Disasters* (1984)

The young Jean-Jacques Rousseau suffered from an obsessive desire to expose his bare buttocks to passing women:

My agitation became so strong that, being unable to satisfy my desires, I excited them by the most extravagant behaviour. I haunted dark alleys and hidden retreats, where I might be able to expose myself to women in the condition in which I should have liked to have been in their company. What they saw was not an obscene object, I never even thought of such a thing; it was a ridiculous object. The foolish pleasure I took in displaying it before their eyes cannot be described.

Confessions (1782)

And finally, two visitors to the Soviet Union recall

...a militiaman directing traffic at the intersection which we were approaching. His pose was, to say the least, bizarre; he had taken his member out of his trousers and was squeezing it at its base with his

right hand. Left, right, stop: the officer was directing the traffic with his penis, which was red as a pepper. The drivers and their passengers were splitting their sides with laughter.

Stern and Stern *Sex in the Soviet Union* (1981)

Feminism

There is no doubt that women have been given a bad time since the unfortunate episode in the Garden of Eden when Eve found herself cast in the role of the temptress:

> *Unto the woman he said, I will greatly multiply thy sorrow and thy conception; in sorrow thou shalt bring forth children; and thy desire shall be to thy husband, and he shall rule over thee.*
>
> Genesis 3:16

Judging by the Bible, the ancient Hebrews regarded women primarily as begetters of sons and seducers of loyal husbands. They had few rights of their own:

> *In the Old Testament women were subject and inferior beings; the Decalogue includes a wife amongst a man's possessions. They could be repudiated, but could not themselves claim a divorce. They could not inherit, nor make a valid vow without the consent of husband or father, and they were severely punished for sexual misconduct, while men were punished only if they violated another husband's rights.*
>
> Judith Armstrong *The Novel of Adultery* (1976)

Some men still think of women as things:

> *If my wife cheated, I'd kill her…I feel I own her, the way I own my car. And I don't lend my car.*
>
> Al Goldstein, (1973)

Some ancient Greeks even questioned the role of women in conception:

> *The mother is not the parent of that which is called her child: but only the nurse of the newly planted seed that grows. The parent is he who mounts.*
>
> Aeschylus *Eumenides* (485 BC)

> *Man is active, full of movement, creative in politics, business and culture… Woman, on the other hand, is passive. She stays at home, as is her nature…Man consequently plays a major part in reproduction; the woman is merely the passive incubator of his seed.*
>
> Aristotle *Politiks* (4th century BC)

See also REPRODUCTION

These ancient views have continued to reverberate throughout Christian history:

> *Let your women keep silence in the churches: for it is not permitted unto them to speak; but they are commanded to be under obedience as also saith the law.*
>
> I Corinthians 14:34

For St Paul, as for many subsequent Christians, sexual intercourse was a debasing activity only tolerated as a means of procreation. The idea that sexual activity is a dangerous rival to religious activity was taken over from primitive religions by the early Church. This led to an insistence on a celibate priesthood, implying that any contact with female sexuality would pollute the ritual purity of the priest:

> *Among all savage beasts, none is found as harmful as woman…*
>
> St John Chrysostom (4th century)

Although most Christians no longer talk like this, neither the Church of Rome nor the Orthodox Churches allow their women to become priests – a position only recently abandoned by the Church of England. Islam, too, places a strong emphasis on masculine supremacy:

> *Men are in charge of women, because Allah hath made the one of them to excel the other...So good women are the obedient.*
>
> Koran

In almost all cultures, women have had to endure an unthinking scorn for their mental and moral qualities:

> *For a man wins no better prize than a good woman,*
> *and none more chilling than a bad one –*
> *always hunting something to devour.*
> *And no matter how strong he is,*
> *she roasts her man without fire,*
> *and hands him over to raw old age.*
> *Woman is the wrath of Zeus, a gift given in place*
> *of fire – cruel countergift!*
> *For she burns a man with cares and withers him*
> *up and brings old age on youth too soon.*
>
> Hesiod *Works and Days* (8th century BC)

> *Girls begin to talk and stand on their feet sooner than boys because weeds grow up more quickly than good crops.*
>
> Martin Luther *Table Talk* (1533)

In most societies, women's inferior status has been codified in law until relatively recently:

> *By marriage the very being or legal existence of woman is suspended, or at least it is incorporated and consolidated into that of a husband.*
>
> Sir William Blackstone *Commentaries on the Laws of England* (1780)

> *In marriage, perhaps more consistently than anywhere else, is revealed the desire to protect; and yet the law enshrines the husband's right to batter, abuse, intimidate and rape at will. Since women were defined as passive, they were afforded few, if any, legal rights.*
>
> Susan Edwards *Female Sexuality and the Law* (1981)
>
> See also RAPE, MARRIAGE

Examples of grotesque unfairness abound. In 3rd-century Rome for example:

> *If a woman had a sexual relationship with someone other than her husband while she was living with him then she was committing adultery. If she set up home with another man then this was a marriage or a concubinage and cancelled her first marriage. But if a man took another wife before his first wife had left the marital home...it was regarded in law not as adultery but as concubinage.*
>
> Aline Rousselle *Porneia* (1983)
>
> See also ADULTERY

and in 20th-century America:

> *Legislation and case law still exist in some parts of the United States permitting the 'passion shooting' by husband of a wife; the reverse, of course, is known as homicide.*
>
> Diane B. Schulder in *Sisterhood is Powerful* (ed. Robin Morgan; 1970)

Pressure for women to be granted equal legal, educational, and political rights grew steadily during the 18th and 19th centuries. The successful battle for women's suffrage, in both Britain and the US, proved a major turning-point:

> *We still wonder at the stolid incapacity of all men to understand that woman feels the invidious distinctions of sex exactly as the black man does those of color, or the white man the more transient distinctions of wealth, family, position, place, and power; that she feels as keenly as man the injustice of disfranchisement.*
>
> Elizabeth Cady Stanton *History of Woman Suffrage* Vol. I (1880)

> *The public roughly seems divided between people who deny the struggle any significance at all, and those who, seeing the significance, attribute it to sexual morbidity and hysteria. The situation with which we are face to face represents indeed a sex war. It is a war which signifies vitality, not decadence.*
>
> Lucy Re-Bartlett *The Coming Order* (1911)

Even in societies where women have won equal rights in law, many women have continued to feel hampered by social expectations and conditioning:

Women are told from their infancy and taught by the example of their mothers, that a little knowledge of human weakness, justly termed cunning, softness of temper, 'outward' obedience and a scrupulous attention to a puerile kind of propriety, will obtain for them the protection of man...

Mary Wollstonecraft *A Vindication of the Rights of Women* (1792)

There was one great snag; even the most forward looking had been conditioned by education, precept and upbringing...Beneath every emancipated cigarette-smoking woman with free-wheeling sexual views there was a lily of the field, a girlish plaything, embryo wife and mother, a rooted conservative, depository of inconsistency and irrationality.

Ronald Pearsall *The Worm in the Bud* (1971)

Traditionally, women have not been expected to initiate sexual contact:

In the case of a lady, she probably first meets the gentleman at a ball, or croquet party, where the excitement has caused everything that surrounds her to appear couleur de rose. The gentleman approaches her and solicits her hand as a partner in a dance...the first step towards intimacy is taken...her prudence whispering that he is – as yet – but a comparative stranger, she endeavours to escape from his attentions. He is not, however, to be thus checked. He tries again, and she, finding it very hard to resist his advantages...at length yields to his solicitations, and joins him for the giddy dance. From this moment the real courtship may be supposed to commence.

Anon. *Cupid's Guide to the Wedding Ring* (1877)

The primary part of the female in courtship is the playful, yet serious, assumption of the rôle of a hunted animal who lures on the pursuer, not with the object of escaping, but with the object of finally being caught.

H. Havelock Ellis *Studies in the Psychology of Sex* (1936)

See also MODESTY

These assumptions have often allowed men to ignore clear signs that their attentions are unwelcome:

Disapproval of sexual harassment tends to focus on demands for sex as a condition of hiring as well as for keeping a job. These are considered serious manifestations of sexual coercion, while generalised staring, commenting, touching and other forms of male familiarity are regarded as annoying and of little consequence.

Lyn Farley *Sexual Shakedown* (1978)

"...it is usual with young ladies to reject the addresses of the man whom they secretly mean to accept, when he first applies for their favour; and that sometimes the refusal is repeated a second or even a third time. I am, therefore, by no means discouraged by what you have just said, and shall hope to lead you to the altar ere long."
"Upon my word, sir," cried Elizabeth, "your hope is rather an extraordinary one after my declaration..."

Jane Austen *Pride and Prejudice* (1813)

In post-war Western societies women have demanded a new egalitarian basis for their relationships with men – one in which the experience is shared rather than the woman 'possessed':

Another characteristic I found of love in healthy people is that they have made no really sharp differentiations between the roles and personalities of the two sexes. That is, they did not assume that the female was passive and the male active, whether in sex or love or anything else. These people were so certain of their maleness or femaleness they did not mind taking on some of the aspects of the opposite sex role.

A. H. Maslow *Motivations and Personality* (1954)

Marriage in modern times is regarded as a partnership of equals and no longer one in which the wife must be the subservient chattel of the husband.

Lord Keith of Kinkel, passing judgment in a rape-within-marriage case (1991)

Male contempt for female sexuality is apparent everywhere – from the most casual dirty jokes to the pronouncements of philosophers and psychoanalysts:

Seven wise men with knowledge so fine,
Created a pussy to their design.
First was a butcher, smart with wit,
Using a knife, he gave it a slit.
Second was a carpenter, strong and bold,
With a hammer and chisel, he gave it a hole.
Third was a tailor, tall and thin,
By using red velvet, he lined it within.
Fourth was a hunter, short and stout,
With a piece of fox fur, he lined it without.
Fifth was a fisherman, nasty as hell,
Threw in a fish and gave it a smell.
Sixth was a preacher whose name was McGee,
Touched it and blessed it and said it could pee.
Last came a sailor, a dirty little runt,
He sucked it and fucked it and called it a cunt.

Anon. *The Creation of a Pussy* (19th century)

According to Freud's notorious theory, when little girls

...notice the penis of a brother or playmate, strikingly visible and of large proportions, they at once recognize it as the superior counterpart of their own small and inconspicuous organ, and from that time forward fall a victim to envy for the penis...The psychical consequences of penis-envy...are various and far-reaching. After a woman has become aware of the wound to her narcissism, she develops, like a scar, a sense of inferiority. When she has passed beyond her first attempt at explaining her lack of a penis as being a punishment personal to herself and has realized that that sexual character is a universal one, she begins to share the contempt felt by men for a sex which is the lesser in so important a respect.

Sigmund Freud *Some Psychical Consequences of the Anatomical Distinction Between the Sexes* (1925)

One motive for this sort of contempt seems to be fear – fear in particular, perhaps, of sexual inadequacy:

Besides, the older you got, the clearer it became that men were basically terrified of women. Some secretly, some openly. What could be more poignant than a liberated woman eye to eye with a limp prick? All history's greatest issues paled by comparison with these two quintessential objects: the eternal woman and the eternal limp prick...Quite terrifying, when you think about it. No wonder men hated women. No wonder they invented the myth of female inadequacy.

Erica Jong *Fear of Flying* (1974)

Most women find the notion of penis envy bizarre, even laughable:

Jealous of male potency we'd dearly love a penis
That's a stupid phallusy spread by men who fear us
A penis is a marvellous *thing, fiddled with in the pocket*
Is it just coincidence it's shaped like a nuclear rocket?...
Maybe men are jealous of us, they come with just one spasm
They will never know the joy of having a TENTH orgasm.

Sensible Footwear 'Penis Envy' (1990)

Women don't have penis envy; men have pussy envy.

Valerie Solanas *SCUM* [Society for Cutting up Men] *Manifesto* (1967)

Men have often chosen to deny female sexuality altogether:

> *The majority of women are not very much troubled with sexual feeling of any kind.*
>
> Dr William Acton *Prostitution Considered in its Moral, Social, and Sanitary Aspects* (1857)

Or to see in it only a reflection of their own needs and desires:

> *Women were not permitted to experience their own sexuality on their own terms. Her orgasm was important for* his *pleasure; bringing a woman to orgasm became a mark of a man's masculinity and virility.*
>
> Sandra Coyno *Women's Liberation and Sexual Liberation* (1979)

> *In 1977 Shere Hite argued that women should choose how to experience their sexuality. The change was 'much deeper than just the idea that "a woman needs an orgasm too".' The definition of women's sexual freedom was not their ability to orgasm 'just like men'. She proposed women move away from the inevitability of intercourse and in particular from 'male orgasm during intercourse as the conclusion of "sex",' towards varieties of imaginative sensuality which stressed the potential for women's expression of sexual loving, affection and pleasure on terms other than the 'male dominated' sex act.*
>
> Cate Haste *Rules of Desire* (1992)

See also ORGASM

A deliberate rejection of the role of 'sex object' is one of the main characteristics of the 20th-century feminist movement:

> *A full bosom is actually a millstone around a woman's neck: it endears her to the men who want to make their mammet of her, but she is never allowed to think that their popping eyes actually see her. Her breasts are only to be admired for as long as they show no signs of their function: once darkened, stretched or withered they are objects of revulsion. They are not parts of a person but lures slung around her neck, to be kneaded and twisted like magic putty, or mumbled and mouthed like lolly ices. The only way that women can opt out of such gross handling is to refuse to wear undergarments which perpetuate the fantasy of pneumatic boobs, so that men must come to terms with the varieties of the real thing.*
>
> Germaine Greer *The Female Eunuch* (1970)

and again from the same book:

> *...I do not mean that large-scale lesbianism should be adopted, but simply that the emphasis should be taken off male genitality and replaced upon human sexuality. The cunt must come into its own...*

It is hardly surprising that some feminist anger should have gone over the top, issuing in a blanket rejection of men and heterosexual relationships:

> *The male is a biological accident: the Y (male) gene is an incomplete X (female) gene, that is, it has an incomplete set of chromosomes. In other words, the male is an incomplete female, a walking abortion, aborted at the gene state...*
>
> *It is now technically possible to reproduce without the aid of males, and to produce only females. We must begin immediately to do so.*
>
> *Being an incomplete female, the male spends his life attempting to complete himself, to become female.*
>
> Valerie Solanas *SCUM* [Society for Cutting up Men] *Manifesto* (1967)

> *No woman needs intercourse, few escape it.*
>
> Andrea Dworkin *Our Blood* (1982)

In the 1970s some radical separatists began to argue that any true feminist commitment led inevitably to lesbianism. In doing so they appeared to endorse the crass chauvinist jibe that all feminists are lesbians:

> *If hostility to men causes Lesbianism, then it seems to me that in a male-domi-*

nated society, Lesbianism is a sign of mental health.

Martha Shelley *Notes of a Radical Lesbian* (1969)

Feminist sexual politics in the 1970s aimed to define a positive female sexuality around the principle 'our bodies are our own'...For some it meant opting out of heterosexual relationships altogether; some women moved into lesbianism because they discovered their real sexual preferences, others because they took the separatist political view that sex with men was a form of collaboration with the oppressor.

Cate Haste *Rules of Desire* (1992)

A lesbian is not considered a 'real woman'. And yet in popular thinking, there is really only one essential difference between a lesbian and other women, that of sexual orientation – which is to say, when you strip off all the packaging, you must realise that the essence of being a 'woman' is to get fucked by men.

Radicalesbians (a political activist group) *The Woman-identified Woman* (1970)

I have met many, many feminists who were not Lesbians – but I have never met a Lesbian who was not a feminist. 'Straight' women by the millions have been sold the belief that they must subordinate themselves to men, accept less pay for equal work, and do all the shitwork about the house. I have met straight women who would die to preserve their chains.

Martha Shelley *Notes of a Radical Lesbian* (1969)

Lesbianism is not a matter of sexual preference, but rather one of political choice which every woman must make if she is to become woman-identified and thereby end male supremacy.

N. Myron and C. Burch *Lesbianism and the Women's Movement* (1975)

...I no longer need a man. Until recently, even as I actively struggled for my liberation, it was with a part of me still reserved for 'men only'. I always thought I would end up having one man. I suppose that is still a possibility, but now it is only one of many. Instead of that, I think about living with women because the emotional and psychological interchange is so satisfying...There are signs that I may yet discover what I like to do, which is very different from trying to figure out what men and society in general expect of me.

Martha Shelley 'Off Our Backs' *Commentary* (Nov. 1970)

See also LESBIANISM

In the Western world, feminism has largely succeeded in eradicating the grosser forms of male oppression. Despite this, there are still sceptics who maintain that the biological and psychological differences between the sexes are not so easily set aside:

A powerful antidote to women's liberation lies in the plain fact of biological function, with all the deep differences in the behaviour and life-experiences which this entails.

Leading article *The Times* (22 Nov. 1970)

The brains of girls and boys are made in a distinctive way that may determine how well they perform in certain specialised tasks. This may mean that we may never see equal numbers of men and women in engineering, or a woman chess master able to beat the best men. In other fields – Professor Kimura suggests medicine, where perceptual skills are important – women may in due course constitute a majority. The fact that sex differences are real does not, of course, justify discrimination. In both sexes the range of ability is wide, with large areas of overlap; and most professions require a blend of skills which can be provided in more than one way.

The Times (12 Sept. 1992)

The success [of feminism] *should have made some men confront the fact that they had no possible self-interest in oppressing women...it should have made some women confront the fact that there are genuine sexual differences which could not be ploughed under by the pursuit of a spurious and depraved conception of equality.*

Bryan Appleyard *The Times* (23 Sept. 1992)

In the early 1990s the debate seems to have become more open-ended (and ill-tempered) than for several years. On the one hand, both men and women have shown an increasing readiness to attack the feminist orthodoxies of the 1970s and 1980s:

Consider the feminist claims to which we have consented: that one half of humanity is inferior, by genetic composition and by natural disposition, to the other half; that the inferior half holds the superior in subjection through the use of economic power and brute force; and that the superior female half is obliged to fight a war of liberation to emancipate itself from the oppressions inflicted by men. Each of these presumptions is false. They are false in logic, false in their assessments of social change and its consequences, false in the deductions and conclusions to which they lead.

Neil Lyndon *No More Sex War* (1992)

I disagree with the current phase of feminism. Women's sexual power is an enormous force. Feminists think only in terms of social power.

Camille Paglia 'Quote Unquote' *Independent* (30 Nov. 1991)

On the other hand, feminists remain understandably resistant to the idea that all the important battles have been won – or to the insinuation that they were fought on the wrong battlefields, using the wrong weapons.

Flagellation

Beating is decent and can even be done in church; sex isn't.

Dr Alex Comfort *The Joy of Sex* (1972)

There are two kinds of flagellant: active flagellants, who either beat themselves (autoflagellants) or other people, and passive flagellants, who allow themselves to be beaten. Autoflagellation is widespread. Nuns do it:

I was for two years a sister of a convent on the French coast. We were compelled there by the rules of the order to flagellate ourselves at least three times a week. It was generally done on rising in the morning. The instrument used was a common domestic birch rod, such as is used in England; and the locality to which it was applied the same. We inflicted on ourselves from twenty to thirty smart strokes of the rod. The Superior paid us a visit on these mornings, and examined our persons, to see that the whipping had been duly inflicted; and in case of an omission, she administered a severe correction herself.

Anon. letter, *Family Herald* (18 Mar. 1848)

Future prime ministers do it:

In 1849 Gladstone also began to scourge himself to counter stimulation from it [pornography]. *By 1851 he was also scourging himself after conversations with prostitutes during which he felt that he had allowed himself to be excessively excited.*

H. C. G. Matthew *Gladstone: 1809–1874* (1986)

Young men in their prime do it:

Many persons not sufficiently acquainted with human nature, and the ways of the world, are apt to imagine that the lech *for flagellation must be confined either to the aged, or to those who are exhausted through too great a devotion to venery: but such is not the fact, for there are quite as many young men and men in the prime and vigour of life, who are influenced by this passion as there are amongst the aged and debilitated.*

George Cannon *Venus School Mistress* (1808)

Even little boys and girls do it:

Self-flagellation is also sometimes practised [by children of both sexes], *and even after puberty, when the genital centres are fully active, it may be adopted by either sex to heighten the solitary pleasure of the sexual impulse in the absence of a person of the opposite sex.*

H. Havelock Ellis *The Psychology of Sex* (1897–1928)

Why do they all do it? For some people, being beaten either by oneself or by someone else is a powerful physical stimulant:

The flagellation which originally served the purpose of self-castigation with early Christian monks and ascetics later became a means of sexual excitement. The increase of pain produced ecstasies. Ultimately the Church was forced to forbid too severe expiatory practices because they frequently led to sexual gratification.

Theodor Reik *Masochism in Modern Man* (1957)

'Tis very probable, that the refrigerated Parts grow warm by the STRIPES, and excite a heat in the seminal matter, and that more particularly from the PAIN of the FLOGG'D Parts, which is the reason that the Blood and Spirits are attracted in a greater Quantity, 'till the Heat is communicated to the Organs of Generation, and the perverse and frenzical Appetite is satisfied.

Johann Heinrich Meibom *On the Use of Rods in Venereal Matters and in the Office of the Loins* (1718)

His inactive torpid machine...could, no more than a boy's top, keep up without lashing.

John Cleland *Fanny Hill: Memoirs of a Woman of Pleasure* (1749)

I meant only the spanking idea. A warm tingling glow without effusion. Refined birching to stimulate the circulation.

James Joyce *Ulysses* (1922)

It seems that most flagellants acquire their taste for the practice in childhood:

I love castigation mightily, I was so us'd to't at Westminster School that I could never leave it off since.

Thomas Shadwell *The Virtuoso* (1676)

At one preparatory school the boys' name for beating was in fact 'stimulation'.

Dr Anthony Storr *Sexual Deviation* (1964)

The first sexual emotions he experienced when, a boy of eight, he witnessed other boys being caned on the fundament. Although he felt compassion for the boys, he yet had a feeling of lustful pleasure pervading his whole body. Some time afterwards he was late for school and on the way the anticipation of a caning on the fundament excited him so much that, for a short time, he could not move and had a violent erection.

P., aged twenty-two, of independent means, heavily tainted by heredity, by accident saw the governess chastising his sister (fourteen years of age) on the fundament. This made a deep impression on him and hence forth he had a constant desire to see and touch his sister's buttocks. When seven years later he became the playfellow of two small girls, one of whom was tiny and lean, the other rather plump. He played the role of the father chastising his children. The lean girl he simply spanked over the clothes. The other, however, allowed him to smack her bare bottom (she was then ten years old). This gave him great sexual pleasure and caused erection.

Richard von Krafft-Ebing *Psychopathia Sexualis* (1886)

Who could have supposed that this childish punishment, received at the age of eight at hands of a woman of thirty, would determine my tastes and desires, my passions, my very self for the rest of my life, and that in a sense diametrically opposed to the one in which they should normally have developed?

Jean-Jacques Rousseau *Confessions* (1782)

We are tainted with flagellomania from our childhood. When will we realise that the fact that we can become accustomed to anything, however disgusting at first, makes it necessary to examine carefully everything we have become accustomed to?

George Bernard Shaw *Misalliance* (1914)

Examples of reciprocal flogging agreements amongst schoolboys are surprisingly common and often seem to have lasting effects:

When I seriously enquir'd of him the Cause of this uncommon plague, his Reply was, I have used my self to it from a Boy. And upon repeating the Question to him, he added, that he was educated with a Number of wicked Boys, who set up this Trade of Whipping among themselves, and purchased of each other these infamous stripes at the expence of their Modesty.

Pico della Mirandola *Disputationes Adversus Astrologiam Divinatricem* (1502)

By the force of a vicious habit gaining ground on him, he practised a vice he disapproved. But it grew more obstinate and rooted in his nature, from his using it from a Child, when a reciprocal frication among his schoolfellows used to be provoked by the titulation of stripes. A strange instance what a Power the force of Education has in grafting inveterate ill habits on our morals.

Ludovicus Coelius Richerius *Lectionum Antiquarum* (1562)

There may, too, be a warm relationship between the willing victim and his equally willing tormentor:

Mr London brought the stick down with all his force, four times, four deliberate, even strokes, and each stroke raised a purple weal under Chummy's shorts...and that is how Chummy came to worship Mr London with all his might.

Chums Annual (1927–28)

When in the end I was beaten I found the experience less dreadful in fact that in anticipation; and the very strange thing was that this punishment increased my affection for the inflicter. It required all the strength of my devotion and all my natural gentleness to prevent my deliberately earning another beating; I had discovered in the shame and pain of the punishment an admixture of sensuality which had left me rather eager than otherwise for a repetition by the same hand.

Jean-Jacques Rousseau *Confessions* (1782)

I think many women will agree with me that there is pleasure in being tightly laced by one's husband. Once my husband asked me to whip him, which I did, severely, having first laced him in a pair of my stays. We have been great friends since, but one of us is sure to get a whipping before long.

Anon. letter, *Society* (23 Sept. 1899)

I had six strokes across the bottom and the effect was amazing. It hurt a lot and I felt very resentful. Then a curious warmth took over and then all my sexual inhibitions seemed to melt away. Afterwards I felt grateful, I even wanted to say 'thank you'.

Anon. interviewee, *Guardian* (28 Nov. 1992)

In this example of Victorian flagellation literature one Dora Doveton is being flogged for the first time by the governess Martinet:

Fear and shame were both gone; it was as though I was surrendering my person to the embraces of a man whom I so loved I would anticipate his wildest desires. But no man was in my thoughts; Martinet was the subject of my adoration, and I felt through the rod *that I shared her passions...Then, too, there was a thrill in a certain part, I knew magnetically, of both our persons, which every fresh lash kept on increasing. The added pang unlocked new floods of bliss, till it was impossible to tell in my case whether the ecstasy was most of pain or pleasure. When the rods were changed, I continued to jump and shout, for she liked that, but – believe me or not – I saw my nakedness with her eyes, and exulted in the lascivious joy that whipping me afforded her.*

George H. Stock *The Romance of Chastisement* (19th century)

But this relationship does not always exist. Some who relish the pain and humiliation of a beating are indifferent to those who inflict it:

There is now alive a Man of a prodigious, and almost unheard of kind of Lechery; For he is never inflamed to Pleasure, but when he is whipt; and yet he is so intent on the Act, and longs for the Strokes with such an Earnestness, that he blames the flogger that uses him gently, and is never thoroughly Master of his Wishes unless the Blood starts, and the Whip rages smartly over the wicked limbs of the Monster.

Pico dello Mirandola *Disputationes Adversus Astrologiam Divinatricem* (1502)

During the last decade of his life he was tormented by demons, and he developed a penchant for being beaten. He maintained a troupe of ten or a dozen young men whose duty it was to flagellate him three times daily, during which operation he was wont to smile joyfully. Masochism may have kept the demons at bay for a while, but Gesualdo soon developed the unusual symptom of being unable to move his bowels unless he was whipped.

William B. Ober, MD *Carlo Gesualdo, Prince of Venosa; Murder, Madrigals & Masochism* (1987)

Some, with less than compliant wives, husbands, or lovers have to resort to prostitutes:

Sir – May I ask whether you or any of your readers have ever heard of a vile practice of birching of men by women who have been paid for their services? I am led to believe that this is now in vogue. If it is, it is a form of vice which should be speedily stamped out. Yours, etc. TRUTH.

Anon. letter, *Town Talk: A Journal for Society at Large* (22 Mar. 1884)

This creature begs this Favour of the Women he is to enjoy, brings her a Rod himself, soak'd and harden'd in Vinegar a Day before for the same Purpose, and intreats the Blessing of a Whipping from the Harlot on his Knees; and the more smartly he is whipt, he rages the more eagerly, and goes the same Pace both to Pleasure and Pain. A singular Instance of one who finds a Delight in the Midst of Torment.

Pico della Mirandola *Disputationes Adversus Astrologiam Divinatricem* (1502)

When Francis comes to solace with his whore,
He sends for rods and strips himself stark naked;
For his lust sleeps, and will not rise before
By whipping of the wench it be awaked.
I envy him not, but wish I had the power
To make myself his whore but one half hour.

Sir John Davies 'Epigram' (17th century)

This unnatural beast gives money to those strumpets which you see, and they down with his Breeches and Scourge his Privities till they have laid his leachery.

London Spy (17th century)

Her [Mrs Theresa Berkley of 28 Charlotte Street, Portland Place] *instruments of torture were more numerous than those of any other governess. Her supply of birch was extensive, and kept in water, so that it was always green and pliant: she had shafts with a dozen whip thongs on each of them; a dozen different sizes of cat-o'-nine-tails, some with needle points worked into them...and currycomb tough hides rendered callous by many years' flagellation. Holly brushes, furze brushes; a prickly evergreen, called butcher's bush; and during the summer, glass and China vases, filled with a constant supply of green nettles, with which she often restored the dead to life. Thus, at her shop, whoever went with plenty of money, could be birched, whipped, fustigated, scourged, needle-pricked, half-hung, holly-brushed, furze-brushed, butcher-brushed, stinging-nettled, curry-combed, phlebotomized, and tortured till he had a belly full.*

George Cannon *Venus School Mistress* (1808)

The 19th-century Mrs Berkley was quite a lady:

The 'Berkley Horse' was in fact not a machine but a folding ladder, fully padded, with holes in the relevant places, to which flagellants could be affixed to receive their whippings at whatever angle they found most titillating...Mrs Berkley made £10,000 from her invention before she died in 1836, an incredible sum...One can imagine the number of passive flagellants there must have been in London at the time.

Ian Gibson *The English Vice* (1978)

The essential equipment of the prostitute has not changed greatly:

The equipment of the prostitute's room, of course, varies according to her own versatility in the performance of perversions;

nearly all have whips, canes, or improvisations for flagellation hidden away in otherwise empty drawers.

C. H. Rolph *Women of the Streets* (1955)

In England, the 18th and 19th centuries saw an unprecedented outpouring of flagellation literature, which must reflect a widespread public obsession with the subject:

The extent to which literature inspired the practice of flagellation is debateable. In the one era of addiction about which we know a good deal – in England from early in the eighteenth century to late in the nineteenth – writing and beating seem to have gone hand in hand. At least the first important book on the subject, A Treatise on the Use of Flogging, *appeared in 1718, about the time we hear of the first London brothels where a man could get a whipping along with a woman. Soon it was so popular that on the Continent it was called 'The English Vice', although this does not mean continentals were less addicted.*

David Loth *The Erotic in Literature* (1962)

Discussion and letters dealing with the art of flogging can be found in periodicals throughout the century, from the respectable Gentleman's Magazine *in the 1730s, to the erotic* Bon Ton Magazine *in the 1790s.*

Peter Wagner *Eros Revisited* (1988)

The Rod should be applied in an Angle of about 45 degrees. For it is a Maxim that this does the Business far more effectively than the most violent perpendicular Impression.

Anon. *Gentleman's Magazine* (Jan. 1735)

There is nothing makes a woman so randy as a good flogging, and nothing so much excites a man as flogging a woman or seeing her flogged.

Anon. *Raped on the Railway* (1894)

Strange to say, the slight spanking had excited a voluptuous feeling in me, and I was anxious to receive the stroke.

Hughes Rebell *The Memoirs of Dolly Morton* (1899)

This sort of thing is all very well for those men and women who enjoy being knocked about – but what about those who are neither adult nor consenting?

It is shameful and abominable that such a punishment should be administered to the buttocks of young boys and girls. It used to be the punishment of slaves. In our colleges I have seen barbarians strip children almost naked and a brute, often drunk, lacerate their flesh with long rods, which made their groins bleed and swell fearfully. The two nerves which join the sphincter to the pubis being irritated, emissions were produced; and this has often happened to young girls.

Voltaire *Dictionnaire philosophique* (1769)

The effect is now so well known that scourging children is entirely abandoned in all well regulated schools and families...Flagellation and denudation are inseparable, and often incite erection in children...It is now totally interdicted in all respectable schools and colleges, and ought also to cease in all families. Medical practitioners should explain the bad effects of this mischievous practice on modesty and on the senses.

Michael Ryan *Prostitution in London, with a Comparative View of that in Paris and New York* (1839)

The first time a schoolmaster ordered me to take my trousers down, I knew it was not from any doubt that he could punish me efficiently enough with them up.

Laurence Olivier, letter to the *Observer* (21 Nov. 1965)

The reason for sometimes forcing schoolboys to lower their trousers for the administration of the punishment is not related to increasing the pain, but to enabling the dominant male to witness the reddening of the buttocks as the beating proceeds, which so vividly recalls the flushing of the primate female hindquarters when in full sexual condition.

Desmond Morris *The Naked Ape* (1967)

The visual effects of flogging are frequently emphasized in flagellation pornography:

Current American magazines emphasize the redness by applying ludicrous patches of rouge to the bottoms of the models who pose for the colour photographs; patches rather than stroke-marks because, it seems, in America table-tennis bats are the preferred instruments of castigation. In modern England the cane holds pride of place in flagellant pornography; and its marks are frequently represented by lipstick strokes laid across the buttocks.

Ian Gibson *The English Vice* (1978)

Flogging *is an Art which teaches us to draw Blood from a Person's Posteriors in such a Manner as may twinge him most severely without Danger of a Mortification...I have seen a Professor foam with Extacy at the sight of a jolly Pair of Buttocks.*

Anon. *Gentleman's Magazine* (Jan. 1735)

I never knew anyone take such delight
When a schoolboy has to be whipped, in the sight,
I believe – his delight is so frank and explicit –
He would rather himself have a whipping than miss it.

Algernon Charles Swinburne *The Whippingham Papers*, 'Reginald's Flogging' (1888)

Despite its clear sexual connotations, flagellation is still sometimes defended as a means of punishment:

People who have the future of our children truly at heart will agree that there is something to be said for the old adage that if one spares the rod one spoils the child.

Patrick Cormack MP *Hansard* (20 Jan. 1976)

Britain is run by people who were beaten at their public schools and don't-think-it-did-them-any-harm.

Corinna Adam 'Beating in Britain' *New Statesman* (29 Nov. 1968)

Some of the birching diehards in the Tynwald have said that the island [of Man] *should break away from the United Kingdom if the British Government were to attempt to enforce a ban on judicial corporal punishment. Perhaps this would be a good idea. In order to boost its revenues, the island could then advertise itself as the world's first holiday centre for unruly young masochists.*

Ian Gibson *The English Vice* (1978)

However, the case against beating in schools and prisons has steadily gained ground:

The cane and the birch are essentially a fool's implements.

George Bernard Shaw *The Times* (23 Aug. 1904)

Those who have studied pathology, as expounded by Continental thinkers, know that the use of the rod, as at present inflicted, is evidence that flagellomania is a real and widespread disease...birching has come to be regarded by medical men in France, Germany, and other parts of the Continent, as a sensuous gratification for people of morbid tastes.

Joseph Collinson *Facts about Flogging* (1907)

Judicial corporal punishment is a specially unsuitable penalty for sexual offences.

Report of the Home Office departmental committee on corporal punishment (Feb. 1938)

I am not convinced that we have yet discovered the proper way to deal with sexual crimes, but I am certain of this – that flogging is no remedy for them, neither is it a deterrent. In fact, in certain circumstances it is an incentive.

J. C. Ede MP *Hansard* (13 Feb. 1953)

In extreme cases the excessive use of corporal punishment could lead to sadism on the part of the teacher, and to masochism on the part of the pupil.

Dennis Canavan MP *Hansard* (20 Jan. 1976)

In Britain the judicial use of corporal punishment was largely discontinued after 1948, while beating in state schools was finally abolished in 1988. These measures may have put an end to the enjoyment of sadistic judges and schoolteachers, but flagellation remains available for those who want it:

...people who play flagellation games and are excited by them bother nobody, provided they don't turn off a partner who finds the scenario frightening.

Dr Alex Comfort *The Joy of Sex* (1972)

Persians and Russians chastize their wives with blows from a stick on the posterior before they perform their marital duty. The bride in Russia would rather be without any other piece of household goods than rods. These rods are never used for punishment, but only for the purpose mentioned.

Thomas Bartolinus *Historiam Anatomicarum and Medicarum* (1661)

The members are mainly married women, who, tired of marriage in its usual form, and the cold indifference which is wont to accompany it; determined by a novel method to re-awaken the ecstasy which they knew at the beginning of their married life. The honourable society to which we refer never has fewer than 12 members. At each meeting 6 are chastized by the other 6. They draw lots for the order of procedure; then either a written speech is read or an extempore one is delivered, on the effects of flagellation, after which the 6 patients take their places and the 6 flagellants begin the practical demonstration. The president of the club hands to each a stout rod, and begins the chastisement herself with any variations she likes, while the others watch.

Bon Ton Magazine (Dec. 1792)

Whatever the precise origin of sexual flagellation in Europe, there can be no doubt that it soon became extremely common, and so it remains at the present day. Those who possess a special knowledge of such matters declare that sexual flagellation is the most frequent of all sexual perversions in England.

H. Havelock Ellis *Studies in the Psychology of Sex* (1897–1928)

I'm all for bringing back the birch, but only between consenting adults.

Gore Vidal *Sunday Times* (16 Sept. 1973)

See also SADISM AND MASOCHISM

Impotence and Frigidity

Inadequate sexual desire, is probably the most prevalent of the sexual dysfunctions.

Helen S. Kaplan *Medical Aspects of Human Sexuality* (Nov. 1979)

Absence of sexual desire or prowess in the male – impotence – and the corresponding female state – frigidity – have been the subject of comment from earliest times. Male impotence, literally a 'lack of power', has been noted for its physical manifestation:

His dagger dangled more limply than an unripe beet and never rose to the middle of his tunic.

Catullus (1st century BC)

It is not necessarily through lack of trying:

She could provoke me to do nothing because my roger would not stand up, with all she could do.

William Byrd *The London Diary* (1718)

The condition has been a source of some amusement to observers:

There was a young fellow named Bliss
Whose sex life was strangely amiss,
For even with Venus
His recalcitrant penis
Would never do better than t
h
i
s

Anon. Victorian limerick

But sufferers from the condition have been moved to more serious poetry, often lamenting former glories:

A Weaver's Beam – the Handle of a Hoe,
A Bowsprit once – now a thing of Dough;
A sorry change, lamented oft with Tears
At Midnight by the Master of the Show.

Behold – the Penis mightier than the Sword,
That leapt from Sheath at any heating Word
So long ago – now peaceful lies, and calm
And dreams unmoved of ancient Conquests scored.

Anon.

This dart of love, whose piercing point, oft tried,
With virgin blood ten thousand maids have dyed;
Which nature directed with such art
That it through every cunt reached every heart –
Stiffly resolved, 'twould carelessly invade
Woman or man, nor ought its fury stayed:
Where'er it pierced, a cunt it found or made,
Now languid lies in this unhappy hour,
Shrunk up and sapless like a withered flower.

John Wilmot, Earl of Rochester 'The Imperfect Enjoyment' (1680)

Another group of sufferers have, according to Sir Richard Burton, a different reaction:

El mourekhi *(the flabby one) – The one who can never get in because it is too soft, and which is therefore content to rub its head against the entrance to the vulva until it ejaculates. It gives no pleasure to woman, but only inflames her passion without being able to satisfy it, and makes her cross and irritable.*

Sheikh Nefzawi *The Perfumed Garden* (trans. Sir Richard Burton)

The Honourable Mrs Catharine Weld was probably 'cross and irritable' when, in 1732, she petitioned for the dissolution of her marriage:

As often as he attempted to have carnal knowledge of his Wife, a Pain struck him cross his Belly, which so contracted his Privy Parts, as to put him in much Torment, and obliged him to desist from further Caresses.

Petition, seeking dissolution of her marriage on the grounds of impotence (1732)

Similarly, Annie Court divorced her husband in 1863; a friend gave this testimony at the hearing:

Despite his teasing her by his caresses and kissings exciting her womanly passions, he had never cohabited with her and could not. He was no man and she might as well sleep with a woman.

In Catholic teaching, failure to consummate a marriage because of impotence is grounds for an annulment. For example:

Today we have declared null and void the marriage between Jean Carré and Jeanne la Hondouron de Lagny, thirteen months after the marriage contract, because of the frigidity, incapacity and impotence of the husband. We have heard the report of Masters Ginbert de Sarseto and Guillaume Boucher Masters of Medicine, and of Michel de Pisis, our sworn surgeon, who reported to us that they examined the aforementioned man and they they found and deemed him incapable of knowing a woman.

Register of Civil Causes of the Episcopal Officiality of Paris (1385)

The Church treated the subject with the same seriousness and sensitivity in 1984:

In 1984, former soldier Stephen Rigby wanted to marry his fiancée Ilana Bradhun, in a Catholic Church. The Nottingham Diocesan Marriage Tribunal refused permission, because Rigby was paralysed and therefore judged to be impotent. The marriage would not be valid.

Kate Saunders and Peter Stanford *Catholics and Sex* (1992)

Impotence involving inability to have an erection is only one aspect of the condition. The inability to achieve penetration as a result of premature ejaculation is also regarded as impotence. Here the problem is not too little desire, but perhaps too much:

But whilst her busy hand would guide that part
Which should convey my soul up to her heart,
In liquid raptures I dissolve all o'er,
Melt into sperm, and spend at every pore.
A touch from any part of her had done't:
Her hand, her foot, her very look's a cunt.

John Wilmot, Earl of Rochester 'The Imperfect Enjoyment' (1680)

James Boswell gave the usual excuse:

Quite agitated. Put on condom; entered. Heart beat; fell. Quite sorry, but said 'A true sign of passion.'

Diary (1764)

Many writers have speculated on the causes of impotence. In medieval times, witchcraft was always a popular explanation:

Impotence through bewitchment was a matter with far-reaching legal and theological as well as medical implications, since it gave rise to the question whether the marriage could be dissolved and whether the man could then remarry. The solution which may seem obvious and on which some consensus emerged, was that dissolution was permitted if the impotence was permanent, while remarriage was allowed if the impotence was selective. Such bewitchment could arise in any of several situations, but one that leapt quickly to the medieval mind was that of the abandoned lover wishing to prevent marriage out of jealousy. Burchard of Worms referred to adulteresses who, on learning that their paramours want to marry other women, used magic to "extinguish the male desire, so that they are impotent and cannot consummate their union with their legitimate wives."

Richard Kieckhefer 'Erotic Magic in Medieval Europe' in *Sex in the Middle Ages* (1991)

Even in 18th-century Holland it was believed:

To make a man impotent, during his wedding night someone had to tie a number of knots in a piece of string while mumbling some words, preferably at the moment bride and groom joined hands. If this knotting were carried out, then the newly wed husband would be unable to do anything in bed, at least not with his wife. The spell would only be broken if the man urinated through his wife's wedding ring. Other antidotes were smearing the bedroom door with wolves' grease or hanging roosters testicles on the bed-end.

Herman Roosenberg *Sexual Beliefs in 18th Century Holland* (1989)

Other suggested causes include lack of practice:

Another cause of impotency is the allowing the parts of generation to remain too long in a state of inaction. Those parts of the body which are most exercised are always found to be better grown, stronger and more fitted for the discharge of their natural function provided the exercise be neither too violent nor too frequent. The parts...which are condemned to rest and inactivity wither and gradually lose their tone, as well as the power of effecting the movements natural to them.

John Davenport *Aphrodisiacs and Anti-Aphrodisiacs* (1869)

Or perhaps lack of opportunity:

A large class of men commonly supposed to be nervous, bashful, or timid are in fact sufferers from an absence of sexual feeling, which may, perhaps, be due to their having been brought up in retired country places, without any female companions.

Dr William Acton *The Functions and Disorders of the Re-Productive Organs* (1857)

Or even, in some people, thinking too much:

Impotency may, however, equally proceed from moral as from physical causes. In this case it consists in the total privation of the sensibility peculiar to the reproductive organs. This insensibility is by no means infrequent in persons whose mental powers are continually in action.

John Davenport *Aphrodisiacs and Anti-Aphrodisiacs* (1869)

Although thinking, in itself, is an unlikely cause of impotence psychological causes are common. Various writers have commented on the difficulties arising from unfamiliarity or from emotional involvement. The fear of failure and the anger and resentment that may result only compound the problem:

El mostahi *(the shame-faced) – This sort of member which is met with sometimes, is capable of feeling ashamed and timid when faced with a vulva which it does not know, and it is only after a little time that it gets bolder and stiffens. Sometimes it is even so much troubled that it remains incompetent for the coitus, which happens in particular when a stranger is present, in which case it becomes quite incapable of moving.*

Sheikh Nefzawi *The Perfumed Garden* (trans. Sir Richard Burton)

Didst thou e'er fail in all thy life before?
When vile disease and scandal lead the way
With what officious haste dost thou obey.
But when great Love the onset does command
Base recreant to thy Prime, thou dar'st not stand...

I sigh, alas! and kiss, but cannot swive.
Eager desires confound my first intent,
Succeeding shame does more success prevent,
And rage at last confirms me impotent.
Ev'n her fair hand, which might bid heat return
To frozen age, and make cold hermits burn,
Applied to my dead cinder, warms no more

Than fire to ashes could past flames restore.
Trembling, confused, despairing, limber, dry,
A wishing, weak, unmoving lump I lie.

John Wilmot, Earl of Rochester 'The Imperfect Enjoyment' (1680)

Nature's support (without whose aid
She can no human being give)
Itself now wants the art to live;
Faintness its slackened nerves invade.
In vain th'enraged youth essayed
To call its fleeting vigour back,
No motion 'twill from motion take.
Excess of love is Love betrayed.
In vain he toils, in vain commands –
Insensible falls weeping in his hands.

In this so amorous, cruel strife
Where love and fate were too severe
The poor Lysander in despair
Renounced his reason with his life…

Aphra Behn 'The Disappointment' (1670s)

Similarly, social reasons have been suggested:

It is a very common phenomenon that men of high distinction are fully virile with women mentally, spiritually, or socially inferior to them, while they fail with women who are their equals.

Sophie Lazarsfield *Rhythm of Life: a Guide to Sexual Harmony for Women* (1935)

There are two other main causes of impotence in men. One is alcohol – the 'brewer's droop' recognized by Shakespeare:

It provokes the desire but, it takes away the performance. Therefore much drink may be said to be an equivocator with lechery.

Macbeth (1605)

The other is simply old age, again lamented by Shakespeare:

Is it not strange that desire should so many years outlive performance?

Henry IV, Part II (1597)

In this respect, some have noted the difference between men and women:

Thirty years ago we were of one heart,
Single-mindedly spending the nights in elegant dalliance
Since then, I've turned old and useless;
Yours too wide, mine too weak.

Yuan-wu

His grandmother is as good as new. Her candlestick is as hard as ever, whereas his candle is increasingly softened and weakened by the weather of age, as the years go by, until at last it can no longer stand, and is mournfully laid to rest in the hope of a blessed resurrection which is never to come…

During 23 days in every month, from the time a woman is 7 years old till she dies of old age, she is ready for action, and competent. Competent every day, competent every night. Also, she yearns for it, longs for it, hankers after it, as commanded by the law of God in her heart. But man is only briefly competent; and then only in moderate measure applicable to the word in his sex's case. He is competent from the age of 16 or 17 thenceforward for 35 years. After 50 his performance is of poor quality, the intervals between are wide, and its satisfactions of no great value to either party.

Mark Twain *Letters from the Earth* (1909)

Yuan-wu and Mark Twain regard this as a matter for regret; others are less charitable:

The ultimate sexist put-down: the prick which lies down on the job. The ultimate weapon in the war between the sexes: the limp prick. The banner of the enemy's encampment: the prick at half-mast. The symbol of the apocalypse: the atomic warhead prick which self-destructs. That was the basic inequity which could never be righted: not that the male had a wonderful added attraction called a penis, but that the female had a wonderful all-weather cunt.

Erica Jong *Fear of Flying* (1973)

Male impotence can, of course, also have physical causes resulting from disease or injury. For example:

> *A study by US doctors estimates that up to 15 per cent of all cases of impotence are caused by injury during intercourse. The study, which appears in the* Journal of Urology, *is the first to demonstrate how pressure or abnormal bending of an erection during intercourse or masturbation can result in chronic impotence. 'Men think their erections are made of concrete,' Irwin Goldstein, leader of the team of researchers, said.*

Independent (30 Oct. 1992)

The traditional male idea that impotence is something to be ashamed of or sniggered about has provoked a reaction from the modern 'men's movement':

> *What's called 'impotence' is another internalization of a perverse system of male-dominant cultural values. Men are taught to believe that a cock is either limp and dysfunctional or erect and functional, and anything in between doesn't have sense unless it's clearly on its way to erection or legitimately on its way to limpness (a legitimacy which can be presumed only if ejaculation has been achieved).*

John Stoltenberg *Refusing to be a Man* (1977)

Lack of sexual desire or activity in the female has also provoked much comment, although it has been less often a subject for humour:

> *When we was wed she turned afraid*
> *Of love and me and all things human;*
> *Like the shut of a winter's day*
> *Her smile went out, and 'twadn't a woman –*
> *More like a frightened fay.*

Charlotte Mew 'The Farmer's Bride' (1915)

In particular, attitudes to frigidity have been complicated by the 19th-century idea that women do not enjoy sex – they do it under sufferance either to satisfy their husbands or to procreate. It was not a case of 'nice girls don't' – more a case of 'nice girls don't want to':

> *As a general rule, a modest woman seldom desires any sexual gratification for herself. She submits to her husband, but only to please him, and, but for the desire of maternity, would far rather be relieved from his attentions.*

Dr William Acton *The Functions and Disorders of the Re-Productive Organs* (1857)

> *So many Englishwomen look upon sexual intercourse as abhorrent and not as a natural fulfilment of true love. My wife considered all bodily desire to be nothing less than animal passion, and that true love between husband and wife should be purely mental and not physical...Like so many Englishwomen she considered that any show of affection was not in keeping with her dignity as a woman and that all lovemaking and caresses should come entirely from the man and that the woman should be the passive receiver of affection.*

Anon. letter to Marie Stopes (4 Apr. 1921)

> *A well-bred woman does not seek carnal gratification, and she is usually apathetic to sexual pleasures. Her love is physical or spiritual, rather than carnal, and her passiveness in regard to coition often amounts to disgust for it; lust is seldom an element in a woman's character, and she is the preserver of chastity and morality.*

O. A. Wall *Sex and Sex Worship* (1932)

See also MARRIAGE

At the beginning of this century the psychoanalysts defined female frigidity in terms that are now generally rejected:

> *The sole criterion of frigidity is the absence of the vaginal orgasm.*

Three Essays on the Theory of Sexuality (1905)

This view persisted among Freudians for 50 years:

> *Whenever a woman is incapable of achieving an orgasm via coitus, provided the husband is an adequate sexual partner, and prefers clitoral stimulation to any*

other form of sexual activity, she can be regarded as suffering from frigidity and requires psychiatric assistance.

Frank Caprio *The Sexually Adequate Female* (1953)

See also ORGASMS

Frigidity is not simply a question for the pathologist and the student of morbid psychology. It is a matter of serious social importance. Conjugal calamity being so frequently brought about by the coldness of one of the pair, it is necessary that the idiosyncrasy should be reckoned with.

Walter Gallichan *Sexual Antipathy and Coldness in Women* (1927)

Frigidity in women is by no means an insignificant phenomenon. It is a social disease that can take on the proportions of an epidemic. The offspring of frigid mothers are exposed to the greatest dangers. It is their fate to swell the infinite host of psychopaths, of those who are ill-equipped for life.

William Stekel *Frigidity in Mothers* (1930)

Others have no doubt where the fault lies:

Man, through prudery, through the custom of ignoring the woman's side of marriage, and considering his own whim as the marriage law, has largely lost the art of stirring a chaste partner to physical love. He therefore deprives her of a glamour, the loss of which he deplores, for he feels a lack not only of romance and beauty, but of something higher which is mystically given as the result of the complete union. He blames his wife's 'coldness' instead of his own want of art.

Marie Stopes *Married Love* (1918)

It takes two persons to make one frigid woman.

Robert Dickinson *A Thousand Marriages* (1932)

There are no frigid women, there are only inexperienced men.

George Lombard Kelly *Sexual Relations in Marriage* (1954)

Indeed, both frigidity and impotence have been seen as weapons in the war between the sexes:

We shall never understand the problem of the frigid woman unless we take into consideration the fact that the two sexes are engaged in a lasting conflict...the social aspect of the problem, too, unveils itself before our eyes. We recognize plainly that dyspareunia (frigidity in women) is a social problem, it is one of woman's weapons in the universal struggle of the sexes.

William Stekel *Frigidity in Woman in Relation to her Love Life* (1926)

There are cases of a woman excluded from a group for no other reason than that one of its leaders proved impotent with her.

Marge Piercy in *Sisterhood is Powerful* (ed. Robin Morgan; 1970)

In modern times it is no longer necessary to resort to hanging roosters' testicles on the bed end to cure impotence. A wide choice of modern witchcraft is available from psychiatrists, sex therapists, agony aunts, and counsellors. Perhaps the advice of a 4th-century Greek physician is still relevant:

To cure male impotence, let the patient be surrounded by beautiful girls or boys. Give him books to read which stimulate him.

Theorus Priscianus

and if it's not as simple as that, perhaps it's as simple as this:

The vast majority of cases of coital frigidity are due simply to the absence of frequent, prolonged coitus.

Dr Mary Jane Sherfey *A Theory of Female Sexuality* (1966)

Most people are agreed that impotence and frigidity are a source of much sadness to those afflicted –

If the body feels no sexual desire it seems to suffer just as the spirit does.

Soranus of Ephesus (2nd century)

Not everyone, however, thinks that a lack of sexual activity is a bad thing in one's life:

> *All this fuss about sleeping together. For physical pleasure I'd sooner go to my dentist any day.*
>
> Evelyn Waugh *Vile Bodies* (1930)

> *Someone asked Sophocles, "How do you feel now about sex? Are you still able to have a woman?" He replied, "Hush, man; most gladly indeed am I rid of it all, as though I had escaped from a mad and savage master."*
>
> Plato *Republic* (4th century BC)

Incest

There'd be no need for an incest taboo if people didn't want to perform incest.

James Oliver *Who Should be Sleeping in Your Bed – and Why* (1988)

Dread of incest is buried deeply in the human unconscious and evokes volatile and unpredictable emotions.

M. Giarretto *Humanistic Treatment of Father-Daughter Incest* (1978)

Two conflicting views of incest, both of which are probably true. Western dread of incest dates back to the Bible, where three specific cases are forbidden:

The nakedness of thy sister...thou shalt not uncover. The nakedness of thy son's daughter, or of thy daughter's daughter, even their nakedness thou shalt not uncover.

Leviticus 18:7–9

St Paul prohibits relationships between step-parents and step-children:

It is reported commonly that there is fornication among you, and such fornication as is not so much as named among the Gentiles, that one should have his father's wife. And ye are puffed up, and have not rather mourned, that he that hath done this deed might be taken away from among you.

I Corinthians 5:1–2

By the Middle Ages sexual transgressions had been placed in a hierarchy of sinfulness:

The evil of adultery surpasses fornication, but is surpassed by incest; for it is worse to sleep with one's mother than with another man's wife.

Gratian *Canon Adulterii Malum* (11th century)

Non-Western societies have also shunned incest:

I have heard that a woman of one's own surname should not be admitted into one's harem. Their children will die young, and though the affection between husband and wife may in the beginning be great, it will soon come to an end. Then both will fall ill.

Counsellor to the Prince of China, quoted in *Tsu-Chuan Chronicle* (722–450 BC)

Among the Cherokees...the sun, a young woman, lived in the east, while the moon, her brother, lived in the west. The young woman had a lover who always visited her in the dark. He came by night and departed before daybreak. She wondered who it could be. To find out, one night she rubbed his face with ashes. When the moon rose the next evening, its face was smeared. Then the sister knew it was her brother who had visited her. She was so ashamed that in future she kept as far away from her brother as possible.

Leo V. Frobenius *The Era of the Sun Gods* (1904)

The view that incest is a universal taboo is common among anthropologists:

The horror of incest is an almost universal characteristic of mankind, the cases which seem to indicate a perfect absence of this feeling being so exceedingly rare that they must be regarded nearly as anomalous aberrations from a general rule.

Edward A. Westermarck *The History of Human Marriage* (1921)

Incest taboos are among the universals of human behaviour. The avoidance of sexual intercourse between brothers and sisters, and between parents and their offspring is everywhere achieved by cultural sanctions. Where incest does occur at low frequency in less closed societies, it is ordinarily a source of shame.

Edmund O. Wilson *On Human Nature* (1978)

However, it has been part of the social order of several cultures:

It is not all that long since, in certain peasant cultures, when the mother died, the oldest daughter took her place in all respects.

Bruno Bettelheim *The Uses of Enchantment* (1976)

There was more incest in the past and it was always fathers and daughters, never brothers and sisters. It happened when mother had too many children, or when mother was ill, or when mother was dead. And very often it didn't matter a bit. The daughter usually proved to be very fond of the father and there would be no sign of upset in the family. No, I think it was quite an understood thing that a daughter would take on a father when the mother was ill or dead.

The magistrate and chairman of the bench in a little English town, quoted by Ronald Blythe in *Akenfield* (1969)

Among the Sinhalese, a father could claim the right of deflowering his own daughter before marriage, asserting a right to the first-fruit of the tree he had planted.

Edward A. Westermarck *The History of Human Marriage* (1921)

Among the tribes of the Upper Congo, it is rare for children that grow up together to fail to marry.

Sir Harry Hamilton Johnston *British Central Africa* (1807)

Among the tribes of British Central Africa there is a curious notion that a man who commits incest with his sister or mother is thereby rendered bullet-proof.

Robert Briffault *The Mothers: a Study of the Origins of Sentiments and Institutions* (1927)

In world history we have such blatant line-breeding 'violations' as the Incan empire, the native Hawaiian royalty, the ancient Persian rulers, the Ptolemaic dynasty in Egypt. None of these aristocratic societies made any secret out of doing in public exactly what was forbidden to commoners in private.
...Cleopatra, for instance, was the issue of at least eleven generations of incest and was herself a sibling partner.

James Twitchell *Forbidden Partners* (1987)

There is also a tradition of sanctioned incest among certain illiterate groups of remote mountain dwellers. This emerges in the hillbilly story of a youth who told his father he wanted to marry a girl in the next valley; he was real proud that she was a virgin too.
"Well now, I don't know," replied his elder, "if she ain't good enough for her own folks, how do I know she's good enough for us?"

David Loth *The Erotic in Literature* (1962)

Margaret Mead was horrified when confronted with the Mountain Arapesh tribesmen of New Guinea:

What, you would like to marry your sister! What is the matter with you anyway? Don't you want a brother-in-law? Don't you realize that if you marry another man's sister and another man marries your sister you will have at least two brothers-in-law, while if you marry your own sister you will have none? With whom will you hunt, with whom will you garden, whom will you go to visit?

Sex and Temperament in Three Primitive Societies (1950)

Scarcity of available partners may explain why certain societies accept incest:

Incest and polyandry are bedmates... Wherever women are scarce, and the males, through isolation, danger, or other causes, are prevented from seeking women of other races or families, polyandry is common; and for precisely the same reasons, incest is common too.

George Ryley Scott *Marriage in the Melting Pot* (1930)

This problem was faced by the daughters of Lot, living in seclusion with their father after God's destruction of Sodom and Gomorrah (and most of the available men):

"Come, let us make our father drink wine, and we will lie with him, that we may preserve seed of our father." And they made their father drink wine that night: and the firstborn went in, and lay with her father; and he perceived not when she lay down, nor when she arose.

Genesis 19:32

Legislators, however, have usually condemned incest:

But when our men and women get past the age for breeding, then we can leave them free to mate as they please, provided that no man mates with his daughter or granddaughter or with his mother or any of her forbears, and no woman with her son or father or their descendents or forbears.

Plato *Republic* (4th century BC)

Interestingly, Plato did not prohibit incest between brother and sister – chiefly because the communal childrearing practised in his Republic would make it impossible for anyone to tell who his or her natural siblings were:

There will be no rule to prevent brothers and sisters cohabiting, if the lot so falls out and Delphi approves.

Plato *Republic* (4th century BC)

Medieval Christian fear of incest became so intense that the prohibition was extended not only to remote blood relations but also to spiritual relations:

The Christian Saxons had regarded it as incestuous to marry a first cousin, arguing that since marriage makes man and wife 'one flesh' to marry a deceased husband's cousin is incestuous. But in the eleventh century the Church beame increasingly obsessed with incest fears and extended the ban to second and finally third cousins. (It was later reduced.) But this was not all. So strongly was the principle of sympathetic contagion embedded, so intense were the fears of incest, that godfathers and godmothers were included in the ban; next, even the relations of the priests who had baptized or confirmed a person; finally, even two persons who had stood sponsor to the same child might not marry each other.

Gordon Rattray Taylor *Sex in History* (1953)

Christian thinking later relaxed and first cousins were allowed to marry:

There was a strong tendency towards endogamy, for families frequently felt that a marriage between cousins could be used to reunite the scattered portions of inheritances disassembled in previous generations. Thus...the notion of incest came to lose all rigour beyond the third degree of kinship.

Georges Duby *Medieval Marriage* (1978)

In some societies

Marriages between first cousins were associated with a higher birth-rate and a markedly greater vitality in the offspring than unions between non-relatives. So much so that the Fijians who still adhere to the ancestral custom of first-cousin marriages are the only ones who succeed in maintaining their numbers, while those who do not intermarry are rather rapidly dying out.

Robert Briffault *The Mothers: a Study of the Origins of Sentiments and Institutions* (1927)

Various theories have been proposed to explain the origins of the taboo:

Anthropology suggests the origin of the taboo lies in the disruption and strife which incest generates in family groupings.

M. D. A. Freeman *The Law and Sexual Deviation* (1964)

Domestic incest is viewed as personally irresponsible and a prime example of antisocial behaviour, engaged in for the sake of individual gratification at the expense of the wider group.

W. Arens *The Original Sin* (1986)

It has been suggested that the origin of the incest taboo was an agreement wrung from the father by the mother when she consented to accept male authority in return for protection of herself and her children. I like this theory but I'll admit it's only speculation, but no wilder speculation than the theory that the incest taboo sprung from the father's own recognition of his desire to sleep with his daughter, or was a compact a tribe wrung from each male member, either to increase their number through marrying out (exogamy) or to discourage inbreeding and hereditary flaws.

Susan Brownmiller *Against Our Wills* (1975)

The large amount of free-floating ceremonies in primitive man, which led to the creation of taboo ceremonies in the widest sense (totem, etc.), produced among other things the incest taboo *as well (or rather: the mother and father taboo)…incest is forbidden* not because it is desired *but because the free-floating anxiety regressively reactivates infantile material and turns it into a ceremony of atonement (as though incest had been, or might have been, desired).*

Carl Jung, letter to Sigmund Freud (17 May 1912)

Fear of genetic defects has been cited as an explanation for prohibition of incest, although many have argued that such fears are unfounded, especially in marriages between cousins:

There is no evidence whatsoever of any ill results accruing to the offspring in consequence of cousinship of parents.

Edward A. Westermarck *The History of Human Marriage* (1921)

The evidence from genetics is that if cousin marriage, or even incest, is pretty common, and has been for some time, we run no greater risk of having infertile or sickly offspring by our cousin or our sister than by anyone else. But if we live in a highly exogamous society like the US and Britain, where even cousin marriage is slightly frowned upon, then our chances of having below-par children will be sensibly higher.

Wayland Young *Eros Denied* (1964)

In Arabia no evil results are anticipated from the union of first cousins, and the experience of ages and of a mighty nation may be trusted. Our physiologists adduce cases to prove that degeneracy inevitably follows breeding in. Either they have theorised from insufficient facts, or civilisation and artificial living exercise some peculiar influence, or Arabia is a solitary exception to a general rule.

Sir Richard Burton *Personal Narrative of a Pilgrimage to Al-Medinah and Meccah* (1856)

In the case of Arab horses inbreeding seems to be beneficial:

I cannot take upon me to say how often an incestuous breed may be carried on before a degeneracy takes place, as I am not aware of that being the case in any instance, and experiment is in favour *of breeding from son to mother, and from father to daughter.*

N. H. Smith *Observations on Breeding for the Turf* (1825)

Consanguinity by itself counts for nothing, but acts solely from related organisms generally having similar constitutions, and having been exposed in most cases to similar conditions.

Charles Darwin *The Descent of Man and Selection in Relation to Sex* (1888)

However, in most societies the avoidance of incest has preceded knowledge of any genetic considerations:

It is perhaps unfortunate that this phenomenon of exogamy is so often referred to as indicating an 'incest taboo'. This immediately implies that it is a comparatively recent, culturally controlled restriction, but it must have developed biologically at a much earlier stage, or the typical breeding system of the species could never have emerged from its primate background.

Desmond Morris *The Naked Ape* (1967)

The incest taboo is enforced in societies that have no knowledge of reproductive causality, let alone of genetic complexity.

James Twitchell *Forbidden Partners* (1987)

The taboo preventing any kind of relationship between a man and his mother-in-law may result from a misunderstanding of consanguinity:

The most widespread and strictest avoidance, which is perhaps the most interesting one for civilised races, is that which restricts the social relations between a man and his mother-in-law.

Sigmund Freud *Totem and Taboo* (1919)

Offspring of incestuous relationships were considered monstrous in classical times:

O how she wept, mourning the marriage bed where she let loose that double brood – monsters – husband by her husband, children by her child.

Sophocles *Oedipus Rex* (c. 430 BC)

Aufillena, to live with one's husband alone is the greatest of compliments one can pay to wives; but it is better for a woman to sleep with anyone at all than conceive by her own father and become the mother of brothers.

Catullus (1st century BC)

OEDIPUS *Marriages! O marriage, you gave me birth, and once you brought me into the world you brought my sperm rising back, springing to light, fathers, brothers, sons – one murderous breed – brides, wives, mothers. The blackest things a man can do, I have done them all!*

Sophocles *Oedipus Rex* (c. 430 BC)

Nevertheless, occurrences of incest continued to be documented in Greek and Roman times:

Alcibiades was once travelling with his friend Axiochus to the Hellespont. In Abydos they wedded a girl in common named Medontis, and lived with her in turns. Afterwards she bore a daughter, of whom they said that they did not know who was the father. When the daughter grew up they also lived with her, and when she was with Alcibiades in bed with her he said she was the daughter of Axiochus, and when she was with Axiochus he said she was the daughter of Alcibiades.

Lysias *De Caede Eratosthenis* (4th century BC)

How vile, Gellius, is he who frolics with mother and sister, keeping all night vigil with clothes removed?

Catullus (1st century BC)

It was his habit to commit incest with each of his three sisters...they say that he ravished his sister Drusilla before he came of age.

Suetonius *The Twelve Caesars* 'Caligula' (1st century AD)

That Nero had an incestuous passion for his mother was accepted by all, and it was said that whenever he travelled with her in a litter he abandoned himself to this pleasure, as the stains on his clothing proclaimed.

Suetonius *The Twelve Caesars* 'Nero' (1st century AD)

Later Western history also provides many incidences, and alleged incidences, of incest:

Throughout Western history it is difficult to determine the extent to which incest was practised in spite of the bans of law and prejudice. Enemies of individuals, groups and nations repeatedly hurled at them the accusation of incest. It does not mean the charges were true. At various times, especially during the Middle Ages and Renaissance, the Church was concerned with the possibility that vows of celibacy might be violated incestuously. Priests were forbidden to live with female relations. When Marozia's grandson, Pope John XII was deposed in 964, he was accused of incest. But since he was also said to be guilty of sacrilege, selling sacred offices, perjury, murder, adultery and turning St John Lateran into a brothel, there may have been some exaggeration...Henry VIII added incest with her brother to the crimes alleged against Anne Boleyn; the only evidence he had was that they had been alone together once.

David Loth *The Erotic in Literature* (1962)

The queen...procured and incited her own natural brother...to violate her, alluring him with her tongue in the said George's mouth, and the said George's tongue in hers.

Part of the charge against Anne Boleyn (1536)

This Examinate being charged to have willed her sonne Phillip Barrenger, beeing of the age of xxiii yeares to lye in bedde with her, denyeth that she hath so doone, other then shee hath willed at some tymes to lye uppon the bedde at her backe. But the saide Phyllipe beeing examined, confesseth and saith, that manye times and of late hee hath layne in naked bed with his owne mother, being willed and commanded to doe of her.

Records of witch trials in Essex, England (1582)

Hic jacet in tumulo Lucretia nomine, sed re Thais, Alexandri filia, sponsa nursus.
Here lies entombed one named Lucretia – in truth Thais, Alexander's daughter, wife, and daughter-in-law.

Epitaph of Lucrezia Borgia (1519)

One of my friends is living with the daughter he has had by his own mother; only a week ago he deflowered a boy of thirteen years, fruit of his commerce with that daughter; in a few years this same boy will marry his mother.

Marquis de Sade, quoted by D. J. Enright in 'The Marquis and the Madame'

Incest has also been a common theme in literature:

Unhappy child! *says she, what miserable chance could bring thee hither? And in the Arms of my own Son, too!* Dreadful girl!, *says she,* why we are all undone! *Married to thy own Brother! Three children, and two alive, all of the same Flesh and Blood! My Son and my Daughter lying together as Husband and Wife! All Confusion and Distraction for ever!* miserable Family! *what will become of us? what is to be said? what is to be done?*

Daniel Defoe *Moll Flanders* (1722)

"Son of my brother," he replied, "you must know that this youth was in love with his half-sister from his earliest days. When they were children I forbade him to see her and consoled myself that they were young and foolish; but when they grew older they committed evil together and I was informed of the outrage...Thenceforth I kept the two apart, but the wicked girl's passion for her brother was as great as his, and their souls willingly yielded to Satan's promptings."

Tales from the Thousand and One Nights
'The Porter and the Three Girls of Baghdad'

Poor Simeon! Ill-fated youth!
Dark the hour, when you first departed.
Darker still the hour that brought you to Buda!
When you made love to the queen,
When you kissed her face.
You made love to your own mother.

'The Foundling Simeon' (15th century Serbian folksong)

Like Oedipus poor Simeon committed incest unknowingly. According to Jeremy Bentham, if

Oedipus had been brought up by his mother he would not have been attracted to her:

> *It is very rare that the passion of love is developed within the circle of individuals to whom marriage ought to be forbidden. There needs to give birth to that sentiment a certain degree of surprise, and sudden effect of novelty. Individuals accustomed to seeing each other from an age which is capable neither of conceiving desire nor of inspiring it, will see each other with the same eyes to the end of life.*
>
> *Theory of Legislation* (1864)

Nor, perhaps, would Lord Byron have formed a liaison with his half-sister Augusta Leigh:

> *What a fool was I to marry – and* you *not very wise – my dear – we might have lived so single and so happy...I shall never find any one like you – nor you (vain as it may seem) like me. We are just formed to pass our lives together, and therefore – we – at least – I – am by a crowd of circumstances removed from the only being who could ever have loved me, or whom I can unmixedly feel attached to...no matter – my voice and my heart are ever thine –*
>
> Lord Byron, letter to Augusta Leigh (17 Sept. 1816)

> *Generally speaking, there is a remarkable absence of erotic feelings between persons living very closely together from childhood. Nay more, in this, as in many other cases, sexual indifference is combined with the positive feeling of aversion when the act is thought of...Hence their aversion to sexual relations with one another displays itself in custom and law as a prohibition of intercourse between near kin.*
>
> Edward A. Westermarck *Ritual and Belief in Morocco* (1926)

Others are undeterred by any such taboos:

> *You mean to say that a lovely girl cannot tempt me because I am guilty of having sired her. That what ought to bind me more intimately to her should become the very reason for my removal from her.*
>
> Marquis de Sade *Eugenie de Franval* (1788)

> *I have never been able to understand how a father could tenderly love his charming daughter without having slept with her at least once.*
>
> Giovanni Jacopo Casanova *Histoire de ma vie* (late 18th century: published 1830)

> *There is nothing more exquisite than carnal connection within the family.*
>
> Marquis de Sade *Philosophy in the Bedroom* (1795)

Is it possible that a taboo as deep-rooted as that against incest may in time disappear in the same way that many other previously rigid prohibitions have done? Some sexual liberals are now prepared to argue for a relaxation of the taboo as it affects consenting adults:

> *Few things are as powerful as a deviation whose time has come. Homosexuality, wife-swapping, open marriage, bisexuality, S & M, and kiddie porn have already had their seasons.*
> *Just as we seem to be running low on marketable taboos, the unspeakable predictably popped up. Incest is a game that every family can play.*
>
> 'The Last Taboo', *Penthouse* article quoted by James Twitchell in *Forbidden Partners* (1987)

However, it seems more likely that the growing recognition of the problem of child abuse will keep the taboo in place for the forseeable future:

> *At any rate, the incest taboo, when it works,* does *protect children, and that is important.*
>
> Susan Brownmiller *Against Our Wills* (1975)

See also CHILD ABUSE

Jealousy

Love is strong as death; jealousy is cruel as the grave.

Song of Solomon 8:6

There are basically two views. One is that jealousy is only natural – an inevitable adjunct of human relationships:

It cannot be emphasized enough that jealousy occurs in everyone's life. Encroachment on an intense love relationship between two partners by external demands, stimuli, and temptations leading to the formation of jealousy's basic configuration, the triangle, is inevitable.

Hildegard Baumgart *Jealousy* (1990)

To us, jealousy is not only inbred in human nature, but it is the most basic, all-pervasive emotion which touches man in all aspects of every human relationship. The origin of this emotion may be found in the past of mankind, when man was wild and primitive. And yet, in jealousy, the intensity and force of this reaction does not diminish with the development of sophistication.

Boris Sokoloff *Jealousy: A Psychological Study* (1948)

In order to be able to love, one must be capable of being envious for some length of time and of continuing to be jealous of the person, *not of his accomplishments.*

Theodor Reik *A Psychologist Looks at Love* (1929)

Never love unless you can
Bear with all the faults of man:
Men will sometimes jealous be,
Though but little cause they see;
And hang the head as discontent,
And speak what straight they will repent.

Thomas Campion 'Never Love' (1595)

The idea that jealousy may even be welcomed as a proof of love is very old:

CHRYSIS *He loves me! But you would not have thought so had you seen him last night, in that insane fury that overcomes him when I but walk in the shadow of another man.*
AMPELIS *But this fury is only proof of his great love...He must be crazy about you. If he weren't, he wouldn't have become excited when he saw you with another lover.*

Lucian *Dialogues of the Courtesans* (2nd century)

The other view is that jealousy under any circumstances is an aberration:

Jealousy signifies a weakness in the capacity to love, a lack of self confidence.

Ernest Jones 'La Jalousie' *Revue Française de Psychoanalyse* (1929)

Jealousy often is an indication of impotence, or of doubts about potency.

Melitta Schmideberg 'Some Aspects of Jealousy and of Feeling Hurt' *Psychoanalytic Review* (1953)

Perfect love must always be the abnegation of jealousy.

F. B. T. C-N. Latymer *Ventures in Thought* (1915)

Perhaps the two views can be reconciled:

Jealousy may be seen as existing on a continuum. On one end is apathy. On the other are intense anxiety and overwhelming suspicion. Only the middle range of this continuum contains what could be called 'normal jealousy'. This is the kind that most people usually experience. When it is in this middle range, it is usually identified as a slightly bothersome but basically harmless human trait, the kind people think of when they find jealousy to be amusing and rather insignificant.

Robert L. Barker *The Green-Eyed Marriage* (1987)

It is clear, however, that carried to extremes, jealousy can be disastrous:

For those who experience abnormal jealousy, the emotion sets up a self-fulfilling prophecy. As their associates try to avoid them, their worst fears of losing love and respect are realized. Rather than improving in the behaviour that led to their rejection, they become even more vigilant, more distrustful. They strive harder to gather evidence to confirm their suspicions in the hope that this will prevent the loss. Yet, they remain highly vulnerable to the loss of everything they most desire – lovers, spouse, family, job, friends and, especially, self-esteem.

Robert L. Barker *The Green-Eyed Marriage* (1987)

He who is consumed by the flame of jealousy turns at last, like the scorpion, the poisoned sting against himself.

Friedrich Nietzsche *Thus Spake Zarathustra* (1883–92)

Many sociological and criminological studies show that there is a significant correlation between pathological jealousy and homicide. Recent FBI statistics show that around 25,000 murders are committed every year in the United States. Of those that are solved, just over one-third (34·5 per cent) of all the victims were spouses, mistresses, lovers, or rivals of the offenders, with real or suspected sexual infidelity a major precipitating factor.

Robert L. Barker *The Green-Eyed Marriage* (1987)

It is only in the absence of love that insane jealousy may progress to such an extent that murder or suicide are the only logical ends of this emotion.

Boris Sokoloff *Jealousy: A Pathological Study* (1948)

The self-tormenting nature of obsessive jealousy has been analysed at great length by Proust:

Now it was another of the faculties of his studious youth that his jealousy revived, the passion for truth…a private and personal truth the sole object of which (an infinitely precious object, and one almost disinterested in its beauty) was Odette's life, her actions, her environment, her plans, her past. At every other period in his life, the little everyday activities of another person had always seemed meaningless to Swann; if gossip about such things was repeated to him, he would dismiss it as insignificant, and while he listened it was only the lowest, the most commonplace part of his mind that was engaged; these were the moments when he felt at his most inglorious. But in this strange phase of love the personality of another person becomes so enlarged, so deepened, that the curiosity which he now felt stirring inside him with regard to the smallest details of a woman's daily life, was the same thirst for knowledge with which he had once studied history. And all manner of actions from which hitherto he would have recoiled in shame, such as spying, to-night, outside a window, tomorrow perhaps, for all he knew, putting adroitly provocative questions to casual witnesses, bribing servants, listening at doors, seemed to him now to be precisely on a level with the deciphering of manuscripts, the weighing of evidence, the interpretation of old monuments – so many different methods of scientific investigation with a genuine intellectual value and legitimately employable in the search for truth…Of course it occurred to him from time to time that Odette's daily activities were not in themselves passionately interesting, and that such relations as she might have with other men did not exhale naturally, universally and for every rational being a spirit of morbid gloom capable of infecting with fever or of inciting to suicide.

Marcel Proust *In Search of Lost Time: Swann's Way* (1912)

Do men and women experience jealousy in the same way?

Jealousy per se is the same everywhere. Its intensity and significance in the life of the individual vary, but not the character of the feeling. The frequently raised question concerning the differences between male and female jealousy can be answered only in terms of its psycho- and sociogenesis, not in terms of what concerns the emotional state per se.

Hildegard Baumgart *Jealousy* (1990)

In the man, jealous aggression tends to concentrate on the partner. The woman more frequently extends the aggression to the rival and third parties.

Daniel Lagache *La Jalousie amoreuse* (1947)

One isn't jealous because one loves a woman very deeply but because one fears the humiliation which would result from her changing; and the proof that this passion is purely egoist is that there is not a single lover who would not agree that he would rather see his mistress dead than unfaithful.

Marquis de Sade *Juliette* (1796)

The main object of jealous aggression is invariably the woman, irrespective of whether she is the partner causing a disappointment or the rival. Thus, a jealous woman will always find extenuating factors responsible for her partner's conduct, whereas a man will not find any excuses for his wife's infidelity.

M. Marcuse *Zur Psychologie der Eigensucht und der Psychopathologie ihres Fehlens* (1950)

The jealousy of female patients was more frequently neurotic and less frequently psychotic than that of male patients. In other words, there is a greater tendency for male patients to fall ill with a grave, delusional type of jealousy as compared with female patients.

Kauko Vauhkonen *On the Pathogenesis of Morbid Jealousy* (1968)

Before a woman introduces her husband or lover to her woman friend, she looks her suspiciously and carefully over, face and body, and tries to find out her possible intentions. It is as if she wants to see her first with the eyes of the man, especially when the other woman is younger and prettier than herself. The feminine sense of hostility and jealous possessiveness will inevitably emerge in this tentative process.

Theodor Reik *Sex in Man and Woman* (1960)

Can jealousy be curbed?

Lycurgus also desired to eliminate jealousy...He made it lawful for the elderly husband of a young wife to allow her the company of a young man of good birth whom he himself esteemed and liked and to authorise intercourse between, so as to obtain a well-connected son, whom he would then treat as his own.

Plutarch *Lycurgus* (1st century AD)

More recently Bertrand Russell thought it could:

There can be no doubt that mutual jealousy, even when there is physical faithfulness, often causes more unhappiness in a marriage than would be caused if there were more confidence in the ultimate strength of a deep and permanent affection.

Bertrand Russell *Marriage and Morals* (1929)

He therefore agreed with his second wife, Dora Black, that:

...husbands should not 'possess' wives, nor wives husbands...

Dora Russell *The Tamarisk Tree* (1975)

He also said:

A man or woman who has been thwarted sexually is apt to be full of envy; this generally takes the form of moral condemnation of the more fortunate.

Bertrand Russell *Why I am Not a Christian* (1957)

However, when Dora had a child by another man he left her, later commenting:

My capacity for forgiveness, and what might be called Christian love, was not equal to the demands I was making on it...I was blinded by theory.

The Autobiography of Bertrand Russell, vol. 1 (1967)

Their daughter pithily remarked:

...calling jealousy deplorable had not freed them from it...both found it hard to admit that the ideal had been destroyed by the old-fashioned evils of jealousy and infidelity.

Kathleen Tait *My Father Bertrand Russell* (1976)

The Russells were only discovering what a long line of writers had found before them: Plato puts these words into the mouth of Socrates, who is, of course, talking about the love of an older man for a young boy:

The lover is of necessity jealous and will do great damage to his beloved, restricting him from many advantageous associations which would do most to make a man of him, and especially from that which would bring his intellect to its capacity – that is, divine philosophy. The lover will have to keep his boy far away from philosophy because of his enormous fear of being despised. And he will contrive to keep him ignorant of everything else as well, so the boy looks to his lover for everything.

Phaedrus (4th century BC)

Echoing the jealousy of an even earlier writer:

You haven't fooled me, boy – I'm on your trail –
you've stolen off to your new fast friends,
and thrown my love away in scorn.
But you were no friend of theirs before.
No, out of them all, I thought it was you I'd made a trusted
mate. And now you hold another love.

Theognis of Megara (6th century BC)

In *A Winter's Tale*, *Cymbeline*, and (especially) *Othello* Shakespeare provided some of the most profound and harrowing pictures of sexual jealousy in literature. In *Othello*, jealousy is memorably personified as

the green-eyed monster which doth mock the meat it feeds on.

Othello (c. 1604)

The widespread use of the colour green to denote jealousy seems to originate in an association of ideas between jealousy and jaundice – a disease that produces a yellow or greenish hue in the skin and whites of the eyes. Sufferers from jaundice were commonly supposed to see everything tinged yellow; sufferers from obsessive jealousy are imagined as afflicted with a similarly distorted vision:

Jealousy, the jaundice of the soul.

John Dryden *The Hind and the Panther* (1687)

Jealousy's eyes are green.

Percy Bysshe Shelley *Swellfoot the Tyrant* (1820)

Dr Ebenezer Brewer has provided a further gloss on Shakespeare's lines about the green-eyed monster –

A greenish complexion was formerly held to be indicative of jealousy, and as all the green-eyed cat family 'mock the meat they feed on', so jealousy mocks its victim by loving and loathing it at the same time.

Brewer's Dictionary of Phrase and Fable (1870)

– while a 19th-century American poet drew this moral from the play:

Young Ladies! – beware of hasty connections;
And don't marry suitors of swarthy complexions;
For though they may chance to be capital fellows,
Depend upon it, they're apt to be jealous!

John Godfrey Saxe *Othello, the Moor. Moral* (1850s)

A miscellany of views to end with:

jealousy…the injur'd lover's hell.

John Milton *Paradise Lost* (1667)

How much are they deceived who vainly strive,
By jealous fears, to keep our flames alive?
Love's like a torch, which if secured from blasts,
Will faintlier burn; but then it longer lasts.
Exposed to storms of jealousy and doubt,
The blaze grows greater, but 'tis sooner out.

William Walsh 'Love and Jealousy' (1690s)

Though he was jealous, he did not show it,
For jealousy dislikes the world to know it.

Lord Byron *Don Juan* (1819–24)

Moral indignation is jealousy with a halo.

H. G. Wells *The Wife of Sir Isaac Harman* (1914)

Lesbianism

Everyone these days, from our pseudonymous girls, to the Smart Sloane, the supermodel, the glamorous TV presenter and the glossy magazine editrix, can be found dining à deux *at Blake's or Bibendum, playing not-so-covert footsie with her girlfriend under the table and hotly* not *denying to everybody afterwards that they had had, are having, or are about to have, an affair. If last year's ultimate fashion accessory was having a baby, then this year's is having a lesbian affair.*

Christa d'Souza *Sunday Times* (7 Feb. 1993)

Homosexual love between women was not, however, invented by Sloanes:

Although the Scriptures made no explicit mention of lesbian sex, rabbinical writers assumed that female homosexuality was forbidden and firmly registered their disapproval of it. Their disapprobation may be linked to the prohibition in Deuteronomy of the wearing of male attire by a woman or of female dress by a man, a practice that the law labelled an 'abomination before God.'

James A. Brundage *Law, Sex and Christian Society in Medieval Europe* (1987)

Lesbianism acquired its name from the Greek island of Lesbos, where the poetess Sappho lived around 600 BC, much of her poetry being inspired by her relationships with her female admirers:

What did Lesbian Sappho teach girls but love?

Ovid *Tristia* II (c. 10 AD)

In ancient Greece, lesbianism was widely accepted:

[Aristophanes] *Women, cut from the second, feminine sex, don't pay the slightest attention to us men. On the contrary, it's women they are inclined to. That's the species to which the darlings of some ladies we know belong!*

Plato *Symposium* (4th century BC)

Once more Eros of the golden hair
hits me with his purple ball,
calls me out to play with the girl
with the flashy slippers.
But she, since she comes from noble
Lesbos, scoffs at my hair,
since it's white, and gapes
for another girl.

Anacreon (6th century BC)

They say that there are women in Lesbos with faces like men, and unwilling to consort with men, but only with women, as though they themselves were men.

Lucian *Dialogues of the Courtesan* (2nd century BC)

...at Sparta love was held in such honour that even the most respectable women became infatuated with girls.

Plutarch *Life of Lycurgus* (1st century AD)

In classical Rome the practice was also widespread. Here is an account by a Dutch poet of one Roman woman (Tullia) showing another (Octavia) what happened on her wedding night:

Then on your back lie down upon the bed,
And lift your petticoats above your head;
I'll shew you a new piece of lechery,

For I'll the man, you shall the woman be.
Your thin transparent smock, my dear remove
That last bless'd cover to the scene of love.
What's this I see, you fill me with surprise,
Your charming beauties dazzle quite my eyes!
Gods! what a leg is here! what lovely thighs!
A belly too, as polish'd iv'ry white,
And then a cunt would charm an anchorite!
Oh! now I wish I were a man indeed,
That I might gain thy pretty maidenhead,
But since, my dear, I can't my wish obtain,
Let's now proceed t'instruct you in the game;
That game that brings the most substantial bliss;
For swiving of all games the sweetest is.
Ope wide your legs, and throw them round my back,
And clasp your snowy arms about my neck.
Your buttocks then move nimbly up and down.
Whilst with my hand I thrust the dildo home.
You'll feel the titulation by and by;
Have you no pleasure yet, no tickling joy?
Oh! yes, yes, now I faint, I die.

Johannes Meursius *The Delights of Venus* (17th century)

However, in Rome

Lesbian relationships excited greater approbium than did male homosexual liaisons, perhaps because upper-class Roman men found lesbianism threatening to their own sexual self-esteem.

James A. Brundage *Law, Sex and Christian Society in Medieval Europe* (1987)

During the Middle Ages lesbianism was regarded as anti-Christian and treated by the Church with its customary brutality:

By AD 1260 severe punishments for lesbianism emanated from the legal school at Orleans – women were to be mutilated for first and second offenses. For a third offense she was to be burned...Fears of lesbianism became entangled with concern over heresies and later with fears about witchcraft and the suppression of non-Christian cults.

Barbara Ponse *Identities in the Lesbian World* (1978)

Sixteenth- and seventeenth-century canon law and theology showed few novelties in their treatment of deviant sexual behaviour. By and large the older condemnations continued in force, and both Catholic and Protestant writers agreed that homosexual acts should be punished severely. Writers and judges seem to have been more concerned with lesbian behaviour in this period than was true earlier. Some scattered sixteenth-century prosecutions for sexual relations between women have come to light in recent years and, while there are not many of them, they greatly outnumber those known from any earlier century in the Middle Ages.

James A. Brundage *Law, Sex and Christian Society in Medieval Europe* (1987)

Violent reactions have persisted among some of the deeply religious:

I remember one time I scratched this girl's back in the middle of the night – I was, you know, nine, and she was twelve, and she asked me to scratch her back. A nun ran in, ripped me off her back, threw me against the lockers, beat the shit out of me and called me a lesbian. I didn't know what a lesbian was.

Cyndi Lauper, on her experiences in a Catholic boarding school (1980s)

From the legal point of view, lesbians have often occupied an anomalous position:

Historically lesbians have lived not so much outside the law, both religious and secular, as beneath it...while men were still condemned to death for homosexual relations, lesbians were simply disqualified from marriage with a priest.

Jane Rule *Lesbian Images* (1975)

Male homosexual acts remained illegal in the UK until the implementation of the recommendations of the Wolfenden Report:

It was not until 1967 that sexual acts between consenting adult males in private were decriminalised, and even then the age of consent remained at twenty-one for gay male sex, whereas heterosexuals (and presumably lesbians) could fuck from the age of sixteen.

Cherry Smith *Lesbians Talk Queer Notions* (1992)

An apocryphal story has it that legislation against lesbian acts was abandoned in the 19th century because Queen Victoria refused absolutely to believe that such things took place.

What, then, is this thing that is spurned by the Church and ignored by the law? How does it affect women?

Men have asked me, 'But what can two women do together?' As though a penis were the 'sine qua non' of sexual pleasure! Man, we can do without it, and keep it going longer, too!

Martha Shelley *Notes of a Radical Lesbian* (1969)

Most female homosexuals merely feel occasional melancholy awareness of their inability to possess a woman as a man. At such times, rather than attempt to find a penis substitute, I think they more often 'lie there wishing perhaps to be a man for a moment'.

Anaïs Nin *Winter of Artifice* (1939)

Women often love each other with as much fervor and excitement as they do men. When this is the case, the emotions awakened heave and swell through the whole being as the tides swell the ocean. Freed from all the grosser elements of passion, as it exists between the sexes, it retains its energy, its abandonments, its flush, its eagerness, its palpitation, and its rapture.

Margaret J. M. Sweat *Ethel's Love Life: A Novel* (1859)

Lesbianism is, and must be accepted as one facet on the continuum scale of human sexual expression...A lesbian relationship is, and must be accepted as, a viable life style.

D. Martin and P. Lyon *Lesbian/Woman* (1972)

The lesbian has a much better knowledge of the female body generally and of the female genitalia in particular than do most males. Her masturbatory caresses, and her caresses generally, tend therefore to be more subtle, more skillful, and more satisfying.

Robert E. L. Masters *The Hidden World of Erotica* (1973)

I have no doubt that lesbianism makes a woman virile and open to any sexual stimulation, and that she is more often than not a more adequate and lively partner in bed than a 'normal' woman.

Charlotte Wolff *Love Between Women* (1971)

Refusal to make herself the object is not always what turns women to homosexuality; most lesbians, on the contrary, seek to cultivate the treasures of their femininity...The truth is that lesbianism is no more perversion deliberately indulged in than it is a curse of fate. It is an attitude chosen in a certain situation – that is at once motivated and freely adopted.

Simone de Beauvoir *The Second Sex* (1949)

Lesbians and female-to-male transsexuals seem to have abnormal levels, at least in part, of testosterone and estradiol (hormones). And if we give them estrogen, their lutenizing-hormone response is lower than that of heterosexual women, suggesting that their brains have been masculinized in some way. The cognitive patterns (the way they think) of their brain, too, may be somewhere intermediate between heterosexual men and heterosexual women. And their body build on the basis of certain measurements, may be closer to that of a man's. It is also possible that they age rather faster than normal women do – rather like men.

Gunter Dorner *Sex and the Brain* (J. Durden-Smith and D. de Simone; 1983)

There is a certain category of women who surpass others in intelligence and subtlety. There is a great deal of the masculine in their nature, to such an extent that in their movements, and in the tone of their voice, they bear a certain resemblance to men. They also like being the active partners. A woman like this is capable of vanquishing the man who lets her. When her desire is aroused, she does not shrink from seduction. When she has no desire, then she is not ready for sexual intercourse. This places her in a delicate situation with regard to the desires of men and leads her to Sapphism. One has to look for the majority of those who possess these qualities amongst the elegant women, those capable of writing and reciting – amongst the cultivated women.

Samau al ibn Yahyâ *Book of Conversation* (12th century)

What is the relationship between feminism and lesbianism?

Lesbianism is one road to freedom – freedom from oppression by men.

Martha Shelley *Notes of a Radical Lesbian* (1969)

Feminism...is about a social, anti-family political movement that encourages women to leave their husbands, kill their children, practice witchcraft, destroy capitalism and become lesbian.

Pat Robertson, candidate for the Republican presidential nomination, quoted in the *New York Times* (1988)

As the question of homosexuality has become public, reformists define it as a private question of who you sleep with in order to sidetrack our understanding of the politics of sex. For the lesbian feminist, it is not private, it is a political matter of oppression, domination, and power.

Charlotte Bunch in *Lesbianism and the Women's Movement* (1975)

Personal perfection in relationships is not a realistic goal under male supremacy. Lesbianism is a necessary political choice, not a passport to paradise.

Leeds Revolutionary Feminist Group *Political Lesbianism: the Case Against Heterosexuality* (1979)

The greatest threat to men is solidarity among women and 'lesbianism' epitomizes that solidarity.

Sidney Abbott and Barbara Love *Is Women's Liberation a Lesbian Plot?* (1971)

In a society which regards men of primary importance to women, lesbians are unlucky. Society thinks, 'poor things, they haven't got any men to cope with or care for'.

E. M. Ettorre *Lesbians, Women and Society* (1980)

For some, lesbianism compels a redefinition of the whole concept of womanhood — even of the word 'woman' itself:

It would be incorrect to say that lesbians associate, make love, live with women, for 'woman' has meaning only in heterosexual systems of thought and heterosexual economic systems. Lesbians are not women.

Monique Wittig in *For Lesbians Only: A Separatist Anthology* (1987)

Women belong to men. Thus a lesbian has *to be something else, a not-woman, a not-man, a product of society, not a product of nature, for there is no nature in society.*

Monique Wittig 'One is Not Born a Woman' *Feminist Issues* (1981)

A lesbian is not considered a 'real woman'. And yet in popular thinking, there is really only one essential difference between a lesbian and other women; that of sexual orientation – which is to say, when you strip off all the packaging, you must realise that the essence of being a 'woman' is to get fucked by men.

Radicalesbians (a political activist group) (1970)

Others are content to see a lesbian as a passionate or not so passionate woman who just happens to fancy other women:

The human race is divided into male and female. Many human beings enjoy sexual relations with their own sex; many don't; many respond to both. This plurality is the fact of our nature and not worth fretting about.

Gore Vidal *Pink Triangle and Yellow Star* (1984)

I have had my passionate attachments among women, which swept like whirlwinds over me, sometimes scorching me with a furnace-blast...I have loved so intensely that the daily and nightly communion I have held with my beloved ones has not sufficed to slake my thirst for them, nor the lavishness of their love for me has been able to satisfy the demands of my exacting nature.

Margaret J. M. Sweat *Ethel's Love Life: A Novel* (1859)

And...she would discuss very different people whom she had been led to believe existed; hard-working honourable men and women...yet lacking the courage to admit their inversion. Honourable, it seemed, in all things save this that the world had forced on them — this dishonourable lie whereby alone they could hope to find peace, could hope to stake out a claim on existence. And always these people must carry that lie like a poisonous asp pressed against their bosoms; must unworthily hide and deny their love, which could well be the finest thing about them.

Radclyffe Hall *The Well of Loneliness* (1928)

Between women, love is contemplative; caresses are intended less to gain possession of the other than gradually to recrate the self through her; separateness is abolished, there is no struggle, no victory, no defeat; in exact reciprocity each is at once subject and object, sovereign and slave; duality becomes mutuality.

Simone de Beauvoir (1974)

Finally, some comments about the appropriate word for a female who is homosexual:

But the word lesbian, possibly the least attractive word in the English language besides moist, conjures up visions of the archetypal man-hating 'diesel dyke' who wears size 26 dungarees, sports a full beard, a pierced nose and looks as if she'd have the back off your washing machine as soon as she walked into your kitchen.

Christa d'Souza *Sunday Times* (7 Feb. 1993)

I never said I was dyke even to a dyke because there wasn't a dyke in the land who thought she should be a dyke or even thought she was a dyke so how could we talk about it.

Jill Johnston *Lesbian Nation: The Feminist Solution* (1973)

'We're here! We're queer! Get used to it!' Some of us are quite happy to call ourselves queer. A once-despised word no longer makes us recoil in fear. Indeed, it is fast becoming a proud symbol of the angry and assertive New Queer Politics of the 1990s.

Peter Tatchell *Independent on Sunday* (26 July 1992)

One of the latest epithets is the SGO (single gender orientation) girl. But whatever word one uses one does sometimes need to identify the concept, the practice, and the people who do it – unless one pretends that it does not exist:

The Soviet Medical Encyclopaedia gives no definition of lesbian love, it merely gives the geographical location of the island of Lesbos.

Stern and Stern *Sex in the Soviet Union* (1981)

Love

Pleasure, which is undeniably the sole motive force behind the union of the sexes, is nevertheless not enough to form a bond between them...if it is preceded by desire which impels, it is succeeded by disgust which repels...That is a law of nature which love alone can alter.

Pierre Choderlos de Laclos *Les Liaisons dangereuses* (1782)

'Which love alone can alter'? What is it that changes sexual desire into something so much more powerful and enduring?

You know very well that love is, above all, the gift of oneself!

Jean Anouilh *Ardèle* (1949)

Nature did not construct human beings to stand alone, since they cannot fulfil her biological purpose except with the help of another; and civilized people cannot fully satisfy their sexual instinct without love. The instinct is not completely satisfied unless a man's whole being, mental quite as much as physical, enters into the relation. Those who have never known the deep intimacy and the intense companionship of mutual love have missed the best thing that life has to give...

Bertrand Russell *Love, An Escape from Loneliness* (1929)

Here are two accounts that emphasize the merging – the oneness – experienced by lovers in the act of love; the first was written nearly 2400 years before the second:

Suppose Hephaestus, with his instruments, to come to the pair who are lying side by side and to say to them, "What do you mortals want of one another?...Do you desire to be wholly one; always day and night in one another's company? for if that is what you desire, I am ready to melt and fuse you together, so that being two you shall become one...and after your death in the world below still be one departed soul, instead of two...?" There is not a man of them who when he heard the proposal would deny or would not acknowledge that this meeting and melting into one another, this becoming one instead of two, was the very expression of his ancient need. And the reason is that human nature was originally one and we were a whole, and the desire and pursuit of the whole is called love.

Plato *The Symposium* (4th century BC)

In a fulfilling sexual act, the two opposite genders, at their most different and separate, simultaneously become one totality, merging with one another in an experience going beyond the capacity of either...It is non-manipulative, non-controlling; the self is offered freely, from generosity and trust, and since there is no demand the return comes equally freely and fully, each emotionally responding and keeping time with the other. Each gives most generously, yet takes most uninhibitedly too, without hedging or bargaining. For a moment, both partners are fully in the present...no longer lost in the concerns of the future or memories of the past.

Robin Skinner *One Flesh: Separate Persons* (1976)

Many poets and philosophers have attempted to define the nature of love and its bewildering effects on men and women:

I bid all men not to shun but to pursue sweet desire; love is the whetstone of the soul.

Alpheus of Mitylene (c. 25 BC)

Love is the only god from whom Hades accepts orders. He feels pity for lovers and for them alone ceases to be inflexible and implacable.

Plutarch *Erotikos* (1st century AD)

Against love there is no remedy, neither a potion, nor powder, nor song; nothing except kissing, fondling, and lying together naked are of assistance.

Longus of Lesbos *Daphnis and Chloe* (c. 200)

Love is a power too strong to be overcome by anything but flight.

Miguel de Cervantes *Don Quixote* (1605–15)

For love, all love of other sights controls,
And makes one little room, an every where.
Let sea-discoverers to new worlds have gone,
Let maps to others, worlds on worlds have shown:
Let us possess one world, each hath one, and is one.

John Donne 'The Good Morrow' (1633)

...this medicine, love, which cures all sorrow
With more...

John Donne 'Love's Growth' (1633)

Love is inevitably consequent upon the perception of loveliness. Love withers under constraint; its very essence is liberty; it is compatible neither with obedience, jealousy, nor fear: it is there most pure, perfect, and unlimited, where its votaries live in confidence, equality and unreserve.

Percy Bysshe Shelley *Queen Mab* (1813)

All mankind love a lover.

Ralph Waldo Emerson *Essays* 'Love' (c. 1840)

For this is one of the miracles of love; it gives – to both, but perhaps especially to the woman – a power of seeing through its own enchantments and yet not being disenchanted.

C. S. Lewis *A Grief Observed* (1961)

Love seeketh not Itself to please,
Nor for itself hath any care,
But for another gives its ease,
And builds a Heaven in Hell's despair.

William Blake 'The Clod and the Pebble' (1794)

Many have stressed the painful, irrational, and selfish nature of love:

Most part of a lover's life is full of agony, anxiety, fear and grief, complaints, sighs, suspicions, and cares (heigh-ho my heart is woe), full of silence and irksome solitariness.

Robert Burton *The Anatomy of Melancholy* (1651)

The arrows of Cupid are various in their effects; some graze our skin, and our hearts languish for years from their creeping poison. But others land with freshly sharpened points, pierce us to the marrow and swiftly kindle the blood.

J. W. von Goethe *Roman Elegies* (c. 1790)

My opinion of love is that it acts upon the human heart precisely as a nutmeg grater acts upon a nutmeg.

Percy Bysshe Shelley, quoted by Richard Holmes in *Shelley: the Pursuit* (1974)

Love is like the lion's tooth.

W. B. Yeats *Words for Music Perhaps* (1931)

Love is a universal migraine,
A bright stain on the vision
Blotting out reason.

Robert Graves 'Symptoms of Love' (20th century)

A handful of kisses and a throb of pleasure – they're not worth any of the pains of love – the unrest, the fever.

Enid Bagnold, in a letter to Frank Harris (20th century)

We often speak of love when we really should be speaking of the drive to dominate or to master, so as to confirm ourselves as active agents, in control of our own destinies and worthy of respect from others.

Thomas Szasz *The Second Sin* (1973)

Love seeketh only Self to please,
To bind another to Its delight,
Joys in another's loss of ease,
And builds a Hell in Heaven's despite.

William Blake 'The Clod and the Pebble' (1794)

The idiom describing the onset of the condition is interesting:

Not for nothing is it called 'falling' in love. You do not climb into love, you fall, you collapse, and invariably everything that makes you a good friend and reliable colleague at work is sacrificed in the quest for some, often unworthy, partner.

Hugo Vickers 'Love' *Independent* (5 June 1993)

Clearly being in love and making love are not at all the same thing:

Love is not born of breasts and bottoms alone.

Graham Masterton *How to Drive Your Man Wild in Bed* (1975)

Sex and love are so different that they belong to distinct realms of research fields; sex to the domain of biochemistry and physiology, love to the domain of the psychology of the emotions. Sex is an urge, love is a desire.

Theodor Reik *A Psychologist Looks at Love* (1954)

For the ancient Greeks the two were quite separate:

As a rule the Greeks distinguished the two deities very clearly. Aphrodite was regarded as the goddess of the physical act of sexual intercourse, while Eros figured as the god of erotic sentiment.

Robert Flacelière *Love in Ancient Greece* (1960)

The Athenians were so far from thinking that Eros had anything to do with carnal union that they erected a statue to him in the Academy, a building dedicated to the virgin goddess Athena, and offered sacrifices to both deities at the same time.

Athenaeus *Deipnosophistae* (2nd century)

A once popular view, now somewhat discredited, is that romantic love was largely an invention of the medieval poets:

Romantic love in Europe appears to have been unknown prior to the appearance in late eleventh century France of the troubadours and trouvères. That is not to say that attachments of this kind did not exist between individuals before that time, but it was not accepted and formalised as a popular conception.

F. Henriques *Love in Action* (1965)

Courtly love essentially involved an idealisation of passionate sexual love, but passionate love was regarded as evil, or at least suspect, by the Church, and declared not to be a proper component of conjugal love; indeed one Church view widely held was that to love one's own wife passionately was adulterous.

Judith Armstrong *The Novel of Adultery* (1976)

There can be no mistake about the novelty of romantic love, our only difficulty is to imagine in all its barrenness the mental world that existed before its coming.... We must conceive of a world emptied of that ideal of 'happiness' – a happiness grounded on successful romantic love which still supplies the motive of our popular fiction.

C. S. Lewis *The Allegory of Love: A Study in Medieval Tradition* (1936)

More recent research suggests that, although it takes different forms in different cultures, romantic love is a universal human phenomenon:

Until recently, there was a tendency to see it as a product of Western medieval culture, aped elsewhere only by elites. But at last December's meeting of the American Anthropological Association, the first-ever session on the anthropology of romance heard that in a survey of 166 cultures, ro-

mantic love had been found in 147 of them.

The Times (11 Feb. 1993)

In the remaining 19, it was assumed that the examining anthropologists had been too inept to recognize the symptoms!

Plainly, there can be sex without love; but can there also be love between men and women without sex, or the desire for it? Some are frankly unconvinced by 'Platonic love':

Oh Plato! Plato! you have paved the way,
With your confounded fantasies to more
Immoral conduct by the fancied sway
Your system feigns o'er the controlless core
Of human hearts, than all the long array
Of poets and romancers: – You're a bore,
A charlatan, a coxcomb – and have been,
At best, no better than a go-between.

Lord Byron *Don Juan* (1819–24)

'Bah!' she said, 'With people like you, love only means one thing.' 'No,' he replied, 'It means twenty things, but it doesn't mean nineteen.'

Arnold Bennett *Journal* (20 Nov. 1904)

The extra-marital affair which consists of sex without love is condemned. The affair which consists of love without sex is not seen as an affair at all.

Two people may love one another, indulge in sexual foreplay in bed, even masturbate one another to orgasm, but do not count it as an affair because the 'normal' sex act is not completed.

Tony Lake and Ann Hills *Affairs* (1979)

Some refuse to make any distinction between the physical act of love and the mental or emotional state:

What is commonly called love, namely the desire of satisfying a voracious appetite with a certain quantity of delicate white human flesh.

Henry Fielding *Tom Jones* (1749)

When people say, 'You're breaking my heart,' they do in fact usually mean that you're breaking their genitals.

Jeffrey Bernard *Spectator* (31 May 1986)

What comes first in a relationship is lust, then more lust.

Jacqueline Bisset (20th century)

Or as Proust's Mme Leroi remarked, when asked for her views on the matter:

Love? I make it constantly but I never talk about it.

Marcel Proust *In Search of Lost Time: The Guermantes Way* (1920–21)

Sometimes love can mean different things for men and women; traditionally, for men, the physical aspect dominates:

Licence my roving hands, and let them go,
Before, behind, between, above, below.

John Donne 'To His Mistress Going to Bed' (17th century)

Love is the delusion that one woman differs from another.

H. L. Mencken *Chrestomathy* (1949)

A woman is a well-served table, that one sees with different eyes before and after the meal.

Honoré de Balzac *The Physiology of Marriage* (1829)

Men imagine their sperm permanently marks a woman they have just made love to.

Emmanuel Reynaud *Holy Virility* (1981)

While for women, the tradition is the opposite:

In an uncorrupted woman the sexual impulse does not manifest itself at all, but only love; and this love is the natural impulse of a woman to satisfy a man.

Johann Fichte *The Science of Rights* (1796)

Girls are taught from childhood that any exhibition of sexual feeling is unwomanly and intolerable…

Mary Scharlieb *The Seven Ages of Woman* (1915)

I do not believe that the normal man's sex needs are stronger than the normal woman's. The average man's undoubtedly are, owing to the utterly false repression of the woman's and the utterly unnatural stimulation of the man's which have been current for so long.

Marie Stopes, in a letter (17 Dec. 1918)

To some extent this dichotomy still persists:

Women still see sex as a relatively unimportant part of an emotional complex. But for many women nowadays, sex is the only affection they get.

Germaine Greer, interviewed in *Woman's Own* (Apr. 1985)

Every 'Mills & Boon' story projects the idea that sex strengthens love. Few women find this in real life.

Irma Kurtz *Over 21* (June 1985)

For some women, sex and love come together most completely in the desire for children:

The sensitive inter-relation between a woman's breasts and the rest of her sex life is not only a bodily thrill, but there is a world of poetic beauty in the longing of a loving woman for the child which melts in mists of tenderness towards her lover.

Marie Stopes *Married Love* (1918)

In Western cultures, love, sex, and the reproductive instinct are traditionally brought together in the institution of marriage:

Love and marriage, love and marriage
Go together like a horse and carriage,
This I tell ya, brother,
Ya can't have one without the other.

Sammy Cahn 'Love and Marriage' (1955)

Although this has not always been the case:

Furthermore, the lover would fervently wish his beloved to remain without marriage, child, or household for as long a time as possible, since it is his desire to reap the fruit that is sweet to himself for as long a time as possible.

Plato *Phaedrus* (4th century BC)

We declare and hold as firmly established that love cannot exert its powers between two people who are married to each other. For lovers give each other everything freely, under no compulsion of necessity, but married people are in duty bound to give in to each other's desires and deny themselves to each other in nothing.

Andrew the Chaplain *The Art of Courtly Love* (1180s)

See also MARRIAGE

Many writers have stressed the transience of love, seeing it as something that either fades away completely or suffers a slow subtle change into something quite different:

O love is gentle and love is hard
Gay as a jewel when first it's new;
But love grows old and waxes cold
And fades away like morning dew.

Anon. 'The Water is Wide'

All through the years of our youth
Neither could have known
Their own thought from the other's
We were so much at one.

But O, in a minute she changed–
O do not love too long,
Or you will grow out of fashion
Like an old song.

W. B. Yeats 'O Do Not Love Too Long' (1904)

Love. Of course, love. Flames for a year, ashes for thirty. He knew what love was...

Giuseppe di Lampedusa *The Leopard* (1956)

Marriage is the tomb of love.

Giovanni Jacopo Casanova *Histoire de ma vie* (late 18th century; published 1830)

No, Mr Lawrence, it's not like that!
I don't mind telling you
I know a thing or two about love,
perhaps more that you do.

And what I know is that you make it
too nice, too beautiful.
It's not like that, you know; you fake it.
It's really rather dull.

D. H. Lawrence *Birds, Beasts and Flowers* (1923)

Marriage from love, like vinegar from wine –
A sad, sour, sober beverage – by time
Is sharpen'd from its high celestial flavour,
Down to a very homely household savour.

Lord Byron *Don Juan* (1819–24)

Although there is an alternative view:

All love at first, like generous wine,
Ferments and frets, until 'tis fine;
But when 'tis settled on the lee,
And from the impurer matter free,
Becomes the richer still, the older,
And proves the pleasanter, the colder.

Samuel Butler 'Love' (17th century)

For some, the mark of true love is precisely its ability to withstand time and change:

I scarce believe my love to be so pure
As I had thought it was,
Because it doth endure
Vicissitude, and season, as the grass;
Methinks I lied all winter, when I swore
My love was infinite, if spring make it more.

John Donne 'Love's Growth' (1633)

But true love is a durable fire,
In the mind ever burning,
Never sick, never old, never dead,
From itself never turning.

Sir Walter Ralegh 'As I Came from the Holy Land of Walsingham' (c. 1600)

...love is not love
Which alters when it alteration finds,
Or bends with the remover to remove.
O no, it is an ever fixed mark
That looks on tempests and is never shaken.

William Shakespeare *Sonnets* (1609)

The passage of time can also lend an enchantment to past love:

Over that love affair, scrappy and clamorous,
Time throws a veil iridescent and glamorous,
Cloaking the sordid, revealing the amorous –
Hiding the ashes but leaving the flame.

Edwin Meade Robinson 'Glamour' (1906)

First loves are undoubtedly special:

I ne'er was struck before that hour
With love so sudden and so sweet,
Her face it bloomed like a sweet flower
And stole my heart away complete.

My face turned pale as deadly pale,
My legs refused to walk away,
And when she looked, what could I ail?
My life and all seemed turned to clay.

And then my blood rushed to my face
And took my eyesight quite away,
The trees and bushes round the place
Seemed midnight at noonday.
I could not see a single thing,
Words from my eyes did start–
They spoke as chords do from the string,
And blood burnt round my heart.

John Clare 'First Love' (1820s)

But sweeter still than this, than these, than all,
Is first and passionate love – it stands alone,
Like Adam's recollection of his fall;
The tree of knowledge has been pluck'd – all's known –
And life yields nothing further...

Lord Byron *Don Juan* (1819–24)

When I was young, I kissed my first woman, and smoked my first cigarette on the same day. Believe me, never since have I wasted any more time on tobacco.

Arturo Toscanini (1957)

Although later experience may induce cynicism even here:

We keep our first lover for a long time – if we do not get a second.

In their first passions, women are in love with their lover; in the rest, with love.

François de la Rochefoucauld *Maximes* (1665)

Perhaps one should also remind oneself that sexual love does not have to be between members of opposite sexes. Just three quotations:

There is no request, however impossible, that the boy he loves can make, which the man wounded by love does not regard it as an absolute necessity to fulfil.

Libanius *Moral Discourses* (c. 367 AD)

And he died – in my arms, in fact peacefully...He'd always said earlier, to me, 'I must die first, before you, because I don't know what I would do without you.'

Peter Pears, describing the death of Benjamin Britten, his lover for forty years (1976)

Hick darling. All day I've thought of you...Oh! I want to put my arms around you, I ache to hold you close. Your ring is a great comfort. I look at it and think she does love me or I wouldn't be wearing it.

Eleanor Roosevelt, in a letter to her lover, Lorena Hickok (1933)

Finally, a suggestion for a chemical basis for love:

Michael Liebowitz of the New York Psychiatric Institute believes that the key to infatuation lies in a brain chemical called phenylethylamine, or PEA, stimulated by attraction.
People who crave emotional relationships but are incapable of keeping them going appear to be addicted to the 'high' achieved by PEA...But nobody can remain infatuated for ever. Dr Liebowitz links this with a growing tolerance to the effects of PEA, or the inability of the body to continue producting it. Among those of us who mature into longer-term relationships, he believes another mechanism operates. Each partner, according to this theory, has the ability to stimulate in the other the production of the body's natural opiates, the endorphins, which produce a sense of stability and tranquility.

The Times (11 Dec. 1992)

This may or may not turn out to be true. In the meantime, St Augustine's advice can hardly be wrong:

Love, and do what you like.

(4th century)

Male Homosexuality

This sort of thing may be tolerated by the French, but we are British – thank God.

Lord Montgomery *Daily Mail* (27 May 1965)

Most human beings nurture a strong antipathy towards other human beings who do not share their beliefs or practices. It is for this reason that race, religion, social class, and intellectual achievement, for example, are so divisive. It also accounts for the strong antagonism that many heterosexual men have for homosexual men.

In the late sixties, a Gallup poll showed that 93% of respondents regarded homosexuality as a sickness; a CBS television poll showed that 76% of respondents felt that homosexuality was a sickness; and a Louis Harris survey showed that 63% of respondents believed that homosexuals were harmful to American life.

Barbara Ponse *Identities in the Lesbian World* (1978)

In Judaeo-Christian cultures, this attitude can be traced back to the Bible:

God gave them up unto vile affections: for even their women did change the natural use into that which is against nature: and likewise also the men, leaving the natural use of the woman, burned in their lust one toward another; men with men working that which is unseemly, and receiving in themselves that recompence of their error which was meet.

Romans 1:26

But the men of Sodom were wicked and sinners before the Lord exceedingly.

Genesis 13:13

And if a man also lie with mankind, as he lieth with womankind, both of them have committed abomination: they shall surely be put to death: their blood shall be upon them.

Leviticus 20:13

The continuing use of these passages to support a blanket condemnation of homosexuality has elicited the following comments from the US writer Gore Vidal:

Elsewhere in the Old Testament, Sodom was destroyed not because the inhabitants were homosexualists but because a number of local men wanted to gang-rape a pair of male angels who were guests of the town. That was a violation of the most sacred of ancient taboos: the law of hospitality. Also, gang rape, whether homosexual or heterosexual, is seldom agreeable in the eyes of any deity…

The authors of Leviticus proscribe homosexuality – and so do all good Christers. But Leviticus also proscribes rare meat, bacon, shellfish, and the wearing of nylon mixed with wool. If Leviticus were to be obeyed in every instance, the garment trade would collapse.

Pink Triangle and Yellow Star (1979)

A more tolerant approach only began to emerge in this century.

Homosexuality between men, though not between women, is illegal in England…Every person who has taken the trouble to study the subject knows that this law is the effect of a barbarous and ignorant superstition in favour of which no rational argument of any sort or kind can be advanced.

Bertrand Russell *Marriage and Morals* (1929)

Homosexuality is assuredly no advantage, but it is nothing to be ashamed of, no vice, no degradation, it cannot be classified as an illness.

Sigmund Freud, letter to a concerned mother (1935)

We confess to a strong personal prejudice in favor of the boy-girl variety of sex, but our belief in a free, rational and humane society demands a tolerance of those whose sexual inclinations are different from our own...

Hugh Heffner 'The Playboy Philosophy' *Playboy* (early 1950s)

No argument which purports to show that homosexuality in general is natural or unnatural, healthy or morbid, legal or illegal, in conformity with God's will or contrary to it, tells me whether any particular homosexual act is morally right or wrong.

K. J. Dover *Greek Homosexuality* (1978)

One would now expect educated opinion to accept that human sexuality can be healthily expressed across a spectrum of appetites from the staunchly heterosexual, through bisexuality, to the exclusively homosexual. Sexual diversity is an integral aspect of the human condition. Because the majority of men are heterosexual and because reproduction and the continuation of the species depend on heterosexual relationships (except in rare instances of artificial insemination), this is always likely to be regarded as the 'normal' end of the spectrum; this is not to say that the minority are abnormal, though they are clearly different:

Blurring the distinction between heterosexuals and homosexuals is profoundly dishonest. Queers are not *the same as heterosexuals. Our sexuality gives many of us experiences and perspectives that are different. That difference is no bad thing, and certainly nothing to apologise for or hide.*

Peter Tatchell *Independent* (26 July 1992)

Or, as John Osborne's Jimmy Porter remarks:

As if I give a damn which way he likes his meat served up.

Look Back in Anger (1956)

I think there is no crime in making what use I please of my own body.

William Brown, on his arrest for homosexuality, in Samuel Stevens *Select Trials* (1726)

We are all fallen beings, and homosexuals are no more fallen than you or me.

Dr David Stacey *Report of the Methodist Church Working Party on Sexuality* (1979)

We do not think it possible to deny that there are circumstances in which individuals may justifiably choose to enter into a homosexual relationship with the hope of enjoying a companionship and physical expression of sexual love similar to that which is to be found in marriage.

'Homosexual Relationships. A Contribution to Discussion', Church of England report (1979)

There's this illusion that homosexuals have sex and heterosexuals fall in love. That's completely untrue. Everybody wants to be loved.

Boy George (1980s)

It seems to me that the real clue to your sex-orientation lies in your romantic feelings rather than your sexual feelings. If you are really gay, you are able to fall in love with a man, not just enjoy having sex with him.

Christopher Isherwood

Although purely homosexual men do not usually produce children, they can be highly creative in other ways – and the world is not short of either fathers or potential fathers:

Jews and homosexuals are the outstanding creative minorities in contemporary urban culture. Creative, that is, in the truest sense: they are the creators of sensibilities. The two pioneering forces of modern sensibility are Jewish moral seriousness and homosexual aestheticism and irony.

Susan Sontag *Notes on Camp* (1964)

There are three kinds of pianists: Jewish pianists, homosexual pianists, and bad pianists.

Vladimir Horowitz

Will he [Wilde] *force me to think that homosexuals have more imagination than the...others? No, but they are more frequently called upon to exercise it.*

André Gide *Journals* (1931)

Had Socrates and Plato not loved young men, what a pity for Greece, what a pity for the whole world. Had Socrates and Plato not loved young men and aimed to please them, each one of us would have been a little less sensible.

André Gide *Journals* (1918)

If Michelangelo had been straight, the Sistine Chapel would have been wallpapered.

Robin Tyler, speech at a gay-rights rally, Washington, (9 Jan. 1988)

However, as one might expect, tolerance of homosexuality is not universal, even in the late 20th century:

We cannot, like Gide, extol homosexuality. We do not, like some, condone it. We regard it as a symptom...

Karl Menninger *The Vital Balance: The Life Process in Mental Health and Illness* (1963)

I will resist the efforts of some to obtain government endorsement of homosexuality.

Ronald Reagan, communication to the publisher of the 'Presidential Biblical Scorecard' (1984)

Homosexuality is treated with greater contempt in the USSR than in any other Western country. The penalty for homosexuality is three to eight years...

I do not believe the Soviet press has ever discussed the problem of homosexuality, generally thought to be a synonym for total perversion. It is a phenomenon which provokes such disgust that people prefer to pass over it in silence. The rare books devoted to sexuality contain at best only a dry definition of what homosexuality is.

Stern and Stern *Sex in the Soviet Union* (1981)

The family as a social institution does not of itself condemn homosexuality, but through its mere existence it implicitly provides a model that renders the homosexual experience invalid.

Kenneth Plummer *Sexual Stigma* (1975)

A local authority shall not
(a) intentionally promote homosexuality or publish material with the intention of promoting homosexuality
(b) promote the teaching in any maintained school of the acceptability of homosexuality as a pretended family relationship.

Section 28 of the Local Government Act (1987–88)

There are still echoes of the 19th-century abhorrence that culminated in the trial and public disgrace of Oscar Wilde:

I am the Love that dare not speak its name.

Lord Alfred Douglas 'The Two Loves' (1892)

It is hateful to me now to speak or write of such things, but I must be explicit. Sodomy never took place between us, nor was it thought or dreamt of. Wilde treated me as an older boy treats a younger one at school, and he added what was new to me and was not (as far as I know) known or practised among my contemporaries: he 'sucked' me.

Lord Alfred Douglas, in a letter to Oscar Wilde's biographer

'The Love that dare not speak its name' in this century is such a great affection of an elder for a younger man as there was between David and Jonathan, such as Plato made the very basis of his philosophy, and such as you find in the sonnets of Michelangelo and Shakespeare...It is

beautiful, it is fine, it is the noblest form of affection. There is nothing unnatural about it. It is intellectual, and it repeatedly exists between an elder and a younger man, where the elder has intellect and the younger has all the joy, hope, and glamour of life before him. That it should be so, the world does not understand.

Oscar Wilde, part of his testimony at his trial (1895)

...the crime of which you have been convicted is so bad that one has to put stern restraint upon one's self to prevent one's self from describing, in language which I would rather not use, the sentiments that must rise to the breast of every man of honour who has heard the details of these two terrible trials...It is no use for me to address you. People who can do these things must be dead to all sense of shame...It is the worst case I have ever tried.

Sir Alfred Wills, sentencing Oscar Wilde to two years hard labour

Should everyone found guilty of Oscar Wilde's crime be imprisoned, there would be a very surprising emigration from Eton, Rugby, Harrow and Winchester to the jails of Pentonville and Holloway.

W. T. Stead *Review of Reviews* (1895)

The laws against male homosexual acts have a long history:

Laws against sodomy have been traced to the Emperor Justinian (483–562 AD*) who believed the act to be the main cause of earthquakes. In English law anal sex is called 'buggery' and has been prohibited since 1533 when Henry VIII reigned. Section 12 of the Sexual Offences Act (1956) states that it 'is a felony to commit buggery with another person or with an animal'.*

Roy Eskapa *Bizarre Sex* (1987)

Every person convicted of the abominable crime of Buggery committed either with Mankind or with any Animal, shall suffer death as a Felon...Owing to the Difficulty of Proof which has been required of the completion of those several Crimes...it will not be necessary to Prove the actual Emission of Seed, but the Carnal Knowledge shall be deemed complete upon Proof of Penetration only.

English Act of Parliament (1828)

However, since the passing of the Sexual Offences Act (1967), homosexual activity in private, between consenting men over 21, has ceased to be a criminal offence in Britain. This change in the law followed the publication of the Wolfenden Report, which stated:

There must be a realm of private morality and immorality which is, in brief and crude terms, not the law's business.

Committee on Homosexual Offences and Prostitution, chaired by John Wolfenden (1957)

This is now the case throughout the EC (the Irish parliament having voted to liberalize the law in 1993). Homosexual acts are still completely illegal in Russia and a number of Eastern European countries.

In the armed services of the UK, homosexual activity remained a criminal offence for many years after it had ceased to be so in civil society:

3624. Homosexuality and other unnatural behaviour
1. Definition. Homosexuality is the unnatural tendency of a man or woman to have sexual inclinations towards a member of his or her own sex. Homosexual acts committed by officers or ratings of the Royal Navy, Royal Marines, QARNNS or WRNS are offences against the Naval Discipline Act *1957 and* Army Act *1955. Furthermore Section 1 of the* Sexual Offences Act *1967, which provides that a homosexual act committed in private by consenting males over the age of 21 should in some circumstances no longer be an offence states that such an act shall continue to be an offence under the Service Discipline Acts.*

Queen's Regulations, Royal Navy (1991)

The situation changed in 1992:

Homosexuality will no longer be a criminal offence in the armed forces...Jona-

than Aitken, the defence minister, emphasised that homosexuality would still be banned in the forces and result in dismissal. He told the Commons that legislation would be introduced in this parliament so that homosexuals would no longer be liable to prosecution under military law and risk a criminal record.

The Times (18 June 1992)

In the US there have been moves to liberalize the remaining regulations against homosexuals serving in the armed forces:

We know there have always been gays in the military. The issue is whether they can be in the military without lying about it.

Bill Clinton, quoted in the *Independent* (17 Nov. 1992)

The Air Force pinned a medal on me for killing a man and discharged me for making love to one.

Leonard Matlovich, former American Air Force sergeant who created a test case to challenge the anti-homosexuality regulations (1975)

Although homosexuality has traditionally been regarded as prejudicial to good discipline in the ranks, several Greek writers took a directly opposite view:

A handful of lovers and loved ones, fighting shoulder to shoulder, could rout a whole army. For a lover to be seen by his beloved forsaking the ranks or throwing away his weapons would be unbearable. He would rather a thousand times die than be so humiliated.

Plato *The Symposium* (4th century BC)

I also love boys; this is more beautiful than languishing in the yoke of marriage; for in murderous battle your friend still stays as a protector at your side.

Seleucus (2nd century BC)

Homosexual relations between heroes were often celebrated in the ancient world. The oldest of religious texts tells of the love between two men, Gilgamesh and Enkidu. When Enkidu died, Gilgamesh challenged death itself in order to bring his lover back to life. In the Iliad, *Gilgamesh's rage is echoed by Achilles when* his *lover Patroclus dies before the walls of Troy.*

Gore Vidal *Pink Triangle and Yellow Star* (1979)

Apart from the military, the other powerful institution to retain an attitude of outright condemnation of homosexuality is the Roman Catholic Church. For the Church

...it is a more or less strong tendency ordered toward an intrinsic moral evil; and thus the inclination itself must be seen as an objective disorder... As in every moral disorder, homosexual activity prevents one's own fulfilment and happiness by acting contrary to the creative wisdom of God.

Sacred Congregation for the Doctrine of the Faith *Letter to the Bishops of the Catholic Church on the Pastoral Care of Homosexual Persons (1986)*

I am a devout Catholic. I am also gay. I became fully aware of my sexual orientation about three years ago when I was fifteen. I can't say that I glorified in the discovery, yet neither was I particularly distressed; it was just me – another one of the facets, the qualities, that make me the person I am.
Paradoxically, perhaps, given the anti-homosexual teaching of the Church, I retained and still retain, the implicit faith and trust in God and Catholicism that I had up to that point. However with the passing of puberty and the first true feelings of sexual awakening encountered by everyone, I realized what a burden had been put on me. While my friends were talking of girlfriends and expressing interest in the female sex, I had to keep quiet and try not to appear conspicuous. Loneliness must be one of the prime characteristics of homosexuality...

Letter, *Catholic Herald* (6 Sept. 1991)

Being a Catholic as well as a homosexual is no easy matter. As usual, the statute-books of Catholic dominated Ireland, where homosexuality is still illegal, reflect the Vatican's attitude. The Church will only sanction sex which can transmit life, so you can imagine what it thinks about

acts between persons of the same sex. In the late seventies, cracks began to appear in the crust of prejudice. These closed ten years later, as part of the world-wide reaction to AIDS. Never mind transmitting life – many in the (Catholic) Church held that homosexuals were transmitting death.

Kate Saunders and Peter Stanford *Catholics and Sex* (1992)

Nor is homosexuality confined to the laity:

Until recently...fewer than 20 per cent of clergy were of homosexual orientation or undetermined in orientation, of which one-fourth, or 5 per cent of total clergy, had a regular sexual acting out with a number of partners. However, Sipe comments, reports of homosexual activity have increased significantly since 1978, in some areas closer to 40 per cent...

Richard Sipe *The Search for Celibacy* (1992)
See also CHASTITY AND CELIBACY

Traditional Christian moralists have often equated homosexuality with the selfish pursuit of pleasure:

As people hovered between God and Self, so they hovered between heterosexuality and homosexuality. If God triumphed, people attained "the home-life for which we are made and in which alone we can find joy and rest". Homosexuals, as we have seen, were defined as Egotists...who seemed to reject the patriarchy of Christianity as they rejected the patriarchy of the family.

Richard Davenport-Hines, paraphrasing the views (1906) of Bishop Cosmo Lang in *Sex, Death and Punishment* (1990)

However, the view that homosexual love is no more than selfish lust is hardly borne out by the evidence:

Love is Blind – and what your dear eyes do not see is that it is you who have given me *everything, from yourself in Grand Rapids! Through* Grimes *and* Serenade *and* Michelangelo *and* Canticles *– one thing after another, right up to this great Aschenbach – I am here as your mouthpiece and I live in your music. And I can never be thankful enough to you and to Fate for all the heavenly joy we have had together for 35 years. My darling, I love you – P.*

A letter from Peter Pears to Benjamin Britten (1971). And a comment by Pears, after Britten's death:

We'd faced up to what was going to come a good deal earlier than this, and he was not in any terror of dying...And he died – in my arms, in fact – peacefully, as far as he could be said to be peaceful when he in fact was very ill...But what was his greatest feeling was sadness and sorrow at the thought of leaving me, his friends, and his responsibilities. He'd always said earlier, to me, "I must die first, before you, because I don't know what I would do without you."

Britten may have written his music for Pears – but the rest of us have benefited greatly. Just as we have from Tchaikovsky, who dedicated his 6th Symphony to his nephew Vladimir (Bob) Davidov, about whom the composer wrote in his diary:

Bob will finally drive me simply crazy with his indescribable fascination...Frightful how I love him!

The love expressed in these brief extracts makes a stark contrast with the harsh pronouncements of those who presume to know what is right, what is a sin, or what is God's will. However, not all Christians take the same view as the Roman Catholic Church:

Homosexual affection can be as selfless as heterosexual affection, and therefore we cannot see that it is in some way morally wrong. An act which expresses true affection between two individuals and gives pleasure to them both does not seem to us to be sinful simply because it is homosexual.

Towards a Quaker View of Sex (1964)

In some non-Christian cultures homosexual behaviour of certain kinds has been widely accepted:

> *The love of boys is as old as humanity.*
>
> J. W. von Goethe *Achilleis* (c. 1790)

For example, in ancient Greece:

> *Boys in the flower of their youth are loved; the smoothness of their thighs and soft lips is adored.*
>
> Solon (594 BC)

> *Happy the man who's got boys for loving and single foot horses, hunting dogs and friends in foreign lands.*
>
> Theognis of Megara (6th century BC)

According to Aristophanes' Dikaios Logos, the ideal young man

> *...will have a robust chest, a clear complexion, broad shoulders, a short tongue, big buttocks, and a small penis.*
>
> *Clouds* (5th century BC)

> *If a beautiful boy of good family finds no lover, this is considered a disgrace, since the reason for it must be in his character.*
>
> Ephoros of Cyme *History of the Greeks* (4th century BC)

> *Well, this is a fine state of affairs, you damned desperado! You meet my son just as he comes out of the gymnasium, all fresh from the bath, and you don't kiss him, you don't hug him, you don't feel his balls! And you're supposed to be a friend of ours!*
>
> Aristophanes *The Birds* (5th century BC)

> *Is it your intention to teach Greek customs [of homosexuality] to that young man lying next to you, since he is so handsome?*
>
> Xenophon *Cyrodaedia* (4th century BC)

> *O what magic comfort are boys to men!*
>
> Euripides (5th century BC)

What happened in ancient Greece to encourage this wholesale inversion of procreative sexuality?

> *To all appearance it was the Dorian invaders of the eleventh century BC who introduced into Greece both the use of iron and homosexual practice...*
>
> *In Greece, though pederasty was forbidden by law in most of the cities, it had become so fashionable that no one troubled to conceal it...Many Greeks, moreover, did not feel in the least ashamed of admitting that homosexuality was held in more honour among them than anywhere else in the world.*
>
> Robert Flacelière *Love in Ancient Greece* (1960)

> *At former epochs, male love-affairs were unknown. In those days it was thought indispensable to couple with women in order to preserve the human race from extinction...Only with the advent of divine philosophy did homosexuality develop. We should be careful not to condemn an invention merely because it came late...Let us agree that the old customs arose from necessity, but that subsequent novelties due to the ingenuity of man, ought to be more highly regarded...*
>
> *Marriage is for men a life-preserving necessity and a precious thing, if it is a happy one; but the love of boys, so far as it courts the sacred rights of affection, is in my opinion a result of practical wisdom. Therefore let marriage be for all, but let the love of boys remain alone the privilege of the wise, for a perfect virtue is absolutely unthinkable in women.*
>
> Attributed to Lucian *Erotes* (2nd century BC)

And what did the boys think of it?

> *The boy does not share in the man's pleasure in intercourse, as a woman does; cold sober, he looks upon the other drunk with sexual desire.*
>
> Xenophon *Symposium* (4th century BC)

> *His kisses, to be sure, are not sophisticated like a woman's, they are no devastating spell of lips' deceit. But he kisses as he knows how – acting by instinct, not technique.*
>
> Achilles Tatius *Leucippe and Cleitophon* (5th century BC)

I am Eurymedon, I am stationed bending forward.

Caption to illustration identifying the about-to-be-buggered young soldier as a representative of the losing side in the Athenian victory over the Persians at the battle of Eurymedon (465 BC)

Apparently only the older participant was expected to enjoy the act:

The Athenian vases clearly show that only the adults were considered to derive satisfaction from pederastic intercourse; the boy usually looks as if he is solving some academic problem.

Professor Jan Bremmer *Greek Pederasty and Modern Homosexuality* (1989)

Although vase paintings can easily be misinterpreted:

...experts sometimes err, e.g. on describing a typical pair of males [on Greek vase paintings] *engaged in intercrural copulation as 'wrestlers', or in taking a scene of homosexual courtship, in which hares are offered as gifts, as 'a discussion of the day's hunting'.*

K. J. Dover *Greek Homosexuality* (1978)

Acceptance of pederasty was, however, by no means universal;

The signs of a kinaidos *are an unsteady eye and knock-knees; he inclines his head to the right; he gestures with his palms up and his wrists loose; and he has two styles of walking – either waggling his hips or keeping them under control. He tends to look around in all directions.*

Aristotle *Virtues and Vices* (4th century BC)

Terrible, terrible, and utterly intolerable, are the practices of the young [homosexual] *men in our city – here, where there are, after all, very good-looking young things in the whore-houses, whom one can see basking in the sun, their breasts uncovered, stripped for action and drawn up in battle-formation by columns.*

Xenarchus *The Pentathlete* (4th century BC)

For it was only yesterday or at best the day before yesterday that the pederast came slinking into our gymnasia, to view the games in which youths then first began to strip for exercise. Quite quietly at first he started touching and embracing the boys. But gradually, in those arenas, he grew wings – and then there was no holding him. Nowadays he regularly insults conjugal love and drags it through the mud.

Plutarch *Erotikos* (1st century AD)

See also CHILD ABUSE

Whether sanctioned or condemned, male homosexuality has been widespread in all human cultures. In ancient Rome:

Men's faces are not to be trusted; does not every street abound in gloomy-visaged debauchees? And do you rebuke foul practices, when you are yourself the most notorious of the Socratic reprobates? A hairy body, and arms stiff with bristles, give promise of a manly soul: but the doctor grins when he cuts into the growths on your sleek buttocks.

Juvenal *Satire II* (2nd century)

He had not the slightest regard for chastity, either his own or others', and was accused of homosexual relations, both active and passive...moreover, a young man of consular family, Valerius Catullus, revealed publicly that he had buggered the Emperor, and quite worn himself out in the process.

Suetonius *The Twelve Caesars* 'Gaius Caligula' (1st century AD)

In the Islamic World:

Know that many eminent men of our time indulge in the frivolous practice of having relations with boys. Several of them have been led to do so by their doctors, who have persuaded them that sexual union with women leads more quickly to old age and to the weakness of age, and causes podagra and haemorrhoids, whereas relations with boys are less harmful.

Samau al ibn Yahyâ *Book of Conversation* (12th century)

The man who experiences no pleasure with women and enjoys more often than not congress with blameworthy men should suspect that there is something wrong with him.

Yahyâ ibn Māsawaih *Aphorisms* (11th century)

In the Far East:

Although it may have been officially proscribed, homosexuality in fact flourished in Buddhist monasteries throughout the centuries. In China the character for hemorrhoids is 'temple illness'; male love is said not to have existed in Japan until it was introduced by Buddhist monks in the ninth century; homosexuality was prevalent in Yellow Hat monasteries in Tibet and was regarded as a virtue, since it meant that a monk had completely conquered sexual attachment to women.

John Stevens *Lust for Enlightenment* (1990)

It was common practice for parents in [ancient] *China to sell their sons into a life of prostitution. Such boys would then be trained in the 'art'. They would have any pubic hair shaved, their anus dilated, their buttocks massaged, be luxuriously dressed and perfumed, and then offered to rich men.*

Richie J. McMullen *Male Rape* (1990)

And in Christian Europe:

Sir J. Mennes and Mr. Batten both say that buggery is now almost as common among our gallants as in Italy, and that the very pages of the town begin to complain of their masters for it.

Samuel Pepys *Diary* (1 July 1663)

Every boy of good looks had a female name, and was recognised either as a public prostitute or as some bigger fellow's 'bitch'. Bitch was the word in common usage to indicate a boy who yielded his person to a lover.

John Addington Symonds *Memoirs*, 'Harrow in 1854' (ed. Phyllis Grosskurth; 1984)

Attitudes and practices have varied so widely that anthropologists have found it hard to agree in their general conclusions:

Actually, no society, save perhaps Ancient Greece, pre-Meiji Japan, certain top echelons in Nazi Germany, and the scattered examples of such special status groups as the berdaches, *Nata slaves and one category of Chuckchee shamans, has lent sanction in any real sense to homosexuality.*

Marvin Opler *Anthropological and Cross Cultural Aspects of Homosexuality* (1965)

In almost two-thirds of the 76 societies that Clellan S. Ford and Frank A. Beach reviewed in Patterns of Sexual Behavior *(1951), homosexual activities were considered acceptable under certain circumstances.*

Encyclopaedia Britannica

Likewise, scientists and psychologists are still unable to decide how far homosexuality is an innate condition and how far it is a tendency acquired later in life. Those who believe that it is morally blameworthy must presumably take the latter view. Freud also thought that homosexual tendencies were acquired:

It is not possible to adopt the view that the form to be taken by sexual life is unambiguously decided, once and for all, with the inception of the different components of the sexual constitution. On the contrary, the determining process continues.

Sigmund Freud *Three Essays on the Theory of Sexuality* (1905)

Freud believed that all young boys have a sexual bond with their mothers, which has to be broken before they can fancy other women. If the bond is not broken, for whatever reason, until the boy has become an adult, the victim will seek a man with whom to have a relationship, in which he plays the part of the mother. This contorted view implies that parents can be responsible for turning their heterosexual sons into homosexuals and also that the orientation is potentially reversible. There is no evidence to support either of these contentions. On the other hand:

Neurobiologists have defined the brain circuits responsible for sex behaviour, and have shown that the sexual differentiation of these circuits takes place pre-natally under the influence of sex hormones such as testosterone...
Geneticists have demonstrated a strong influence of heredity on sexual orientation in both men and women.
In my own research, published a year ago, I described structural differences between gay and straight men in the anterior hypothalamus, the brain region most centrally involved in the production of typical male sex behaviour.

Simon LeVay 'Are Homosexuals Born and Not Made?' *Guardian* (9 Oct. 1992)

This does not constitute firm evidence, but it does suggest that sexual orientation may be determined prenatally. Before this can be established, the relevant genes, and the way they work, will have to be identified.

Although scientific opinion appears to be moving in this direction, a number of writers have recently come to question the very legitimacy of 'homosexual' and 'heterosexual' as distinct categories of sexual orientation. Such terms, it is argued, owe more to the compulsive desire of 19th-century scientists to categorize and label than to the realities of human experience.

In 1992, when the patriots among us will be celebrating the five-hundredth anniversary of the discovery of America by Christopher Columbus, our cultural historians may wish to mark the centenary of an intellectual landfall of almost equal importance of the conceptual geography of the human sciences: the invention of homosexuality by Charles Gilbert Chaddock...An early translator of Krafft-Ebing's classic medical handbook of sexual deviance, the Psychopathia sexualis, *Chaddock is credited by the* Oxford English Dictionary *with having introduced 'homo-sexuality' into the English language in 1892 in order to render a German cognate twenty years its senior. Homosexuality, for better or for worse, has been with us ever since. Before 1892 there was no homosexuality, only sexual inversion.*

David M. Halperin *One Hundred Years of Homosexuality* (1990)

Sexual inversion, the term used most commonly in the nineteenth century, did not denote the same conceptual phenomenon as homosexuality. 'Sexual inversion' referred to a broad range of deviant gender behaviour, of which homosexual desire was only a logical but indistinct aspect, while 'homosexuality' focused on the narrower issue of sexual object choice.

George Chauncey *Sexual Inversion to Homosexuality* (1983)

Homosexuality appeared as one of the forms of sexuality when it was transposed from the practice of sodomy into a kind of interior androgyny, a hermaphroditism of the soul. The sodomite had been a temporary aberration; the homosexual was now a species.

Michel Foucault *History of Sexuality* (1979)

The artificial categories 'heterosexual' and 'homosexual' have been laid on us by a sexist society.

Allen Young *Out of the Closets: Voices of Gay Liberation* (1972)

If the categories 'homosexual/heterosexual' and 'gay/straight' are the inventions of particular societies rather than real aspects of the human psyche, there is no gay history.

John Boswell *Revolutions, Universals, and Sexual Categories* (1982)

The word ['homosexual'] *itself is a bastard term compounded of Greek and Latin elements.*

H. Havelock Ellis *Sexual Perversion: Studies in the Psychology of Sex* (1922)

In the centuries of Rome's great military and political success, there was no differentiation between same-sexers and other-sexers; there was also a lot of crossing back and forth of the sort that those

Americans who do *enjoy inhabiting category=gay or category=straight find hard to deal with.*

Gore Vidal *Pink Triangle and Yellow Star* (1979)

There is probably no sensible heterosexual alive who is not preoccupied with his or her latent homosexuality.

Norman Mailer *Advertisement for Myself* (1970)

I am claiming that there is no such thing as 'homosexuality itself' or 'heterosexuality itself.' Those words do not name independent modes of sexual being, leading some sort of ideal existence apart from particular human societies, outside of history or culture. Homosexuality and heterosexuality are not the atomic constituents of erotic desire, the basic building-blocks out of which every person's sexual nature is constructed. They just represent one of the many patterns according to which human living-groups, in the course of reproducing themselves and their social structures, have drawn the boundaries that define the scope of what can qualify – and to whom – as sexually attractive.

David M. Halperin *One Hundred Years of Homosexuality* (1990)

Many of these ideas are associated with a radical new tendency known as the New Queer Politics:

The New Queer Politics looks beyond *equality, and challenges the assumption that lesbian and gay desire is an intrinsically minority sexual orientation. It argues that everyone is potentially homosexual (and heterosexual). While some biological factors may predispose individuals to a sexual preference, all the psychological and anthropological evidence suggests that sexuality is primarily culturally conditioned, and is not rigidly compartmentalised. None of us is wholly attracted to one sex or the other. We are all a mixture of desires. Some we express, others we repress.*

Peter Tatchell *Independent* (26 July 1992)

In 1992 the *Cassell Concise English Dictionary* supplied a new definition of the word 'queer', traditionally applied abusively to homosexuals:

queer (kwiə), *a.* (*esp. N Am.*) also applied by lesbians and gay men to themselves as a means of confirming their identity as a group in/out of society.

The defiant adoption of this term reflects the uneasiness that many homosexuals have begun to feel with the word 'gay' (itself adopted in the early 1970s in an attempt to dispel the medical associations that 'homosexual' had by then acquired):

We feel angry and disgusted, not gay. Using 'queer' is a way of reminding us how we are perceived by the rest of the world. It's a way of telling ourselves we don't have to be witty, charming people who keep our lives marginalised and discreet in the straight world. 'Queer' can be a rough word, but it is also a sly and ironic weapon we can steal from the homophobe's hand and use against him.

NYQ (Jan. 1992)

In Spring 1990 two activist groups formed to set out a 'new queer agenda' for gay politics – Queer Nation in New York and OutRage! in London. OutRage! staged a mass kiss-in in Piccadilly Circus and a 'queer wedding' in Trafalgar Square, to provide sensational headlines for the tabloid press. The attitude to straight society is overtly confrontational:

Queer denotes a very radical break from the old order. It sticks two fingers up at the sanitisation of lesbian and gay identities by authority figures within the [gay] *community…Queer emerged out of the AIDS epidemic in the US but seems to reflect many of the energies that powered gay liberation and subsequently got respectabilised…*

OutRage! (June 1990)

It's time to put our cocks and cunts on the line, to smash once and for all the lie that we're all the same, that we want to be like the gay and straight zombies out there who watch propaganda TV, who believe the lies in the Sun *and the* Guardian, *who think they've got a right to judge us, our bodies, our lovers, our lives… Queer means to fuck with gender. There are straight queers, biqueers, tranny queers, lez queers, fag queers, SM queers, fisting queers in every single street in this apathetic country of ours.*

Anon. leaflet, 'Queer Power Now' (1991)

Queer is a symptom, not a movement, a symptom of a desire for radical change.

Keith Alcorn (1992)

I get angry that queer is becoming another form of political correctness. If you say you're queer, then everyone else can be shouted down. 'They're the baddies because they're lesbian and gay pinkos and we're the radical queers with attitude.'

Paul Burston (1992)

While there is resistance to the word queer, it is useful to remember that there were also battles over 'gay', which was not a term without contradictions. In the early 70s, gay too was characterised as radical and oppositional. By the 80s, lesbians felt the term had rendered them invisible and the addition of 'lesbians and' became a necessary part of naming. For some people who have come out since the beginning of the AIDS epidemic, there is a tendency to associate 'gay' with AIDS and to fail to identify with its happy subtext…

Queer promises a refusal to apologise or assimilate into invisibility. It provides a way of asserting desires that shatter gender identities and sexualities, in the manner some early Gay Power and lesbian feminist activists once envisaged. Perhaps it will fail to keep its promise, but its presence now in the early 90s marks the shape of the territory to come with an irrevocable and necessary passion.

Cherry Smyth *Lesbians Talk Queer Notions* (1992)

Marriage

What is marriage for?

To achieve order and regulation in sexual behaviour some form of marriage is necessary. Marriage assures the sexual rights of the partners in each other, and ensures the creation and care of a family to inherit property and to help perpetuate the society.

F. Henriques *Love in Action* (1965)

Marriage is a social device for regulating heterosexual activity, preventing socially disruptive competition, and establishing the mutually advantageous responsibilities of the spouses and their offspring.

Paul Gebhard et al. *Pregnancy, Birth and Abortion,* Institute for Sex Research (1958)

Marriage is the destiny traditionally offered to women by society. It is still true that most women are married, or have been, or plan to be, or suffer from not being.

Simone de Beauvoir *The Second Sex* (1972)

Marriage is insurance for the worst *years of your life. During your best years you don't need a husband.*

Helen Gurley Brown *Sex and the Single Girl* (1962)

Marriage is the beginning and the pinnacle of all culture. It makes the savage gentle, and it gives the most cultivated the best occasion for demonstrating his gentleness. It has to be indissoluble: it brings so much happiness that individual instances of unhappiness do not come into account.

J. W. von Goethe *Elective Affinities* (1790)

The marriage certificate is proof of heterosexual normality. Many young people need it, to convince themselves and others that they are OK.

Thomas Szasz *The Second Sin* (1973)

By having a wife and children to be proud of a man shows that he is a fully qualified male, able to display his virility, and the fact that he is a normal adult.

Tony Lake and Ann Hills *Affairs* (1979)

We have courtesans for our pleasure, concubines for our daily personal service, and married women to bear us children and manage our house faithfully.

Plato *Laws* (4th century BC)

Wives are young men's mistresses, companions for middle age, and old men's nurses.

Francis Bacon *Essays* 'Of Marriage and Single Life' (c. 1625)

The traditional Christian view of the matter is bleakly unromantic:

First, It was ordained for the procreation of children, to be brought up in the fear and nurture of the Lord, and to the praise of His holy Name.

Secondly, It was ordained for a remedy against sin, and to avoid fornication; that such persons as have not the gift of contin-

ency might marry, and keep themselves undefiled members of Christ's body.

Thirdly, It was ordained for the mutual society, help, and comfort, that the one ought to have of the other, both in prosperity and adversity.

Book of Common Prayer 'Solemnization of Matrimony' (1662)

Marriage is the preservative of Chastity, the Seminary of the Commonwealth, seed-plot of the Church, pillar (under God) of the world, right hand of providence, supporter of Lawes, states, orders, offices, gifts and services; the glory of peace, the sinewes of warre, the maintenance of policy, the life of the dead, the solace of the Living, the ambition of virginity, the foundation of Countries, Cities, Universities, succession of families, Crownes and Kingdomes.

Daniel Rogers *Matrimonial Honour* (1642)

Such attitudes have their origin in the teaching of St Paul, who grudgingly allowed marriage on the grounds that it was preferable to fornication:

Nevertheless, to avoid fornication, let every man have his own wife, and let every woman have her own husband.

I Corinthians 7:2

But if they [the unmarried and widows] *cannot contain, let them marry: for it is better to marry than to burn.*

I Corinthians 7:9

Even within marriage, the medieval church attempted to control the frequency of sexual contact:

The Church regulated sexual activity within marriage, forbidding it on all feast days and fast days (of which there were 273 in the seventh century, though this had shrunk to 140 by the sixteenth century) on Sundays and in periods when the wife was deemed to be unclean (during menstrual periods, during pregnancy, during breast-feeding and for forty days after childbirth).

Jeffrey Richards *Sex, Dissidence and Damnation* (1990)

This menstrual taboo goes back to Old Testament times, when it may have begun as an attempt to maintain desert hygiene.

And if a woman have an issue, and her issue in her flesh be blood, she shall be put apart seven days: and whosoever toucheth her shall be unclean...and if it be on her bed, or on anything whereon she sitteth, when he toucheth it he shall be unclean...And if any man lie with her at all...he shall be unclean seven days; and all the bed whereon he lieth shall be unclean.

Leviticus 15:19–25

The belief that the only legitimate purpose of sex was procreation encouraged the view that the pleasure – and even the consent – of the wife were irrelevant:

Boys and girls should be taught that nothing can justify sexual intercourse unless there is mutual inclination. This is contrary to the teaching of the Church, which holds that, provided the parties are married and the man desires another child, sexual intercourse is justified however great may be the reluctance of the woman.

Bertrand Russell *Why I am Not a Christian* (1957)

A husband cannot be guilty of rape upon his wife for by their mutual matrimonial consent and contract the wife hath given up herself in this kind to her husband, which she cannot retract.

Sir Matthew Hale, quoted by R. H. Small in *History of the Pleas of the Crown* (1847)

Which contrasts with the more civilized view of the Roman jurist Ulpian:

It is not consummation but consent which makes marriages.

Digest of Justinian (533)

There has been much debate about the advantages and disadvantages of marriage from the sexual point of view:

Marriage is surely the only institution where sex without love and love without sex are accepted.

Tony Lake and Ann Hills *Affairs* (1979)

You weep, utter miserable words, look round curiously, are jealous, often touch me, often kiss me. This is the behaviour of a lover; but when I say, 'I am going to bed' and you dally, there is nothing of the lover at all about you.

Philodemus of Gadara (1st century BC)

Personally I know nothing about sex because I've always been married.

Zsa Zsa Gabor 'Sayings of the Week' *Observer* (16 Aug. 1987)

...the deep, deep peace of the double bed after the hurly-burly of the chaise-longue.

Mrs Patrick Campbell, quoted by Alexander Woollcott in *While Rome Burns* (1934)

It is easier to be a lover than a husband, for the same reason that it is more difficult to show a ready wit all day long than to produce an occasional bon mot.

Honoré de Balzac *The Physiology of Marriage* (1829)

The trouble with my wife is that she is a whore in the kitchen and a cook in bed.

Geoffrey Gorer *Exploring the English Character* (20th century)

Today the Duke returned from the wars and pleasured me twice in his topboots.

Duchess of Marlborough, in a letter (1700s)

For some married women sex has always been something to be endured rather than enjoyed:

I am happy now that Charles calls on my bedchamber less frequently than of old. As it is, I now endure but two calls a week and when I hear his steps outside my door I lie down on my bed, close my eyes, open my legs and think of England.

Lady Alice Hillingdon *Journal* (1912)

This quotation is sometimes, erroneously, attributed to Queen Victoria. In the 19th century it does seem to have been assumed that sexual relations were suffered by women to gratify the strange animal passion that only men experienced. Although Victorian ladies wanted (and had) babies, conceiving them was regarded as the unsavoury price to be paid for this pleasure:

She assured me that she felt no sexual passions whatever. Her passion for her husband was of a platonic kind, and far from wishing to stimulate his frigid feelings, she doubted whether it would be right or not. She loved him as he was, and would not desire him to be otherwise except for the hope of having a family. I believe this lady is the perfect ideal of an English wife and mother.

Dr William Acton *Functions and Disorders of the Re-productive organs* (1857)

Such an upbringing was designed to prepare a girl for the duties of wifehood, from which was notably absent any notion of active participation in her husband's sexual pleasure. During the height of the reign of prudery and suppression which dominated the America of the nineteenth century...there was a common assumption that women were more 'passive receptacles' that 'the full force of sexual desire' was seldom known to a virtuous woman.

Judith Armstrong *The Novel of Adultery* (1976)

Indeed, not only was sex undesirable, it could be positively dangerous:

Amative excesses, even in mature age, and under lawful conditions, produce exhaustion, and so cause disease. Good, pious, loving husbands and wives kill each other with kindness, make their lives wretched, and give birth to short-lived, suffering children.

T. L. Nicholls *Esoteric Anthropology* (1860)

Because of the prevalence of such attitudes amongst respectable Victorian women, many

19th-century husbands had to look elsewhere to find their pleasure:

In marital sexual relations it was often as incumbent upon men as it was upon women to conceal satisfaction in the act...He was compelled to recourse to prostitutes in order to enjoy sex without inhibition.

Glen Petrie *A Singular Iniquity* (1971)

However, there were exceptions. Here is the Rev. Charles Kingsley writing to his wife in 1843 to suggest that in heaven, perhaps, their sexual bliss would be uninterrupted:

A more perfect delight when we be naked in each other's arms clasped together toying with each other's limbs, buried in each other's bodies, struggling, panting, dying for a moment. Shall we not feel then, even then, that there is more in store for us, that those thrilling writhings are but dim shadows of a union which shall be perfect.

Quoted in S. Chitty *The Beast and the Monk: A Life of Charles Kingsley* (1974)

While the American spiritualist Ida Craddock believed that a sexual heaven on earth was available to those who accepted her doctrine of Social Purity:

The nude embrace comes to be respected more and more, and finally reverenced, as a pure and beautiful approach to the sacred moment when husband and wife shall melt into one another's genital embrace, so that the twain shall be one flesh, and then, as of old, God will walk with the twain in the garden of bliss 'in the cool of the day' when the heat of ill-regulated passion is no more.

Right Marital Living (1899)

Perhaps it was Marie Stopes who did more than any other person this century to re-establish marital sex as something that women, too, should enjoy:

It should be realized that a man does not woo and win a woman once and for all when he marries her: he must woo her before every separate act of coitus, for each act corresponds to a marriage.

Married Love (1918)

Certain problems appeared to be much more common among the genteel upper and middle classes:

The wide prevalence of premature ejaculation in British men of the professional and upper classes has surprised me. I have little evidence of its existence as a 'problem' in the homes of manual workers, and incline to think it much rarer than among the 'black-coated'. Among Public School and University men it is one of the marital difficulties oftenest brought to my notice.

Marie Stopes *Enduring Passion* (1928)

Another factor was simple ignorance of the physiology of reproduction and sex:

It has now become widely recognized that many applications for separation orders, in the early years of marriage particularly, are due to ignorance of the physical basis of marriage.

Secretary-General of the British Social Hygiene Council *Sunday Times* (12 May 1935)

A serious deterrent to free discussion of sex matters in marriage between doctor and prospective entrants, except those of the more educated classes, is the candidate's ignorance of simple anatomical and physiological terms. Whatever the Old Kent Road's equivalents of 'vagina' and 'orgasm' may be, the inhabitants are shy of using them to the doctor.

W. C. Fowler *Lancet* (1947)

If not knowing a great deal about human anatomy is one serious obstacle to a satisfying married life, not knowing anything at all about one's future spouse's sexual tastes is another. Until the sexual revolution of the late 20th century, young women were taught to see their virginity as their most treasured possession. Without it a girl was virtually unmarketable as a bride. This created a number of problems:

To keep one's self and/or one's suitors at a high pitch of emotional and sexual excite-

ment for five to ten years, from the beginning of dating to marriage, and meanwhile to abstain from coitus is, biologically speaking, a most unnatural as well as difficult task.

Paul Gebhard et al. *Pregnancy, Birth and Abortion,* Institute for Sex Research (1958)

One attempt to provide engaged couples with a chance to learn something about each other's sexual needs was the curious practice of bundling, formerly observed in many rural areas:

Bundling. *The curious and now obsolete New England custom of engaged couples going to bed together fully dressed and thus spending the night. It was a recognized proceeding to which no suggestion of impropriety was attached. The same custom existed in Wales and the remote parts of Scotland.*

Brewer's Dictionary of Phrase and Fable (1870)

The practice was not quite as innocent as this suggests:

The evidence in this case [Harris v. Lingard, 1699–1701] *allows us to find out exactly what happened during these all-night bundling sessions. A clear code of conduct was supposed to apply. Men were allowed to lie on the beds of women, but not get into bed with them without their permission. Once there, the men were allowed to fondle the women's breasts, and even their bellies, but not to touch their genitals. Much, if not all, of this activity took place in public, with sister, maid, and sometimes mother looking on, and occasionally in the same bed.*

Lawrence Stone *Uncertain Unions* (1992)

A bundling couple went to bed
with all their clothes, from foot to head,
that the defense might seem complete
each one was wrapped in a sheet.

But O! This bundling's such a witch,
The man of her did catch the itch,
And so provoked was the wretch
that she of him a bastard catch'd

'A New Bundling Song' (1785), quoted by H. R. Stiles in *Bundling: It's Origins etc.* (1869)

This unfortunate lady was by no means unique:

By the eighteenth century, however, the old moral controls on bundling were clearly breaking down, the proof being the rise in the bastardy rate between 1690 and 1790 from 6 to 20 per cent of all first births, and the even more startling explosion of pre-nuptial conceptions. By the late eighteenth century consummation and conception normally preceded – and indeed precipitated – marriage, as shown by the fact that a third of all brides were pregnant on their wedding day, and over half of all first births were conceived out of wedlock.

Lawrence Stone *Uncertain Unions* (1992)

If bundling prospective marriage partners with their clothes on is no longer fashionable, its unclothed equivalent is:

Pre-marital sexual experience is generally becoming more accepted, and is also a means of discovering whether or not couples are sexually compatible or not, without running the risk of pregnancy. On the whole, it is argued, this should make for better marriages, not worse ones.

Tony Lake and Ann Hills *Affairs* (1979)

Over eight in every ten births to some women under the age of 20 are outside marriage…the proportion of births outside marriage has more than doubled [over the last ten years] *to reach three in ten of all births…*

Social Trends, HMSO (1993)

Whether or not premarital sex makes for better marriages is an open question. It should, at least, prevent this kind of deception:

Any woman who shall impose upon, seduce, and betray into matrimony any of His Majesty's subjects by virtue of her scents, paints, cosmetic washes, artificial teeth, false hair, iron stays, hoops, high-heeled shoes, or bolstered hips, shall incur the penalty against witchcraft, and the marriage ...shall be null and void.

English Act of Parliament (17th century)

Not to mention this:

John Ferren, gent., sen., of St. Andrews, Holborn, br., and Deborah Nolan, ditto, spr. The supposed John Ferren was discovered after the ceremony was over to be in person a woman.

Entry in Fleet Marriage Register (1 Oct. 1747)

Even with the greater freedom to experiment permitted today, the problem of choosing the right spouse can remain acute. Here is some proverbial advice:

The first wife is matrimony, the second company, the third heresy.

Marry in haste, and repent at leisure.

Marry in May, rue for aye.

Marry in Lent, and you'll live to repent.

Who marrieth for love without money hath good nights and sorry days.

More helpful, perhaps, is the personal advice offered by writers through the ages, starting with the 'father of literature':

Lead a wife to thy hearthstone at the right age, neither much below nor much above thirty years. Such is the proper time to marry. A woman should marry in the fifth year after puberty. Marry a virgin, that thou mayst train her in discretion. Prefer one who dwells close by. But consider all her circumstances well beforehand, lest after marriage thou become a laughing-stock to thy neighbours. There is no better stroke of luck for a man than a good wife and no worse fate than a bad one.

Hesiod *Works and Days* (8th century BC)

This carpenter had married a new wife
Not long before, and loved her more than life.
She was a girl of eighteen years of age.
Jealous he was an kept her in a cage,
For he was old and she was wild and young;
He thought himself quite likely to be stung.
He might have known, were Cato on his shelf,
A man should marry someone like himself;
A man should pick an equal for his mate.
Youth and age are often in debate.
However, he had fallen in the snare,
And he had to bear the cross as others bare.

Geoffrey Chaucer *The Canterbury Tales*
'The Miller's Tale' (late 14th century)

Furthermore, in choosing wives and husbands, they [the Utopians] *observe earnestly and straightly a custom which seemed to us very fond and foolish. For a grave and honest matron sheweth the woman, be she maid or widow, naked to her wooer: and likewise a sage and discreet man exhibiteth the wooer naked to the woman. At this custom we laughed, and disallowed it as foolish. But they, on the other part, do greatly wonder at the folly of other nations, which in* buying a colt *(whereas a little money is in hazard) be so chary and circumspect, that though he be almost all bare, yet will not buy him, unless the saddle and all the harness be taken off – least under those coverings be hid some gall or sore. And yet in* choosing a wife, *which shall be a pleasure or displeasure to them all their life after, they be so reckless, that all the residue of the woman's body being covered by clothes, they esteem her scarcely by one hand breadth (for they can see no more but her face)...*

Sir Thomas More *Utopia* (1516)

The ten properties of a woman: Ye.i. is to be merry of chere, ye.ii. to be wel placed, ye.iii. to haue a broad forhed, ye.iiii. to haue brod buttocks, ye.v. to be hard of ward, ye.vi. to be easy to leap upon, ye.vii. to be good at long journey, ye.viii. to be wel sturring under a man, ye.ix. to be always busy wt ye mouth, ye.x. euer to be chewing on ye bridle.

Fitzherbert's *Boke of Husbandry* (1568)

He was reputed one of the wise men, that made answer to the question, when a man should marry? A young man not yet, an elder man not at all.

Francis Bacon *Essays* 'Of Marriage and Single Life' (1625)

He that get a wench with child and marry her afterwards is as if a man should shit in his hat and then clap it on his head.

Samuel Pepys *Diary* (1663)

No man should marry until he has studied anatomy and dissected at least one woman.

Honoré de Balzac *La Physiologie du Mariage* (1829)

To marry a man out of pity is folly; and, if you think you are going to influence the kind of fellow who has 'never had a chance, poor devil', you are profoundly mistaken. One can only influence the strong characters in life, not the weak; and it is the height of vanity to suppose that you can make an honest man of anyone.

Margot Asquith *The Autobiography of Margot Asquith* (1922)

The prerequisite for a good marriage is the licence to be unfaithful.

Carl Jung *Memories, Dreams, Reflections* (1962)

The married state can lead to extremes of joy and misery:

More than any other form of relationship, marriage carries our hopes for a warm, fulfilling, safe, confiding, mentally and physically satisfying bond with another person. Yet in practice marriage causes more bitterness, resentment, disappointment and inarticulate pain than all our other 'relationships' put together. For countless people, what is confidently embarked upon as an exclusive mutual alliance against an indifferent or hostile world, a search for a haven of warmth in a cold and competitive society, turns out to be a journey into a totally unexpected, private and unanalysable hell...

David Smail *An Alternative to Therapy* (1987)

Unfortunately, it does not seem that the greater acceptance of prenuptial experiment in our own day has led to happier or more stable marriages. In the UK, the number of divorces increased sixfold between 1961 and 1990. On the other hand:

If one adopts the reasonable criteria of durability, marriages in the mid twentieth century were more stable than at any other time in history. Indeed it looks very much as if modern divorce is little more than a functionable substitute for death. The decline of the adult mortality rate after the 17th Century, by prolonging the expected duration of marriage to unprecedented lengths, eventually forced Western society to adopt the institutional escape hatch of divorce.

Lawrence Stone *The Family, Sex and Marriage in England 1500–1800* (1977)

As recently as the last century bad marriages could be remedied very simply in some rural cultures:

Samuel Whitehouse, of the parish of Willenhall, in the county of Stafford, this day sold his wife, Mary Whitehouse, in open market, to Thomas Griffiths, of Birmingham, value one shilling. To take her with all faults.

Entry in the register of the Bell Inn, Birmingham (31 Aug. 1773)

Moreover, even in the late 20th century:

Marriage still remained the most holy of institutions in America; even the rising rate of divorce seemed chiefly to be for the purpose of remarriage.

Andrew Sinclair *The Better Half: The Emancipation of the American Woman* (1965)

And a further point, the importance of which can hardly be overestimated when one thinks of the devastation that is inflicted on the lives of young children when their parents divorce:

We ought to recognize the childless marriage as a separate thing from the procreative marriage, instead of stupidly treating them as if they were one and the same thing. We ought to recognize that regulations which are perfectly reasonable in the one are absurd and irrational in the other.

Judge Ben Lindsey *The Companionate Marriage* (1953)

Perhaps the last word should go to the cynics, however:

There are only two days on which a woman can refresh thee, on the day of marriage and when she is buried.

Hipponax of Ephesus (*c* 540 BC)

There is no heaven but women, nor no hell save marriage.

Thomas Webbe (1660s)

How happy a thing were a wedding
And a bedding,
If a man might purchase a wife
For twelve month, and a day;
But to live with her all a man's life
For ever and ay,
'Til she grow as grey as a Cat,
Good faith, Mr Parson, I thank you for that.

Thomas Flatman *The Batchelor's Song* (1674)

Many a man wants a wife, but more want to get rid of one.

Henry Fielding *Don Quixote in England* (1734)

There's doubtless something in domestic doings
Which forms, in fact, true love's antithesis;
Romances paint at full length people's wooings,
But only give a bust of marriages;
For no one cares for matrimonial cooings,
There's nothing wrong in a connubial kiss:
Think you, if Laura had been Petrarch's wife,
He would have written sonnets all his life?

Lord Byron *Don Juan* (1819–24)

Marriage is essentially rather to be termed a tragic condition than a happy condition.

H. Havelock Ellis *Sex in Relation to Society* (1920s)

I married beneath me, all women do.

Nancy Astor, quoted in *The Dictionary of National Biography* (1901)

A man in love is incomplete until he has married. Then he is finished.

Zsa Zsa Gabor *Newsweek* (28 Mar 1960)

If women are to effect a significant amelioration in their condition, it seems obvious that they must refuse to marry.

Germaine Greer *The Female Eunuch* (1971)

Few men are naturally monogamous to the extent that they can be satisfied with one women all their lives.

Graham Masterton (1975)

Marriage *n. The state or condition of a community consisting of a master, a mistress and two slaves, making in all, two.*

Ambrose Bierce *The Devil's Dictionary* (1911)

Masturbation

Masturbation is also known as onanism or the sin of Onan. Onan was a character in the Old Testament who was urged by his father, Judah, to have intercourse with the widow of his brother Er, in accordance with the levirate law (from Latin *levir*, a brother-in-law).

> *And Onan knew that the seed should not be his; and it came to pass, when he went in unto his brother's wife, that he spilled it on the ground, lest that he should give seed to his brother.*
>
> Genesis 38:9

This obscure phrase to 'give seed to his brother' refers to the levirate teaching that any sons born of such a union would be regarded as sons of the dead brother. Onan, unwilling to be a party to this practice, refused to make his brother's wife pregnant.

> *Onan's device was not auto-erotic, but an early example of withdrawal before emission, or coitus interruptus.*
>
> H. Havelock Ellis *The Psychology of Sex* (1933)

In a desert community in which the men had as many wives as they needed to produce as many sons as they could, both withdrawal before emission and masturbation would be seen as a waste of a most valuable human resource. As a Latin poet later put it:

> *What you are losing between your fingers, Ponticus, is a human being.*
>
> Martial (1st century AD)

Whatever the precise nature of Onan's offence, he had broken the levirate law:

> *And the thing which he did displeased the LORD: wherefore he slew him also.*
>
> Genesis 38:10

That was the end of Onan – until he cropped up a few thousand years later as the name of Dorothy Parker's canary (so called, she claimed, because of *his* habit of spilling his seed on the ground).

It was not, however, the end of the view that masturbation was in some way wrong. This has persisted throughout the Christian era. For most Christians any form of sexual satisfaction outside marriage is regarded as sinful:

> *Be not deceived: neither fornicators...nor effeminate, nor abusers of themselves...shall inherit the kingdom of God.*
>
> I Corinthians 6: 9–10

It was St Paul, probably more than anyone else, who was responsible for converting the desert frugality of the Old Testament into two thousand years of Christian sexual guilt. By the 19th century it was firmly established as a part of the Christian ethos that masturbation – usually disparagingly called self-abuse – was both sinful and dangerous.

> *Onanism is a frequent accompaniment of insanity and sometimes causes it.*
>
> Bucknill and Tuke *Psychological Medicine* (1878)

> *Masturbation may be a forerunner of mania, of dementia and even of senile dementia; it leads to melancholy and suicide; its consequences are more serious in men than in women: it is a grave obstacle to cure in those of the insane who frequently resort to it during their illness... Masturbation is recognized in all countries as a common cause of insanity.*
>
> Jean Etienne Esquirol *Des Maladies mentales* (1838)

Masturbation produces seminal weakness, impotence, dysury, tabes dorsalis, pulmonary consumption, dyspepsia, dimness of sight, vertigo, epilepsy, hypochondriasis, loss of memory, managlia, fatuity, and death.

Benjamin Rush *Medical Inquiries and Observations upon Diseases of the Mind* (1812)

Neither plague, nor war, nor smallpox, nor a crowd of similar evils, have resulted more disastrously for humanity than the habit of masturbation: it is the destroying element of civilized society.

Editorial, *New Orleans Medical & Surgical Journal* (1850)

Solitary vice is dangerous and deplorable because it was learnt, not instinctual. Boys are innocent of masturbation until inspired to foul practices by other boys who spread corruption through the school.

Rev. Edward Lyttelton *Prevention of Immorality in Schools* (1887)

Talk in the dormitories and the studies [at Harrow School] *was incredibly obscene. Here and there one could not avoid seeing acts of onanism, mutual masturbation, the sports of naked boys in bed together. There was no refinement, no sentiment, no passion; nothing but animal lust in these occurrences. They filled me with disgust and loathing.*

John Addington Symonds *Memoirs*, 'Harrow in 1854' (ed. Phyllis Grosskurth; 1984)

It is called in our schools 'beastliness', and this is about the best name for it...should it become a habit it quickly destroys both health and spirits; he becomes feeble in body and mind, and often ends in a lunatic asylum.

Robert Baden-Powell *Scouting for Boys* (1908)

It cheats semen getting its full chance of making up the strong manly man you would otherwise be. You are throwing away the seed that has been handed down to you as a trust instead of keeping it and ripening it for bringing a son to you later on.

Robert Baden-Powell *Rovering to Success* (1922)

Naturally enough for a young Victorian, he [Gerard Manley Hopkins] *thought of sins as largely sexual, and the most recurrent he recorded were concerned with masturbation. So painfully did it nag at his conscience that he used a repetitive abbreviation, 'O.H.' to indicate when he had fallen into old habits; the phrase seems to have been used both for completed masturbation and for stimulating acts not followed by climax. Even nocturnal emissions seemed sinful, particularly when, as he indicated, they occurred in half-sleep or in the morning. At the end of his journal he made a recapitulation of his involuntary emissions, obviously not quite believing they could be innocent. The obsession would verge on the comic if it were not so patently agonizing to him.*

Robert Bernard Martin *Gerard Manley Hopkins: A Very Private Life* (1991)

The Victorians were so appalled by the idea of masturbation, that extreme measures were often taken to effect a 'cure':

The prepuce is drawn well-forward, the left forefinger inserted within it down to the root of the glans, and a nickel plated safety pin introduced from the outside through the skin and mucous membrane, is passed horizontally for half an inch or so past the tip of the left finger and then brought out through the mucous membrane and skin so as to fasten from the outside. Another pin is similarly fixed on the opposite side of the prepuce. With the foreskin looped up, any attempt at erection causes painful dragging on the pins and masturbation is effectually prevented. In about a week some ulceration of the mucous membrane will allow greater movement and will cause less pain...but the patient is already convinced that masturbation is not necessary to his existence, and a moral as well as a material victory has been gained.

F. R. Sturgis *Treatment of Masturbation* (1900)

During the course of the post-Christian 20th century this view has gradually changed. But the psychiatrists have not been all of one mind:

It sometimes happens that in boys the first excitation of the sexual instinct is caused by a spanking, and they are thus incited to masturbation. This should be remembered by those who have the care of children.

Richard von Krafft-Ebing *Psychopathia Sexualis* (1886)

Masturbation occasions a heavy burden of guilt, because in the unconscious mind it always represents aggression against someone.

Karl Menninger *Man Against Himself* (1938)

A married lady who is a leader in the social purity movements and enthusiast for sexual chastity, discovered through reading some pamphlets against solitary vice that she herself had been practising masturbation for years without knowing it. The profound anguish and hopeless despair of this woman in the face of what she believed to be the moral ruin of her whole life cannot well be described.

H. Havelock Ellis *The Psychology of Sex* (1933)

Freud tended to the view that neurasthenia could follow upon excessive masturbation: it is nowadays felt that it would be more correct to say that neurasthenia is an outcome of insufficient orgasm, if anxieties and guilt disturb the satisfactory character of the masturbation.

Robert J. Campbell *Psychiatric Dictionary* (1940)

And even D. H. Lawrence, often considered the early 20th-century high-priest of liberated sex, was against it:

Instead of being a comparatively pure and harmless vice, masturbation is certainly the most dangerous sexual vice that a society can be afflicted with, in the long run...But in masturbation there is nothing but loss. There is no reciprocity. There is merely the spending away of a certain force, and no return. The body remains, in a sense, a corpse, after the act of self-abuse. There is no change, only deadening.

D. H. Lawrence *Pornography and Obscenity* (1929)

However, since the war there has been a volte-face:

A 1979 survey, sponsored by the American Academy of Family Physicians, with 900 physicians responding – revealed that 2 per cent of the doctors believed that masturbation caused 'physical harm'.

American Medical News (6 July 1979)

Masturbation: the primary sexual activity of mankind. In the 19th century it was a disease: in the 20th century, it's a cure.

Thomas Szasz (1946)

Masturbation: the preferred mode of sexual gratification for those who prefer the imaginary to the real...Masturbation is more a matter of self-control than of self-love.

Thomas Szasz *The Second Sin* (1973)

Today, there are parents who are alarmed when they discover that their adolescent boy is not masturbating. Several parents who have consulted me about such adolescents are quite concerned that the young person's sexual development is not proceeding normally.

Abram Kardiner *Sex and Morality* (1955)

You know, you might think me weird or crazy, but I have often masturbated my male patients. It seems to calm them and they sleep better, especially the older men. I usually do this for men who cannot do it for themselves. It is a sort of charity.

American nurse, quoted by Roy Eskapa in *Bizarre Sex* (1987) which is reminiscent of an earlier physician who administered masturbation as a cure for hysteria:

Following the warmth of the remedies and arising from the touch of the genital required by the treatment, there followed twitchings accompanied at the same time by pain and pleasure after which she emitted turbid and abundant secretions. From that time on she was freed of all the evil she felt.

Galen (2nd century)

The Roman Catholic Church does not, however, share the medical view. Its primary teaching body, the Magisterium, was still quite certain of its ground in the mid-1970s:

both the Magisterium of the Church...and the moral sense of the faithful have declared without hesitation that masturbation is an intrinsically and seriously disordered act...Even if it cannot be proved that scripture condemns this sin by name, the tradition of the Church has rightly understood it to be condemned in the New Testament when the latter speaks of 'impurity', 'unchasteness' and other vices contrary to chastity.

Sacred Congregation for the Doctrine of the Faith *Declaration on Certain Questions Concerning Sexual Ethics (1975)*

The truth about the incidence of masturbation was finally revealed by Alfred Kinsey, an American biologist who became director of the Indiana University Institute of Sex Research:

Out of a total of 5300 white American males questioned, 92% admitted to masturbating.

Alfred Kinsey et al. *Sexual Behaviour in the Human Male* (1948)

More recent studies have indicated that the figure is closer to 100%. However, Kinsey had confined his study to men. Attitudes to female sexuality, at this time, were still tainted with the Old Testament view that the sexual life of a woman was an accessory to the procreative needs of a man. Kinsey changed this with his second study:

Out of a total of 5940 white American women questioned, 62% admitted to masturbating...
We have recognised very few cases, if indeed there have been any outside of a few psychotics, in which either physical or mental damage had resulted from masturbatory activity.

Alfred Kinsey et al. *Sexual Behaviour in the Human Female* (1953)

Later research has established that a considerable number of the women questioned were too ashamed to admit to masturbating, believing that their solitary sexual exploits were unique. Shere Hite, another American sexologist, found a higher percentage:

Of 1844 women questioned 82% said they masturbated, 3% did not answer, and 15% said they did not masturbate.

Shere Hite *The Hite Report* (1976)

Some further quotations from the Hite Report reveal that for some women the practice has no associated guilt:

Masturbation seems to have so much to recommend it – easy and intense orgasms, an unending source of pleasure...

Nor does the masturbator have to be a teenager:

Yes, I enjoy masturbation...But it is for physical reasons, these days, and also during periods when my lover would be away. At present, I am getting old (age sixty), and I masturbate as a matter of course when I feel the need of it.

But for others the guilt has persisted:

At about eight I made a very feeble attempt at masturbation, at which I was caught by my mother, who gave me a very long lecture on how this would cause me to become insane. This was my last attempt at masturbation until seven years ago, when I had my first orgasm, I am now fifty-one.

One telling comment on masturbation in women:

Girls can have orgasms 100 per cent of the time, but only when they're on their own.

Cathy Hopkins *Girl Chasing – How to Improve Your Game* (1989)

before a few poetic effusions in praise of dildoes of one sort or another:

Just at sixteen her breasts began to heave...
Yet scarce knows what the titillation means.
All night she thinks on Man, both toils and sweats,
And dreaming frigs, and spends upon the sheets;
But never knew the more substantial bliss,
And scarce e'er touched a man, but by a kiss.
Her virgin cunt ne'er knew the joys of love
Beyond what dildoes or her finger gave...
Come this way, I've a pretty engine here,
Which us'd to ease the torments of the fair;
This dildo 'tis, with which I oft was wont
T'assuage the raging of my lustful cunt.
For when cunts swell, and glow with strong desire,
'Tis only pricks can quench the lustful fire;
And when that's wanting, dildoes must supply
The place of pricks upon necessity.

Johannes Meursius *The Delights of Venus* (17th century)

Twelve dildoes meant for the support
Of aged lechers of the Court...
Some were composed of shining horns,
More precious than the unicorn's.
Some were of wax, where ev'ry vein,
And smallest fibre were made plain,
Some were for tender virgins fit,
Some for the large falacious slit,
Of a rank lady, tho' so torn,
She hardly feels when child is born.

Samuel Butler 'Dildoides' (17th century)

I love my little cucumber
So long, so firm, so straight,
So sad, my little cucumber,
We cannot propagate.

Anon. poem in *Top Priority* (ed. S. Walsh; 1891)

One does not have to be Christian, however, to feel guilty about sex.

In medieval times, Jewish elders declared masturbation to be a heinous crime. According to the strictest Orthodox rules, men should not even touch their penises; even while urinating a man was required to direct his penis by lifting the scrotum. Women were allowed to examine their own genitals, but only to detect how close they were to their periods.

Roy Eskapa *Bizarre Sex* (1987)

Better bad aim than bad habits.

Jewish potty-training slogan, quoted by Thomas Szasz in *Sex: Facts Frauds and Follies* (1980)

Thou shalt not practise masturbation either with hand or with foot.

Talmud

In the USSR masturbation is a stigma of moral dissoluteness and at the same time a survival of, or something introduced from, bourgeois society. This prejudice is not only held by psychologists and doctors which would be a lesser evil, but it is also shared by the great bulk of Soviet people, which produces, one suspects, absurd and tragic conflicts.
One of my patients requested a divorce when he learned that his wife masturbated...as a child.

Stern and Stern *Sex in the Soviet Union* (1981)

Nor do you have to be heterosexual:

Most homosexuals find their man-to-man sex unfulfilling so they masturbate a lot...Carrots and cucumbers are pressed into service...Sometimes the whole egg in the shell finds itself where it doesn't be-

long. Sausages, especially the milder varieties, are popular. The homosexual who prefers to use his penis must find an anus. Many look in the refrigerator. The most common masturbatory object for this purpose is a melon. Cantaloupes are usual, but where it is available, papaya is popular.

Dr David Reuben *Everything You Always Wanted to Know About Sex, But Were Afraid to Ask* (1969)

Whether it makes you feel guilty or not, it is now something that can be openly joked about:

When you wake up in the morning and you're feeling grand,
And you've such a funny feeling in your seminary gland,
And you haven't got a woman — what's the matter with your hand
As you revel in the joys of copulation.

'Cats on the Rooftops', marching song sung by British troops during World War I to the tune of 'Do ye ken John Peel'

Masturbation is the thinking man's television.

Christopher Hampton *The Philanthropist* (1970)

WOMAN *You are the greatest lover I have ever known.*
WOODY ALLEN *Well, I practice a lot when I'm on my own.*

Love and Death (1975)

Don't knock it, it's sex with someone you love.

Woody Allen *Annie Hall* (1975)

Which is a more explicit rendering of Oscar Wilde's:

To love oneself is the beginning of a lifelong romance.

In February 1976, the Appeal Court upheld convictions on two men convicted of gross indecency with each other where the evidence was that policemen in a public lavatory in Hereford had peeped under the doors of two adjoining cubicles and seen two men each masturbating in their own cubicle but looking at the other through a hole in the intervening wall. What a way to earn your living!

Fenton Bresler *Sex and the Law* (1988)

The debating society at my school was discussing the motion 'That the present generation has lost the ability to entertain itself'. Rising to make my maiden speech, I said with shaky aplomb, "Mr. Chairman – as long as masturbation exists, no one can seriously maintain that we have lost the ability to entertain ourselves." The teacher in charge immediately closed the meeting.

Kenneth Tynan

Masturbation, for most men and women, is now out of the closet:

It would take the seriousness out of things like the Bay of Pigs or the Cuban Missile Crisis if you could just imagine JFK in the back of the bathroom door whacking it to Miss July once in a while.

Lenny Bruce, quoted by Earl Wilson in *The Showbusiness Nobody Knows* (1966)

We're all wankers underneath...if we were honest about ourselves we'd know we're all wankers under the table...I'm a wanker, I have known the pleasures of the palm...Why can't we be honest? Once we acknowledge everyone's a wanker it'll be easy – suddenly all authority figures disappear. You've got a bank manager, right, won't give you a ten quid overdraft. Look him in the eye – you're a wanker aren't you? All world leaders — Gorbachov – wanker; Pope – wanker; even Mrs Thatch must occasionally slip the claw under the elastic. All world leaders — Churchill – wanker; Napoleon – wanker...Until we come to terms with how small and irrationally paranoid we are – how scared of our feelings, how scared of our functions we are...we've got to remember that the people who lead us are just as farty as us – the people who destroy the environment – they're just gits like us – they think they're Gods...

Ben Elton (1990)

Masturbation has featured prominently in several works of literature, most notably in Philip Roth's *Portnoy's Complaint*, in which a young Jewish New Yorker gives his psychiatrist a hilarious account of the guilt his mother has made him feel:

> *Doctor Spielvogel, this is my life, my only life, and I'm living it in the middle of a Jewish Joke! I am the son in the Jewish joke – only it ain't no joke! Please, who crippled us like this? Who made us so morbid and hysterical and weak?...why, alone on my bed in New York, why am I still hopelessly beating my meat? Doctor, what do you call this sickness I have? Is this the Jewish suffering I used to hear so much about? Is this what has come down to me from the pogroms and the persecution?...Oh my secrets, my shame, my palpitations, my flushes, my sweats!...Doctor, I can't stand any more being frightened like this over nothing! Bless me with manhood! Make me brave! Make me strong! Make me whole! Enough being a nice Jewish boy, publicly pleasing my parents while privately pulling my putz! Enough!...*
> *I believe that I have already confessed to the piece of liver that I bought in a butcher shop and banged behind a billboard on the way to a barmitzvah lesson...That-she-it wasn't my first piece. My first piece I had in the privacy of my own home, rolled around my cock in the bathroom at three-thirty – and then again on the end of a fork, at five-thirty...So. Now you know the worst thing I have ever done. I fucked my own family's dinner.*

Philip Roth *Portnoy's Complaint* (1967)

> *I lie back on the bed and haul up my dress. Yank down my bloomers. Stick the looking glass tween my legs. Ugh. All that hair. Then my pussy lips be black. Then inside look like a wet rose.*
> *It a lot prettier than you thought, ain't it? she say from the door.*
> *It mine, I say. Where the button?*
> *Right up near the top, she say. The part that stick out a little.*
> *I look at her and touch it with my finger. A little shiver go through me. Nothing much. But just enough to tell me this the right button to mash. Maybe.*

Alice Walker *The Color Purple* (1983)

> *If I touched myself, you'd get excited and then you'd make love to me?*
> *Chance did not understand. 'I would like to watch you,' he repeated...*
> *She returned to the bed. She stretched out on her back and let her hand run over her body; languidly, she crept froglike toward her belly. She swayed back and forth and shoved her body from side to side as if it were pricked by rough grass. Her fingers caressed her breasts, buttocks, thighs. In a quick motion, her legs and arms wrapped around Chance like a web of sprawling branches. She shook violently: a delicate tremor ran through her. She no longer stirred; she was half-asleep.*

Jerzy Kosinski *Being There* (1971)

> *A perverse nature can be stimulated by anything. Any book can be used as a pornographic instrument, even a great work of literature if the mind that so uses it is off-balance. I once found a small boy masturbating in the presence of the Victorian steel-engraving in a family Bible.*

Anthony Burgess *A Clockwork Orange* (1962)

Here, the son of a Lowestoft fisherman recalls his boyhood before World War I:

> *Another boy took out his large cock, the first I'd seen with hair round it, spat in his hand, and started to masturbate in the proper manner. After a minute or two he said he was tired and asked me to do it for him, which I did with pleasure. Thus began one of the happiest periods of my life; the real beginning of my happy life; the first awakening to knowledge of the pleasure and warmth in other people's bodies and affection; the realization that physical contact consolidates and increases the pleasure and happiness to be*

got from mutual affection...It was all open and uncomplicated...Whenever in our wanderings we came to a secret place, a wood, a shed or a deserted building, we would merrily wank away...Nowadays, for some reason or other, this traditional experience is thought to be undesirable...We continued happily and unworried for a long time, until the sort of people one finds in the fringes of church life, noticing the dark rings under our eyes, warned us that boys who played with themselves went mad and had to be locked away. This was a typical mean, dirty-minded trick, for they had been boys themselves and knew it was not true. In any case it didn't stop us. Henceforth we wanked and worried, whereas formerly we had experienced nothing but satisfaction and contentment.

Harry Daley *The Small Cloud* (1986)

Sylvia, the fair, in the bloom of fifteen,
Felt an innocent warmth as she lay on the green;
She had heard of a pleasure, and something she guessed
By the towzing, and tumbling, and touching her breast.

John Dryden 'Sylvia the Fair' (1699)

In his *On the Science of Onanism* (1879), Mark Twain attributed a number of satirical comments about masturbation to various historical characters:

Give me masturbation or give me death.

(Homer)

To the lonely it is company, to the forsaken it is a friend; to the aged and to the impotent it is a benefactor; they that are penniless are yet rich, in that they still have this majestic diversion.

(Julius Caesar)

Self-negation is noble, self-culture is beneficent, self-possession is manly, but to the truly grand and inspiring soul they are poor and tame compared to self-abuse.

(Michelangelo)

It is the bulwark of virginity.

(Elizabeth I)

But perhaps the last word should go to Diogenes:

I wish to heaven, that I could satisfy my hunger when my stomach barks for food by rubbing it.

Modesty

Most cultures have agreed that a degree of sexual reserve is admirable or attractive in women:

> *The one who is distinguished for beauty is considered less worth desiring than one renowned for modesty.*
>
> Ephoros of Cyme *History of the Greeks* (4th century BC)

The concept of modesty is rarely introduced into discussions of male behaviour, being seen as an intrinsically female quality. For some writers – mostly but not exclusively male – modesty is such an essential aspect of femininity that the woman who tries to do without it risks losing any claim to respect:

> *And if we consider Modesty in this sense, we shall find it the most indispensible requisite of a woman; a thing so essential and natural to the sex, that even the least declination from it, is a proportional receding from womanhood, but the total abandoning of it ranks them among brutes, nay sets them as far beneath those, as an aquir'd vileness is below a native. I need make no collection of the verdicts either of the Philosophers or Divines in the case, it being so much an instinct of nature, that tho too many make a shift to suppress it in themselves, yet they cannot so darken the notion in others, but that an Impudent woman is lookt on as a kind of monster; a thing diverted and distorted from its proper form.*
>
> Richard Allestree *The Ladies' Calling* (17th century)

> *Chastity, perfect modesty, in word, deed and even thought, is so essential, that, without it, no female is fit to be a wife. It is not enough that a young female abstain from everything approaching towards indecorum in her behaviour towards men; it is, with me, not enough, that she cast down her eyes, or turn aside her head with a smile, when she hears an indelicate allusion; she ought to appear not to understand it, and to receive from it no more impression than if she were a post.*
>
> William Cobbett *Advice to Young Men* (1829)

There are, however, mixed opinions as to whether modesty is a natural quality in women or the product of conditioning. Many have taken the former view:

> *Modesty is the companion of Virtue, it always resides in a mind naturally Pure, it prevents us from observing indelicate occurrences, it will not permit us to listen to improper conversation.*
>
> Wilmot Serres *Olivia's Letter of Advice to Her Daughter* (1808)

> *Though Louisa is the most remote from prudery, of any woman I know, easy and accessible to the other sex, and cheerful, lively and unconstrained, in her conversation with them, yet she really has so great a share of true, female delicacy, that the most licentious man living would not dare to use a double entendre in her company, or give the conversation an improper turn. Nor is it, that she has reduced rules of propriety to a system. She has really a native feeling, which vibrates to the most distant touch of what is proper and be-*

coming, and would tremble, like the sensitive plant, where any thing, that could strain the delicacy of her mind, was conveyed in the most distant allusion.

Rev. John Bennet *Letters to a Young Lady* (1789)

Others feel that modesty needs to be taught:

Even if it could be denied that a special feeling of pudeur was natural to women, would it be any the less true that, in society, their lot ought to be a domestic and retired life, and that they ought to be raised in principles that suit it? If the timidity, pudeur, and modestie which are proper to them are social inventions, it is essential for society that women acquire these qualities; it is essential that they be cultivated in women, and any woman who disowns them offends good morals.

Jean-Jacques Rousseau *Emile, ou de l'Education* (1762)

The Multitude will hardly believe the excessive Force of Education, and in the difference of Modesty between Men and Women ascribe that to Nature, which is altogether owing to early instruction: Miss is scarce three Years old, but she is spoke to every Day to hide her leg, and rebuk'd in good earnest if she shows it; while Little Master at the same Age is bid to take up his coats, and piss like a man.

Bernard Mandeville *The Fable of the Bees: or Private Vices, Publick Benefits* (1723)

To characterize any account of modesty as conventional is not to say that it is simple. Writers of popular conduct books and philosophers alike long insisted on the importance of female modesty, even as they contradicted one another – and themselves – on the nature of virtue. It is a commonplace of the advice literature that the women's modesty is instinctive, but the very existence of the literature testifies to the belief that the 'instinct' must be elaborately codified and endlessly discussed: woman's 'natural' modesty must be strenuously cultivated that argument goes, lest both sexes fall victim to her natural lust.

Ruth Bernard Yeazell *Fictions of Modesty* (1991)

Although there is probably an instinctive element to sexual shyness (in both men and women), conventions of modesty differ widely from one culture to another. As one English anthropologist noted of his experiences in Africa:

In this land of nudity, which I have known for seven years, I do not remember once having seen an indecent gesture on the part of either man or woman... It may safely be asserted that the negro race in Central Africa is much more truly modest, is much more free from vice, than are most European nations.

H. H. Johnston *British Central Africa* (1897)

In some remote regions of Islam it is said, a woman caught unveiled by a stranger will raise her skirt to cover her face.

Raymond Mortimer *Colette* (20th century)

In large parts of the Islamic world rigid notions of female modesty have been enshrined in law. Offenders can expect severe punishment; in some countries male vigilantes are permitted to administer an on-the-spot beating without trial.

In Saudi Arabia, the strictest Islamic country, a form of sexual apartheid is imposed in which women are never permitted to be seen by a man who is not a member of the immediate family... Under Saudi law, the veil must be kept on at all times; some women do not even remove them to sleep.

The Times (19 Aug. 1992)

Yet in recent years many Westernized Muslim women have voluntarily adopted the veil for a variety of cultural and personal reasons:

Veiling among young Muslim women may be a statement of identity in a hostile and racist world... For some young Asian women it may also be a form of rebellion against the commercialisation of women's bodies in Western culture, a stand taken against pornography, sexual harassment and rape. Enveloped in a veil or with their hair hidden by a scarf, robes down to their ankles, women believe that they avoid being a sex object.

The Times (19 Aug. 1992)

Many writers have argued that the conventions of female modesty serve to incite as much as to repel male desire. A degree of reserve, it is claimed, makes the relations between men and women more exciting, adding a frisson to the art of seduction:

Courtship resembles very closely, indeed, a drama or game; the aggressiveness of the male, the coyness of the female, are alike unconsciously assured in order to bring about in the most effectual manner the ultimate union of the sexes. The seeming reluctance of the female is not intended to inhibit sexual activity either in the male or in herself, but to increase it in both. The passivity of the female, therefore, is not a real, but only an apparent passivity, and this holds true of our own species as much as of lower animals.

H. Havelock Ellis *Studies in the Psychology of Sex* (1936)

The maid, who modestly conceals
Her beauties, while she hides, reveals;
Give but a glimpse, and fancy draws
Whate'er the Grecian Venus was.
From Eve's first fig-leaf to brocade,
All dress was meant for fancy's aid,
Which evermore delighted dwells
On what bashful nymph conceals.

Edward Moore *Fables for the Female Sex* (1744)

The pleasures and frustrations of anticipated gratification have inspired a good deal of poetry:

Doing, a filthy pleasure is, and short;
And done, we straight repent us of the sport:
Let us not then rush blindly on unto it,
Like lustful beasts, that only know to do it:
For lust will languish, and that heat decay.
But thus, thus, keeping endless holiday,
Let us together closely lie and kiss,
There is no labour, no shame in this:
This hath pleased, doth please, and long will please, never
Can this decay, but is beginning ever.

Petronius *Satyricon* (1st century AD)

Had we but world enough, and time,
This coyness, Lady, were no crime,
We would sit down and think which way
To walk and pass our long love's day.
Thou by the Indian Ganges' side
Shouldst rubies find: I by the tide
Of Humber would complain. I would
Love you ten years before the Flood.
And you should, if you please, refuse
Till the conversion of the Jews.

Andrew Marvell 'To His Coy Mistress' (17th century)

Mark but this flea, and mark in this,
How little that which thou deny'st me is;
Me it sucked first, and now sucks thee,
And in this flea, our two bloods mingled be:
Confess it, this cannot be said
A sin, or shame, or loss of maidenhead,
Yet this enjoys before it woo,
And pampered swells with one blood made of two,
And this, alas, is more than we would do.

John Donne 'The Flea' (1633)

She felt my lips' impassioned touch –
'Twas the first time I dared so much,
And yet she chid not;
But whispered o'er my burning brow,
'Oh, do you doubt I love you now?'
Sweet soul! I did not.

Warmly I felt her bosom thrill,
I pressed it closer, closer still,
Though gently bid not;
Till – oh! the world hath seldom heard
Of lovers, who, so nearly erred,
And yet, who did not.

Thomas Moore 'Did Not' (19th century)

"I saw you take his kiss!" "'Tis true".
"O, modesty!" "'Twas strictly kept:
He thought me asleep; at least I knew
He thought I thought he thought I slept."

Coventry Patmore 'The Kiss' (19th century)

Some have taken a frankly cynical attitude:

Since maids, in modesty, say 'No' to that
Which they would have the profferer construe 'Ay'.

William Shakespeare *The Two Gentlemen of Verona* (*c.* 1594)

Let those who never tried, believe
In woman's chastity!
Let her who ne'er was asked, receive
The praise of modesty!

Anon. (19th century)

Historically, women have had to tread a difficult line between being considered too forward on the one hand and absurdly or hypocritically prudish on the other:

Safe, in the golden Mean, with Caution steer,
Fair Nymph, nor be too gay, nor too austere;
Distant, as far from Prude, as from Coquet,
Form your Deportment between both compleat.

Thomas Marriott *Female Conduct: Being an Essay on the Art of Pleasing. To be Practised by the Fair Sex, Before, and After, Marriage* (1759)

Excessive modesty is always open to ridicule:

She might not have had the bearing of a queen, but she exuded such sensuality in every department – eyes so tender and languid, such a pretty mouth, a bosom so firm and shapely, and the remainder designed to provoke such desire – that there were very few beautiful women in all Paris more capable of appealing to a man. But Madame de Sernenval for all her physical attractions had a capital moral failing: insupportable prudery, tiresome devoutness, and such a ridiculously exaggerated brand of maidenly modesty that her husband found it quite impossible to persuade her to appear in the circles he frequented. Taking bigotry to an extreme, Madame de Sernenval was rarely willing to spend a whole night with her husband and even in those moments she deigned to grant him, she did so only with excessive reservations and a night-gown which was not to be raised. A buckler of sorts tastefully positioned at the portals of the temple allowed access thereto only on the express condition that all unseemly gestures not to mention carnal conjoining were forbidden.

Marquis de Sade *Tales and Fabliaux of the 18th Century, by a Provençal Troubadour*, 'The Prude, or the Unexpected Encounter' (1787)

Some have argued that women should maintain strict standards of decorum in public while abandoning all restraint in the bedroom:

The daughter-in-law of Pythagoras said that a woman who goes to bed with a man ought to lay aside her modesty with her skirt, and put it on again with her petticoat.

Michel de Montaigne *Essays* (late 16th century)

He sayde, a woman cast her shame away
When she cast of hir smok.

Geoffrey Chaucer *The Canterbury Tales* (late 14th century)

Others have insisted that the demands of modesty are paramount even here:

When undressing, when arising, be mindful of modesty and take care not to expose to others anything that morality and nature require to be concealed.

Desiderius Erasmus *Adagia* (16th century)

As a general rule, a modest woman seldom desires any sexual gratification for herself. She submits to her husband, but only to please him; and but for the desire of maternity, would far rather be relieved from his attentions.

Dr William Acton, quoted by S. Marcus in *The Other Victorians* (1964)

Few people today would find such an attitude – which seems to deny women the right to any sexual feelings – either healthy or attractive. The modern consensus seems to be that an exaggerated reticence on sexual matters leads only to frustration and unhappiness. Many feel that even the slightest hint of prudery is to be avoided:

> *If the creator had not meant us to enjoy sex he would not have constructed our bodies specifically to derive enjoyment from lovemaking.*
>
> Robert Chartham *Sex Manners for Men* (1967)

An attitude anticipated by the sceptical Montaigne:

> *How is man wronged by the genital act, which is so natural, so necessary and so just, that he should not dare to speak of it but with shame, and should exclude it from serious and gentle conversation? Shall we say boldly: kill, rob, betray, but that – only in whispers?*
>
> Michel de Montaigne *Essays* (late 16th century)

Monogamy and Polygamy

Bigamy is having one wife too many. Monogamy is the same.

Anon. (19th century), quoted by Erica Jong in *Fear of Flying* (1973)

The pros and cons of monogamy, both for the wife and the husband, have been argued throughout the history of mankind. In Western cultures, monogamy is now virtually the only acceptable form of marriage.

The one common thread running through a variety of contemporary issues, surrogate motherhood, the remarriage of divorcees in church, changes in sexual ethics, is whether monogamous marriage must be maintained as an absolute and inflexible model, or whether it can survive the making of exceptions. Arguments commonly supposed to be about morality are in fact about monogamy, whose origins in the Judaeo-Christian tradition are far from clear.

Clifford Longley *The Times* (21 Jan. 1985)

In the early books of the Old Testament polygyny (a type of marriage in which one man may have many wives) is regarded as normal and acceptable:

The Bible reflects, without recommending, a polygamous society…Polygamy became general in the luxurious courts of the first Jewish kings…

Cecil Roth and Geoffrey Wigoder *The New Standard Jewish Encyclopedia* (1970)

And he [Solomon] *had seven hundred wives, princesses, and three hundred concubines…*

I Kings 11:3

It is an ancestral custom of ours to have several wives at one time.

Flavius Josephus *Antiquitates Judicae* (c. 70 AD)

This type of polygamy still occurs in some Muslim and African societies:

If you are afraid that you will not treat orphans justly, then marry such women as may seem good to you, two, three, or four. If you feel that you will not act justly, then one.

Koran (7th century)

Only between the age of fifty and his death at sixty-two did Muhammad take other wives, only one of whom was a virgin, and most of them were taken for dynastic and political reasons. Certainly the Prophet's record was better than that head of the Church of England, Henry VIII.

Geoffrey Parrinder *Mysticism in the World's Religions* (1976)

According to one Egyptian psychologist, legal polygamy may act as a deterrent to men considering starting an affair:

The fact that you're allowed to marry another woman, in addition to your wife, makes you hesitate about having an affair with another woman.

Dr Muhammed Sha'alan, quoted by Anthony Clare in *Lovelaw* (1986)

In the West, the Mormon Church continues to regard polygyny as a sacred institution:

I believe in the principle of plural marriage just as sacredly as I believe in any other institution which God has revealed.

I believe it to be necessary for the redemption of the human family from the low state of corruption into which it has sunken...this sacred principle of plural marriage tends to virtue, purity, and holiness.

Eliza R. Snow, at a Mass Meeting in Salt Lake City (16 Nov. 1878)

The ancient Thracians also practised polygyny:

The Thracians who live among the Crestonaeans observe the following customs: Each man among them has several wives; and no sooner does a man die than a sharp contest ensues among the wives upon the question, which of them all the husband loved most tenderly; the friends of each eagerly plead on her behalf, and she to whom the honour is adjudged, after receiving the praises both of men and women, is slain over the grave by the hand of her next of kin, and then buried with her husband. The others are sorely grieved, for nothing is considered such a disgrace.

Herodotus *History of the Persian Wars* (5th century BC)

Polyandry (marriage between one woman and many men) has also occurred in various societies. It is still the custom of the Nyinba Indians of Nepal that one woman marries some or all of the brothers in a family.

With one or two husbands always away on herding or trading trips, one husband will always be at home to care for the wife... We think polyandry is just like insurance for the wife. If one husband is no good or leaves his wife, there's always another brother.

Maila Dai, quoted in the *Observer* (18 Oct. 1992)

The Christian tradition of monogamy follows Roman rather than Judaic practice:

Roman law assumed monogamy; so strong and basic was this assumption that classical Roman law simply ignored the possibility of bigamy.

James A. Brundage *Law, Sex and Christian Society in Medieval Europe* (1987)

The laws of inheritance seem to have been a factor in sustaining Christian monogamy:

There had come to be so deep a bond of common interest between landlords seeking an orderly system of inheritance and the Church trying to enforce Christian monogamy, that the aristocracy was prepared for most purposes to be subject to the jurisdiction of the Church – not only in fits of penitence, but actually when making marriage treaties affecting their inheritances and standing in the world. This was largely because legitimate monogamy had come to be the heart of the system of inheritance, as it was the heart of the Church's idea of marriage as an institution. Doubtless the two affected each other, perhaps quite profoundly – but they would hardly have done so if there had not been a bond of common interest.

Christopher Brooke *The Medieval Idea of Marriage* (1989)

Others have advocated a monogamous lifestyle using arguments based on custom, nature, or health factors:

Monogamy is, has been, and will remain the only true type of marriage.

Bronislaw Malinowski 'Marriage' *Encyclopædia Britannica*

All unreasonable beasts and flying fowles, after they have once united and linked themselves togither to any one of the same kinde, and after they have espoused themselves the one to the other, will never after joyne themselves with any other, till the one be dissolved from the other by death. And thus they keep the knot of matrimonie to the end.

Philip Stubbes *The Anatomie of Abuses* (1583)

If a couple have had a monogamous totally faithful sexual relationship with each other, the risks of HIV infection will have been eliminated.

Roger Gaitley and Philip Seed *HIV and AIDS* (1989)

and have criticized polygamy as immoral or inconvenient:

If the purpose of dinner is to nourish the body the man who eats two dinners at a sitting may perhaps attain greater enjoyment but not his object, since the stomach will not digest two dinners.
If the purpose of marriage is the family the person who seeks to have a number of wives or husbands may possibly obtain much pleasure therefrom, but will not in any case have a family.

Leo Tolstoy *War and Peace* (1865–69)

The principal causes of polygamy and polyandry are an exaggerated fondness for variety and a pride in owning what others do not possess. The need for variety is such that often the worse is preferred only because it is different from the better. The curiosity that was Eve's downfall is still one of the most fertile sources of sin.

Paolo Mantegazza *The Sexual Relations of Mankind* (1894)

Polyandry is no good. There's too much work for one woman – it's too hard trying to take care of many husbands equally.

Nomdyol, a Nyinba, quoted in the *Observer* (18 Oct. 1992)

Yet monogamy has also found doubters and detractors:

Nothing can well be more alien from the animal instincts of mankind than the lifelong union of one man and one woman in holy matrimony.

Bishop James Edward Lowell Welldon *Forty Years On* (1935)

Christian monogamy and its assumption of fidelity, is as fallacious as the Catholic concept of the chastity of priests.

Sir Nicholas Fairburn *Spectator* (4 July 1992)

If a man always couples with the same woman, her vital essence will gradually grow weaker, and in the end she will be in no condition to give the man benefit. Moreover the woman herself will become emaciated.

Yü-fang-pi-chüch *I-hsin-fang* (c. 600)

In monotonous absorption with each other, the married couple destroy each other; each, perhaps, falsely imagining that the other demands such murderous excess.

T. L. Nicholls *Esoteric Anthropology* (1860)

I never was attached to that great sect,
Whose doctrine is, that each one should select
Out of the crowd a mistress or a friend,
And all the rest, though fair and wise, commend
To cold oblivion, though it is in the code
Of modern morals, and the beaten road
Which those poor slaves with weary footsteps tread,
Who travel to their home among the dead
By the broad highway of the world, and so
With one chained friend, perhaps a jealous foe,
The dreariest and the longest journey go.

Percy Bysshe Shelley *Epipsychidion* (1821)

In pious times e'er priest craft did begin,
Before polygamy was made a sin:
When man, on many, multiply'd his kind
Ere one to one was, cursedly, confin'd;
When Nature prompted, and no law deny'd
Promiscuous use of concubine and bride.

John Dryden *Absolom and Achitophel* (1681)

They say that for one man to be tied to one woman, or one woman to one man, is a fruit of the curse; but, they say, we are freed from the curse, therefore it is our liberty to make use of whom we please.

John Holland *The Smoke of the Bottomles Pit* (1652)

Take wise King Solomon of long ago;
We hear he had a thousand wives or so.

And would to God it were allowed to me
To be refreshed, aye, half as much as he!

Geoffrey Chaucer *The Canterbury Tales* 'The Wife of Bath's Tale' (late 14th century)

There have been different views as to which of the sexes is best suited to monogamy. Some people have claimed that women are naturally polyandrous:

Woman's destiny is to be wanton, like the bitch, the she-wolf, she must belong to all who claim her. Clearly it is to outrage the fate Nature imposes upon women to fetter them by the absurd ties of a solitary marriage...

Women are not made for one single man; 'tis for men at large Nature created them. Listening only to this sacred voice, let them surrender themselves, indifferently, to all who want them: always whores, never mistresses, eschewing love, worshipping pleasure.

Marquis de Sade *Philosophy in the Bedroom* (1797)

Women's inordinate orgasmic capacity did not evolve for monogamous, sedentary cultures. It is unreasonable to expect that this inordinate sexual capacity could be, even in part, given expression within the confines of our culture...

Mary Jane Sherfey *The Nature and Evolution of Female Sexuality* (1972)

Women of good family, beautiful, and well married do not stay within the moral bounds...There is not a man they would not go to...And when women cannot come on to a man, they even fall lustfully on one another, for they will never be true to their husbands...So soon as a woman sees a handsome man, her vulva becomes moist...

The Râmâyana (c. 400 BC)

Others claim it is men who are naturally polygynou:

Man is by nature polygamic whereas woman as a rule is monogamic, and polyandrous only when tired of her lover. For the man, as has been truly said, loves the woman, but the love of the woman is for the love of the man.

Sir Richard Burton 'Terminal Essay' in his translation of *The Thousand and One Nights* (19th century)

Women are more naturally monogamous than men. It is a biological necessity. When promiscuity prevails, they will always be more often the victims than the culprits. Also domestic happiness is more necessary to them than to us, and the quality by which they most easily hold a man, their beauty, decreases every year after they come to maturity.

C. S. Lewis 'We have no right to happiness' *Saturday Evening Post* (1963)

Feminists would be unlikely to accept this argument:

Many women today both in and out of the feminist networks have come to see women's enclosure in monogamy as the primary location of female subordination, and so have pressed for a more comprehensive understanding of its roots in history and culture.

Susan Dowell *They Two Shall Be One* (1990)

If women are to effect a significant amelioration in their condition it seems obvious that they must refuse to marry.

Germaine Greer *The Female Eunuch* (1970)

Monogamic association is the most desirable form of association. But the desirability of that intelligent and difficult relation vanishes entirely when it is coercively imposed upon a woman who repudiates it.

Robert Briffault *Sin and Sex* (1931)

The first class antagonism which appears in history coincides with the development of the antagonism between man and woman in monogamous marriage, and the first class oppression with that of the female sex by the male. Monogamy was a great historical advance, but at the same time it inaugurated, along with slavery and private wealth, that epoch, lasting until today, in which every advance is likewise a relative regression, in which the well-being and development of the one group are attained by the misery and repression of the other

Friedrich Engels *The Origin and History of the Family, Private Property and the State* (1884)

As a footnote, it is worth mentioning that anthropologists recognize two forms of monogamy: *absolute monogamy* in which one man has one wife and that is that, and *serial monogamy* in which one man has one wife at one time – divorcés and widowers of both sexes being free to remarry. Timothy Leary, using slightly different terminology, has the point:

The US has evolved from a culture of traditional monogamy to one of consecutive marriage or serial polygamy.

Timothy Leary *Neuropolitics* (1977)

Accursed from birth they be
Who seek to find monogamy,
Pursuing it from bed to bed –
I think they would be better dead.

Dorothy Parker *Reuben's Children* (1937)

Morality

Debate about sexual morals tends to become polarized, with people taking one of two basic positions. One approach attempts to lay down detailed rules about what is and what is not permitted, often on arbitrary grounds:

It is unnatural carnal copulation for a person to take into his or her mouth or anus the sexual organ of another person or animal; or to place his or her sexual organ in the mouth or anus of another person or of an animal; or to have carnal copulation in any opening of the body, except the sexual parts, with another person; or to have carnal copulation in any opening of the body of an animal.

US Code of Military Justice, Article 125 (1954)

The other approach condones anything that happens between consenting adults in private, provided that no one suffers as a result of it:

If anyone wants to engage in any kind of sexual activity with any consenting partner, that is their business...I don't feel that legality should have anything to do with it. There are certain bodily functions of mine which I will not allow to be supervised.

Madalyn Murray O'Hair, Interview (1965)

What's so normal, natural, fulfilling about heterosexuality? Natural is what feels good, normal is feeling ordinary, fulfilled is when you just did what you felt like doing. Anyone can be any or all of these things and no one except themselves can possibly know whether or not they are. What is it that makes heterosexuals feel so insecure about themselves that they can allow no alternative sexuality? How solid are the foundations upon which they build their moral values?

Angela Stewart-Park and Jules Cassidy *We're Here* (1977)

I am fortunate in not experiencing moral shock or disgust at any genital act whatsoever, provided that it is welcome and agreeable to all the participants (whether they number one, two, or more than two).

K. J. Dover *Greek Homosexuality* (1978)

Others are dissatisfied with both these approaches:

It has become almost impossible to think clearly or constructively about sex, since sexual satisfaction is the pivot around which our commercial culture turns, the sacred central axiom of a dogma of gratification which will not allow itself to be questioned or criticized. To suggest, for instance, that sex should be for *anything other than itself...is to invite immediate dismissal from the community of rational beings, even to occasion worried concern for the state of one's mental health.*

Where once sex may have been surrounded by a moralism of prudish disapproval, it is now hedged about with, if anything, an even more thornily impenetrable if quite different moralism, i.e. one which permits no challenge to the creed that everyone shall be permitted to enjoy themselves in any way they choose — 'whatever turns you on'...We use each other to satisfy needs so personal as to be almost autistic, and sex becomes a kind of suspicious bartering of incompatible self-indulgences rather than the unifying joy which sexual rhetoric proclaims.

David Smail *Taking Care, an Alternative to Therapy* (1987)

At one time it was almost universally assumed that the law had a duty to enforce standards of sexual morality:

Whatever is against good morality and decency, the principles of our law prohibit.

Lord Mansfield (1774)

The law has rarely been given this role in other areas of human life:

Sex laws...are unique in one important respect. Whereas all other laws are basically concerned with the protection of person or property, the majority of sex laws are concerned solely with maintaining morality. The issue of morality is minimal in other laws: one can legitimately evict an impoverished old couple from their mortgaged home or sentence a hungry man for stealing food. Only in the realm of sex is there a consistent body of law upholding morality.

Encyclopaedia Britannica

In South Africa the so-called 'Immorality Acts' forebade sexual intercourse between the races until the mid 1980s:

Woman to man, they lie,
He not quite white
As she, nor she
So black as he.

Save where her stomach curves
His flesh and hers,
Commingling, match.
Eyes catch,

That dare not meet
Beyond the night,
Though their alternate
Thighs, locked tight,

Defy you to discriminate
Between his skin and hers.
To him Pass Laws
Apply; she knows no night.

Alan Ross 'In Bloemfontein' (20th century)

In most Western societies it is now generally accepted that the law should not intrude into the sexual behaviour of consenting individuals in private. Although some older 'moral' legislation remains on the statute books, in practice the law is concerned almost entirely with the issue of consent and of avoiding affront to public decency.

The law has some interesting things to say about what constitutes consent:

Although 'consent' is a common word, it covers a wide range of states of mind in the context of intercourse between a man and a woman, ranging from actual desire on the one hand to reluctant acquiescence on the other. There is a difference between consent and submission; every consent involves a submission, but it by no means follows that a mere submission involves consent.

Lord Justice Dunn, Appeal Court Hearing (1981)

If a man has sexual intercourse with a girl under sixteen, whether or not with her consent, it is usually an offence; but there is absolutely no law preventing a woman having sex with a boy under sixteen. The only problem is that, if she so much as touches him other than is absolutely necessary for the act of sex itself, she commits an indecent assault for which she can be sent to prison for ten years.

Fenton Bresler *Sex and the Law* (1988)

People are beginning to question whether it is right that if a girl of fifteen who is thoroughly mature, who is attractive and who provokes a young man of eighteen into making advances to her and having intercourse with her, he should be branded a criminal. There is a strong case for mak-

ing the test the actual maturity of the woman and not her age.

Judge Neil McKinnon, interviewed after conditionally discharging a 22-year-old man who had had intercourse with a 15-year-old girl (1976)

Nowadays, most judges take the view, and rightly take the view, that when there is a virtuous friendship which ends in unlawful sexual intercourse, it is inappropriate to pass sentences of a punitive nature. What is required is a warning to the youth to mend his ways. At the other end, a man in a supervisory capacity who abuses his position of trust for his sexual gratification, ought to get a sentence somewhere near the maximum allowed by law, which is two years imprisonment.

Lord Justice Lawton, R. v. Taylor (Mar. 1977)

It is submitted that in principle a boy under fourteen must be presumed incapable of buggery with an animal but can be guilty of buggery with a male person if the allegation is that he was the passive partner, but not if the allegation is that he was the active partner.

Archbold *Criminal Pleading, Evidence and Practice*

Religious leaders, even those who are celibate, have never been shy of laying down rules for sexual behaviour. Here, for example, are two out of a total of 42 sins denied by chanting priests on behalf of the soul of a dead person:

I have not committed sodomy; I have not masturbated.

Book of the Dead (2700 BC)

And here are some Christian views:

Paul's letters show far greater concern with sexual issues than the Gospel writers attributed to Jesus. Paul considered sex a major source of sin and a frequent impediment to the Christian life. Although he did not place sexual offences at the top of his hierarchy of sins, they nonetheless occupied a prominent place in Paul's thoughts. He considered illicit sex almost as serious as murder.

James A. Brundage *Law, Sex and Christian Society in Medieval Europe* (1987)

A comparison of the two ethical systems in the West since the seventeenth century reveals some significant differences in the realm of sexual ethics. Catholic ethics remains faithful to patristic tradition: sexuality is justified only by procreation and marriage is inferior to celibacy. Protestant ethics affirms that sexuality cannot be bad because God created man as a sexed being: what is evil is the lust which can make it unnatural.

Erich Fuchs *Sexual Desire and Love* (1979)

In so far as the generation of offspring is impeded, it is a vice against nature which happens in every carnal act from which generation cannot follow.

St Thomas Aquinas *Opuscula* (13th century)

Promiscuous intercourse, unnatural passions, violations of the marriage bed, and improper acts to conceal the consequences of irregular connexions, clearly come under the head of vice.

Thomas Malthus *Essay on the Principle of Population* (1798)

That loathsome monster – licentiousness – crawls, tracking the earth with his fetid slime and poisoning the atmosphere with his syphilitic breath.

US Protestant clergyman (1820s), cited in Mary P. Ryan *Cradle of the Middle Class* (1981)

Modest people are ordinarily pure in thought and deed. Knowledge of evil does not keep people from evil. Our predecessors got along without all the sex instruction that is now ruining so many under the pretext of educating them. The purest and healthiest nations of the world have been those least acquainted with sex knowledge.

Father Martin J. Scott *Marriage Problems* (1926)

A fair conclusion from a study of the Old and New Testaments is this: while the

Bible condemns adultery, incest, prostitution, and sexual licentiousness or promiscuity, it is not at all clear that it ever condemns all premarital coitus as sinful, much less premarital petting and sex play.

John F. Dedek *Contemporary Sexual Morality* (1972)

In the realm of human sexuality, I, as a churchman, feel moved to confess that a great deal of the blame for preserving, if not indeed creating, the fears and guilt of sex which permeate our culture, lies at our feet.

Robert L. Treese *Homosexuality: A Contemporary View of the Biblical Perspective* (1972)

The Christian view of sex is that it is, indeed, a form of holy communion.

John Robinson, Bishop of Woolwich (1961), giving evidence for the defence in the prosecution of Penguin books for publishing *Lady Chatterley's Lover*

Sometimes religious authorities become so exercised by carnal thoughts that they lapse into unintelligibility:

the deliberate use of the sexual faculty outside normal conjugal relations essentially contradicts the finality of the faculty.

Vatican declaration 'On Certain Questions Concerning Sexual Ethics' (1976)

A condition that also afflicts others:

Sex must be rescued from the traffic between powerful and powerless, masterful and mastered, sexual and neutral, to become a form of communication between potent, gentle tender people, which cannot be accomplished by denial of heterosexual contact.

Germaine Greer *The Female Eunuch* (1970)

The [sexual] *act is not the problem but the mind is the problem, the mind which says it must be chaste. Chastity is not of the mind. The mind can only suppress its own activities and suppression is not chastity. Chastity is not a virtue, chastity cannot be cultivated...you cannot become chaste. You will know chastity only when there is love, and love is not of the mind nor a thing of the mind.*

J. Krishnamurti *The First and Last Freedom* (1954)

Psychologists and sexologists, too, have views about morals:

Man puts himself at once on a level with the beast if he seeks to gratify lust alone, but he elevates his superior position when by curbing the animal desire he combines with the sexual functions ideas of morality, of the sublime, and the beautiful.

Richard von Krafft-Ebing *Psychopathia Sexualis* (1886)

The truly healthy state for the neurotic is sexual immorality...It seems to me, however, that sexual repression is a very important and indispensable civilizing factor, even if pathogenic for many inferior people. Still, there must always be a few flies in the world's ointment. What is civilization but the fruit of adversity?

Carl Jung, in a letter to Sigmund Freud (25 Sept. 1907)

Suppression of the natural sexuality of the child, particularly of its own genital sexuality, makes the child apprehensive, shy, obedient, afraid of authority, good and adjusted in the authoritarian sense; it paralyses the rebellious forces because any rebellion is laden with anxiety; it produces, by inhibiting sexual curiosity and sexual thinking in the child, a general inhibition of thinking in the child; and of critical faculties. In brief, the goal of sexual suppression is that of producing an individual who is adjusted to the authoritarian order and will submit to it in spite of all misery and degradation.

Wilhelm Reich *Function of the Orgasm* (1942)

The publicly pretended code of morals, our social organization, our marriage customs, our sex laws, and our educational and religious systems are based upon an assumption that individuals are much alike sexually and that it is an equally simple matter for all of them to confine their behaviour to the single pattern which the mores dictate... It is not possible to insist that any departure from the sexual mores, or any participation in socially taboo activities, always, or even usually, involves a neurosis or psychosis, for the case histories abundantly demonstrate that most individuals who engage in taboo activities make satisfactory social adjustments.

Alfred Kinsey et al. *Sexual Behaviour in the Human Male* (1948)

Sexual restrictions protect the structure of society against the onslaught of sexually highly excited individuals, that is, people 'on heat'. At the same time they protect the individual and allow him to enjoy a modicum of sexual pleasure in comparative peace and security.

M. Balint *Problems of Human Pleasure and Behaviour* (1957)

The revolution in sexual attitudes can only go so far before it becomes a direct threat to the fundamental structure of society.

Ann Hills and Tony Lake *Affairs* (1979)

Any ambiguity such as transvestism, hermaphrodism, transsexuality, or homosexuality is moulded into 'normal' appropriate gender behaviour or is relegated to the categories of sick, dangerous or pathological.

M. Brake *Sexual Divisions and Society* (1976)

But politicians, lawyers, religious leaders, and psychiatrists are not the only ones to have opinions. Here are some other views. Some bemoan what they see as a decline in standards:

I do know what the world's coming to and that's a fact. It's coming to complete moral and mental disintegration. We all know that sex orgies, flagellation, homosexuality and procuring have gone on since the beginning of recorded time, but never before has it been so widely and vulgarly and lasciviously publicised.

Noël Coward *Diaries* (1963)

While others rejoice at the new freedom:

The change in eroticism which we experience today has been conditioned by the fall of Christian morality. The act of intercourse no longer carries with it the taste of the forbidden fruit, since the peeping Tom of Nazareth on his cross no longer hangs above the marital bed. Freedom has arrived.

J. J. Beljon *Waar ge Kijkt...Erotiek* (1967)

Or protest at the denigration of sex by false moralists:

It is the brutal and inferior morality which simply allows the sexes to come together for purposes of procreation, and the higher, the human civilized morality which allows intercourse without reference to propagation.

David Goodman Croly *Truth About Love* (1872)

What! Vulgar! The instinct that creates immortal souls vulgar! Who dare stand up amid Nature, all prolific and beautiful, whose pulses are ever bounding with the creative desire, and utter such sacrilege! Vulgar indeed! Vulgar, rather, must be the mind that can conceive such blasphemy.

Victoria Claflin Woodhull (1870)

Are we not brutes to call the act that makes us, 'brutish'?

Michel de Montaigne *Essays* 'On Virgil' (late 16th century)

Some women are justifiably outraged by the double standards that have often prevailed:

Nothing could be more grotesquely unjust than a code of morals, reinforced by laws, which relieves men from responsibility for irregular sexual acts, and for the same acts drives women to abortion, infanticide, prostitution and self-destruction.

Suzanne Lafollette *Concerning Women* 'Women and Marriage' (1926)

Neither in men nor women could the sexual act [in Victorian times] *be entirely divorced from guilt, if enjoyed – though, clearly, the guilt was more intense in women.*

Glen Petrie *A Singular Iniquity* (1971)

All witchcraft comes from carnal lust, which is in women insatiable... Woman is more carnal than a man, as is clear from her many carnal abominations.

Heinrich Kraemer and Johann Sprenger *Malleus Malleficarum* (1486)

While for some, observing the changes or trying to explain them is enough:

It could be said that the advance of civilization has not so much moulded modern sexual behaviour, as that sexual behaviour has moulded the shape of civilization.

Desmond Morris *The Naked Ape* (1967)

But jealousy, I believe, has been the most potent single factor in the genesis of sexual morality. Jealousy instinctively becomes anger, and anger, rationalised, becomes moral disapproval.

Bertrand Russell *Why I am Not a Christian* (1957)

For others, the whole issue has become a bore:

As I grow older and older,
And totter towards the tomb,
I find that I care less and less
Who goes to bed with whom.

Dorothy L. Sayers 'That's Why I Never Read Modern Novels' (1975)

Finally a few one-liners on sexual morality — both platitudinous:

All sentiments of morality and modesty rest on conventionality.

August Forel *Sexual Ethics* (1908)

Sex is no more impure and base than it is noble.

Robert Briffault *Sin and Sex* (1931)

and pithy:

Morality is only expediency in a long white dress.

Quentin Crisp *How to Have a Lifestyle* (1975)

An orgy looks particularly alluring seen through the mists of righteous indignation.

Malcolm Muggeridge *The Most of Malcolm Muggeridge*, 'Dolce Vita in a Cold Climate' (1966)

and an indisputable 19th-century US proverb:

A stiff prick has no conscience.

Nudity

JOURNALIST *Didn't you have anything on?*
M.M. *I had the radio on.*

Marilyn Monroe (attrib; 20th century)

Attitudes towards nudity are determined by a complex range of factors – some personal, some cultural, and some dependent on the particular circumstances in which it occurs:

Modesty depends on the custom of covering or exposing certain parts of the body, and people who live in a state of nature are as much ashamed of clothes as we are ashamed of nudity.

Auguste Forel *Sexual Ethics* (1908)
See also MODESTY

Moreover, nudity, like all else, is subject to the vagaries of fashion:

It is not long ago since it was ridiculous amongst the Greeks, as it still is among most of the non-Greeks, for men to allow themselves to be seen naked.

Plato *Republic* (4th century BC)

At some points in history attitudes to bodily display have been highly censorious:

I see silken clothes, if these can be called clothes, with which the body or only the private parts could be covered; dressed in them, the woman can hardly swear with a good conscience that she is not naked. These clothes are imported at considerable expense from most distant countries, only that our women may have no more to show their lovers in the bedroom than in the street.

Seneca *De Benficiis* (1st century AD)

Bishop William Durantis (1237–96) thought that decent artists should follow what he described as the Greek practice of representing persons only from the waist up 'in order to remove occasion for foolish thoughts.' Moralists even cautioned husbands and wives...not to look upon one another's naked bodies, lest they arouse the spirit of lust which was inappropriate in the marital relationship. The contrast with the celebration of nudity in ancient art and its subsequent reappearance in renaissance art after about 1400 is striking.

James A. Brundage *Law, Sex and Christian Society in Medieval Europe* (1987)

No knight, under the estate of a Lord...nor any other person, use or wear...any Gowne, Jaket, or Cloke, but it be of such length as it, he being upright, shall cover his privy members and buttokkes.

Petition of the House of Commons (15th century)

In other times and places nudity has been much more widely accepted. In ancient Ireland and medieval France, for example:

Nudity was no cause for shame: not only were warriors normally naked, except for their accoutrements, but women also undressed freely: thus the Queen of Ulster and all the ladies of the Court, to the number of 610, came to meet Cuchulainn, naked above the waist and raising their skirts 'so as to expose their private parts', by which they showed how greatly they honoured him...

The daughters of the nobility thought it an honour to parade naked in front of Charles V.

Gordon Rattray Taylor *Sex in History* (1953)

And amongst the supposedly straitlaced Victorians

Nude swimming in rivers was popular and commonplace. At Worcester a barge was moored in the River Severn for use by the bathers. When complaints were received about nude men wading ashore to dry themselves by running on the bank, the authorities of 1868 did not forbid the bathing – but provided an attendant to prevent 'unnecessary or indecent exposure'.

Phil Vallack *Naked As The Day* (1985)

In Western societies the conventions surrounding nudity are fairly complex. Most people find no difficulty in undressing in a doctor's surgery because the medical context rules out any sexual connotations. Other settings, such as a life class, may similarly render nudity asexual and unthreatening. People also tend to be noticeably more relaxed about nudity while abroad on holiday – unfamiliar surroundings seem to legitimize a shedding of everyday inhibitions. There is also an element of safety in numbers:

Women are afraid to come [to the nudist camp], *but they lose their fear the first time – as soon as they have seen that the other women are ugly, too.*

Frances and Mason Merrill *Among the Nudists* (1931)

Nudity is now accepted on the stage and the cinema screen to an extent that would have seemed unthinkable 30 years ago:

It was Sidney Lumet's glum The Pawnbroker *in 1965 that reminded mainstream America what a white woman's breasts looked like...In 1966's* Blow Up, *Michelangelo Antonioni broke the pubic hair barrier in a troilism session between David Hemmings, Gillian Hills and Jane Birkin (hot debate persists as to whose hair you see), while the first white penis in pictures was probably Robert Forster's in* Medium Cool *in 1969, pipping Alan* [Bates] *and Ollie* [Reed] *in* Women In Love *by a few months.*

Kim Newman 'Sex in the Movies' *Empire* (May 1993)

In Britain, however, the use of nudity in advertising is still strictly controlled, as this might seem too obviously exploitative:

We can't allow nudity to advertise something irrelevant, like chocolates.

IBA annual report (1974)

The cultural and psychological meanings of nudity are clearly far from simple. On the one hand it is associated with ideas of innocence and freedom – and on the other with shame, lust, and humiliation. Both poles are present in the Adam and Eve story:

And they were both naked, the man and his wife, and were not ashamed.

Genesis 2:25

And the eyes of them both were opened, and they knew that they were naked; and they sewed fig leaves together, and made themselves aprons...and Adam and his wife hid themselves from the presence of the Lord God.

Genesis 3:7–8

The two attitudes constantly reappear in the debate about the moral effects of nudity:

Shame has its beginnings in public nakedness.

Cicero *Tusculanae Disputationes* (1st century BC)

Nudity in itself is chaste as nature; it is holy, being from God, and it does not need to conceal its existence.

Father Antonin Gilbert Sertillanges *L'Art et la morale* (1925)

Many have argued that a greater acceptance of nudity would actually improve sexual morals, because it would make prurience and titillation redundant:

Their [the Tahitians] *continual state of nakedness has kept their minds free from the dangerous preoccupation with the 'mystery' and from the excessive stress which among civilized people is laid upon the 'happy accident' and the clandestine and sadistic colours of love. It has given their manners a natural innocence, a perfect purity.*

Paul Gauguin *Noa Noa* (1947)

In the 20th century this view has been highly popular with the advocates of organized nudism:

The practice of nudism would no doubt be the best means of rendering simple and easy the sexual education of the young, while keeping them from the curiosities, the fevers of imagination, and the incertitude before the sustained mystery that are at the origin of all perversions.

Dr Pierre Vachet, quoted in Frances and Mason Merrill *Among the Nudists* (1931)

To call attention to the organs of sex by means of the taboo upon nudity is deliberately to incite sexual precocity in the child.

Maurice Parmelee *Nudity in Modern Life* (1929)

The sexual sentiment of modesty very often becomes unhealthy and is then easily combined with pathological sexual conditions.

Auguste Forel *The Sexual Question* (1909)

On these grounds, some enthusiasts have advocated a nudist revolution throughout society:

We shall get rid of our clothes eventually, because of the contradictions and conflicts inherent in their nature.

It will indeed be a short time only before a person who wears more than a loincloth on Fifth Avenue will be stigmatized as indecent and degenerate.

John Langdon-Davies *Future of Nakedness* (1929)

In practice, most societies have reached a compromise with nudism, permitting it within certain designated areas:

The nudist colony of Paris has addressed a letter to the Prefect of Police asking his permission to extend their activities to the city itself. Hitherto they walked around 'in naturalibus' on a discreet little island in the Seine. This is not enough. It's not likely, in spite of the moving appeal on behalf of the pores, that the Prefect will grant the request. Even a Prefect of Police must take into account the slow evolution of fashion.

New York Evening World (28 June 1930)

Are the naturists right in claiming that there is no inherent link between nudity and eroticism? Some are sceptical:

Sex is the main factor which attracts anyone to nudity, whatever ostensible reasons may be given out to the world.

George Ryley Scott *The Common Sense of Nudism* (1934)

The statistics given below suggest that many *are* attracted to nudism for voyeuristic reasons:

One of the chief problems of the organisers of a family Sun- and Air-Bathing Society is the unattached man, the freelance, who wishes to join but has no woman companion to bring. Applications for membership from such men very greatly exceed the total number of applications from women – in fact, for every one hundred men who apply only ten women write in. Yet the Sun-Bathing Society has laid it down as a rule that men who wish to join must be accompanied by a woman, or by a child or children, though, on the other hand, a woman is encouraged to bring a girl friend rather than a man.

The Sun-Bathing Review: Journal of the Sun Societies (1933)

On the other hand, the clothed or partially clothed human body can often be more erotic than the same body naked:

The greatest provocations of lust are from the apparel.

Robert Burton *Anatomy of Melancholy* (1621)

John Hall [17th century English radical] *argued the case for female nudism, not as a symbol of regained innocence, but because nakedness would be less provocative than the clothes which women wore.*

Christopher Hill *The World Turned Upside-down* (1972)

No woman so naked as one you can see to be naked underneath her clothes.

Michael Frayn *Constructions* (1974)

Clothes often have the effect of drawing attention to the parts they are supposed to hide:

Early man wore the little he thought necessary not because of modesty, but because of a vanity which we can have little doubt he possessed. The too sufficient bamboo of the pygmy and the plainly insufficient tassel of the Australian cannot by any manner of juggling or optimism about human nature be explained as a desire to avoid offending the innate delicacy of the female of the species. To our way of thinking, the men would be better without them, for their presence on an otherwise naked body must produce the same effect as one word of italics upon a page of ordinary type.

John Langdon-Davies *Future of Nakedness* (1929)

Attitudes to nudity during the sexual act also vary. For some, full nakedness is a prerequisite of total intimacy:

You wear a nightgown, robe and girdle,
even in hot weather;
I like sleeping with a woman in the
altogether.
I want kisses long drawn out, lips parted,
tongues meeting:
Yours could just as well be your
grandmother's morning greeting.
You think we should be in total darkness
when we're screwing:
I prefer light; I like to see what I am
doing.

Martial *Epigrams* 'Wife, There are Some Points' (1st century AD)

Stark naked as she stood before mine eye,
Not one wen in her body could I spy,
What arms and shoulders did I touch
and see,
How apt her breasts were to be pressed by
me.
How smooth a belly and under her waist
saw I?
How large a leg, and what a lusty thigh!
To leave the rest, all like me passing well,
I clinged her naked body, down she fell,
Judge you the rest, being tired she bade
me kiss,
Jove send me more such afternoons as
this.

Ovid *Elegy V* (1st century BC; trans. by Christopher Marlowe)

Full nakedness! Cast off your linen white
and closely clinging, limb to limb unite;
Off with these flimsy veils: while they are
on
Between us stand the walls of Babylon.
Join breast to breast, our lips together seal,
And ne'er shall blabbing tongues our joy
reveal.

Paulus Silentarius (6th century)

Full nakedness, all joys are due to thee,
As souls unbodied, bodies unclothed must
be,
To taste whole joys.

John Donne 'To His Mistress Going to Bed' (17th century)

In some cultures and classes, however, the taboo on nakedness is even stronger than the taboo on illicit sex:

Well informed persons assure me that these girls [of the servant class] *are much less diffident about engaging in coitus than about being seen naked.*

Sigmund Freud, letter to Carl Jung (14 June 1907)

Others are simply shy:

In all our time together, I don't remember seeing him naked. But I was just as shy about my own body. However, this modesty did not prevent us from having a good time sexually. We satisfied each other and would lie in each others arms for a long time afterwards, delighting in our proximity. It was not exhausting, frenzied love-making but gentle and tender, an absolutely happy state.

Sheilah Graham *The Real F. Scott Fitzgerald* (1967)

Perhaps the whole question of nudity is more aesthetic than moral. Some maintain that the human form is beautiful and ought not to be hidden away like a shameful secret:

We allow women who have a beautiful head of hair, a beautiful face, a beautiful bosom to show off those parts of their bodies; why are we so unjust to those whose beauty resides not in those parts but in others?

Lorenzo Valla (14th century)

My Love in her attire doth show her wit,
It doth so well become her;
For every season she hath dressings fit,
For Winter, Spring, and Summer.
No beauty doth she miss
When all her robes are on:
But Beauty's self she is
When all her robes are gone.

Anon. 'Madrigal' (17th century)

To an Italian, proud of his Roman tradition, nudism appears as an artistic return to the pagan glorification of life for the sake of the beauty of the body and the world.

Anon., quoted in Frances and Mason Merrill *Among the Nudists* (1931)

How idiotic civilization is! Why be given a body if you have to keep it shut up in a case like a rare, rare fiddle?

Katherine Mansfield *Bliss and Other Stories* (1920)

Others argue that the undraped human form is by no means always a pleasant sight:

Many of the advocates of nudism start out with the popular assumption that the human body, and especially the female human body, is a thing of charm. They deny that the perfect body is ugly. True. But what about the imperfect body?

The greatest enemy of nakedness is the ugliness of man and woman.

George Ryley Scott *The Common Sense of Nudism* (1934)

The total exposure of the human body is undignified as well as an error of taste.

Adolf Hitler (1930s)

It would seem that no matter how much fashions change, nor how far and wide the public debate ranges, nudity is largely accepted or rejected on the basis of individual preference and desire; people accept the level of nudity at which they feel comfortable in particular circumstances:

It is the part of wisdom to utilize clothing whenever it is needed, and not to misuse it when more can be gained from going without.

Maurice Parmelee *Nudity in Modern Life* (1929)

Of course, opinions will continue to differ about when clothes can be profitably and properly dispensed with. While many non-naturists can see the appeal of nude swimming or sunbathing, for example, it is probable that nude ping-pong will remain a minority taste. Perhaps the most convincing illustration of the wisdom of Parmelee's suggestion is the point made by Sir Robert Helpmann when asked whether the fashion for nudity would extend from the theatre to the world of dance:

No, you see there are portions of the human anatomy which would keep swinging after the music had finished.

Sir Robert Helpmann (1980s)

Oral Sex

Two definitions:

fellatio *n.* oral stimulation of the penis. [Latin *fellātus,* past participle of *fellāre* to suck]

cunnilingus, cunnilinctus *n.* stimulation of the female genitals by the lips and tongue [Latin *cunnus* vulva, *lingere, linctum,* to lick]

Cassell's English Dictionary (1962)

There is ample evidence that both men and women derive intense satisfaction from receiving *and* administering such stimulation:

I do feel powerful when he does it. I feel quite powerful. Sort of...the Amazon mentality – all-powerful woman. I'm exerting power, I'm rewarding him. The giving of pleasure is a powerful position, and the giving of oral sex is a real, real, pleasure.

Anon. businesswoman, quoted by Morton Hunt in *Sexual Behaviour in the 1970s* (1974)

It means so much to him, Candy kept thinking, so much, as he meanwhile got her jeans and panties down completely so that they dangled now from one slender ankle as he adjusted her legs and was at last on the floor himself in front of her, with her legs around his neck, and his mouth very deep inside the fabulous honeypot.

T. Southern and M. Hoffenburg *Candy* (1958)

It is beautiful to think
that each of these clean secretaries
at night, to please her lover, takes
a fountain into her mouth
and lets her insides, drenched in seed,
flower into landscapes

John Updike *Seventy Poems* (1972)

The daughter of a local high official has an interesting abnormality. An acquaintance of mine, who used to visit the girl's family, soon saw that the girl did not conduct herself as an 18 year old daughter of a highly respectable family should, and persuaded her to visit him at his flat. But as he was about to perform the sexual act, the girl suddenly took his member into her mouth. There was nothing very peculiar about that, but the girl, who had not been intact for some years, said that no other method of sexual intercourse gave her the slightest pleasure, whereas this method she found intensely enjoyable. Cunnilingus did not interest her, either.

Magnus Hirschfeld *Sexual Anomalies and Perversions* (1966)

The next moment I was with her in bed and on her; but she moved aside and away from me. "No, let's talk," she said...To my amazement she began: "Have you read Zola's latest book Nana*?" "Yes," I replied. "Well," she said, "you know what the girl did to Nana?" "Yes," I replied with sinking heart. "Well," she went on, "why not do that to me? I'm desperately afraid of getting a child, you would be too in my place, why not love each other without fear?" A moment's thought told me that all roads lead to Rome and so I assented and soon I slipped down between her legs. "Tell me please how to give you most pleasure," I said and gently, I opened the lips of her sex and put my lips on it and* *my tongue against her clitoris. There was nothing repulsive in it; it was another and more sensitive mouth. Hardly had I kissed it twice when she slid lower down in the bed with a sigh whispering: "That's it; that's heavenly!"*

Frank Harris *My Life and Loves* (1923)

His libertine fingers caressed the portico of the temple which was unlocked by sensuality in response to his desires. Then the divine kiss which he was allowed was duly planted and savoured for a full hour.

Marquis de Sade *Tales and Fabliaux of the Eighteenth Century, by a Provencal Troubadour* (1787)

Licked into shape – my tongue, old soak
And glutton, swears it's long lost count
Of hours spent playing, stroke by stroke,
The cough-sweet game beneath the
Mount:

Well-licked, yes – bitter, though, and grim
That red laugh cut in your brown skin,
Your pretty, teasing, cheeky quim:
So like the lips of Harlequin.

Paul Verlaine *Femmes* (1890)

The pleasure derived from the act may be psychological as well as physical:

One can imply, by performing oral/genital contact, that nothing about the loved one is offensive. In other words, the proximity of the excretary apparatus to the genitalia can be conceived of as a chivalrous challenge, the acceptance of which expresses some such sentiment as: 'See how much I love you – if I am prepared to do this.' Putting one's mouth to the genital regions, breaching the hygiene taboos and conventions of decency, is in fact a gesture of intimacy that transcends coitus itself...

More even than coitus, oral/genital contact caters for the desire to see, and come into intimate contact with, another's body. It is possible, in daylight, to seduce and make love to a woman without seeing anything but her face. It is, of course, not possible to perform cunnilingus without learning a good deal about a woman's intimate anatomy.

Paul Ableman *The Mouth* (1969)

The association of the genitals with uncleanness may explain the long history of disapproval of both fellatio and cunnilingus. In the Classical world:

There was one type of sexual behaviour which was absolutely disgraceful...This behaviour...was fellatio. The historian needs no excuse for bringing it up since Greek and Roman texts refer constantly to it, and it is our business to give our own society a sense of the relativity of values. Fellatio was a very dirty word and we read about cases where disgraceful fellators try to hide their infamy under the lesser shame of pretending to be passive homosexuals.

Philippe Ariès and André Bejin *Western Sexuality* (1982)

Romans considered it disgraceful for a free man to adopt the passive role in anal intercourse...The passive role in fellatio was even more strongly disapproved: again, the objection was not to the act itself, but to what was felt to be the incongruity of a free man acting the role customarily assigned to a slave or servant boy. No such disapproval appears to have attached to the man who performed cunnilingus on a woman...

In a tortuously worded decree of 342 the emperors Constantius and Constans prohibited sexual relations between man and wife in any fashion that did not involve penetration of the vagina by the penis. The intent, clearly enough, was to outlaw anal and oral sex between married persons, as well as other kinds of deviant sexuality.

James A. Brundage *Law, Sex and Christian Society in Medieval Europe* (1987)

Laws against oral sex, even between married couples, have remained on the statute books well into this century (in some US states they have yet to be revoked):

I regret to say that we of the FBI are powerless to act in cases of oral-genital intimacy, unless it has in some way obstructed interstate commerce.

J. Edgar Hoover, quoted by Irving Wallace et al. in *Intimate Sex Lives of Famous People* (1981)

A husband was performing cunnilingus on his wife in the privacy of their bedroom. One of three children in the family, unaware of the sexual activity of the parents, opened the door and observed what was going on. The child, frightened by what he had seen, ran to a neighbour with the story. The police were called and the husband arrested. He readily admitted the act and stated that he did not see anything wrong with it. He further said that the wife did not object to what he was doing and that, in fact, she encouraged him. Armed with this confession, a conviction was obtained and the man sentenced to prison for five years.

Frank Caprio and D. R. Brenner *Sexual Behaviour: Psycho-legal Aspects* (1961)

Others simply don't fancy it:

Sprinkled through the legalese was a Latin term, fellatio, *that had quite a few flappers heading for a dictionary. It seems Mrs. Chaplin did not want to perform this 'abnormal, against nature, perverted, degenerate and indecent act' (as described by Lita's lawyers) while Chaplin encouraged her, 'Relax, dear – all married people do it.'*

Kenneth Anger, referring to Lita Grey Chaplin's 42-page bill of divorcement from Charlie Chaplin (1927) in *Hollywood Babylon* (1975)

Nature didn't intend it, or she wouldn't have put teeth in our mouths. And she'd have made mouths longer or penises shorter.

German prostitute, quoted by Robert E. L. Masters in *The Hidden World of Erotica* (1973)

You know the worst thing about oral sex? The view.

Maureen Lipman (1990)

In particular, some women instinctively recoil from the idea of having a man ejaculate in their mouth:

Unless the ejaculation is an unusually powerful one, gagging probably does not admit of a physiological explanation. That there is a rejection, of the act, of the other person, of the semen, and that the rejection is unconscious (conscious rejection manifesting itself by the individual spitting out the ejaculate) is in many cases clear. It often happens that the individual fully intends and strongly desires to ingest the semen, and has no conscious reluctance of any kind to do so, and yet there is gagging and perhaps vomiting.

Robert E. L. Masters *The Hidden World of Erotica* (1973)

Everybody I know has a different idea of love. One girl I know said, 'I knew he loved me when he didn't come in my mouth'.

Andy Warhol *From A to B and Back Again* (1975)

Some girls do and some don't like the man to go all the way and ejaculate (if they love him very much, that may make all the difference, but not always). Those who don't can easily stop just short of getting him there...Others once they are used to it don't find the experience complete unless their lover does ejaculate. John Hunter wrote, "The semen would appear both by smell and taste to be a mawkish kind of substance: but when held in the mouth it produces a warmth similar to spices."

Dr Alex Comfort *The Joy of Sex* (1972)

Men have, if anything, even more reason to feel vulnerable during the act:

'Put it in your mouth,' he said. 'Yes, as you would a delicious thing to eat.' I like to broaden my mind when I can and I did as he suggested, swallowing it

up entirely and biting it off with a snap. As I did so my eager fellow increased his swooning to the point of fainting away, and I, feeling both astonished by his rapture and disgusted by the leathery thing filling up my mouth, spat out what I had not eaten and gave it to one of my dogs. The whore from Spitalfields had told me that men like to be consumed in the mouth, but it seems to me a reckless act, for the member must take some time to grow again.

Jeanette Winterson *Sexing the Cherry* (1989)

She bent down and, taking it in her lips, sucked it and moved up and down. Suddenly the white sperm squirted out like living silver; she took it in her mouth and could not swallow it fast enough. At first it was sperm and then it became an unceasing flow of blood. Hsi-men Ch'ing had fainted and his limbs were stiff outstretched.

Wang Shih-Chen *Chin P'ing Mei (The Golden Lotus)*

Less obviously, cunnilingus can involve genuine risks for the woman:

There are several authentic hazards to oral sex and these must be specified. The most important is that of 'air embolism' and the rule it exacts is 'never blow air into a girl's vagina'. This can lead to rapid death as a number of documented cases have shown.

Paul Ableman *The Mouth* (1969)

For male homosexuals, fellation is one of the most customary means of gratification:

The little pissoir under the bridge had become the scene of a frenzied homosexual saturnalia. No more than two feet away the citizens of Holloway moved about their ordinary business. I came, squirting come into the bearded man's mouth, and quickly pulled up my jeans. As I was about to leave, I heard the bearded man hissing quietly, 'I suck people off! Who wants his cock sucked?'

Joe Orton, diary entry (March 1967) published in *The Orton Diaries* (1986)

Among the New Guinea Sambia...an aberrant bachelor is one who does not offer his penis to be sucked by prepubescent boys.

G. H. Herdt *Guardians of the Flutes* (1981)

Emperor Tiberius taught children to play between his legs while he was in his bath. Those who were still very young he set at fellatio, the practice best suited to their inclination and age.

Suetonius *Lives of the Twelve Caesars* (c. 100 AD)

Andy sighed, 'Oh for God's sake shut up and enjoy yourself!' And he took Benson into his mouth and began to suck on him in a way that Benson had always reserved for Strawberry mivvies.

Michael Carson *Sucking Sherbet Lemons* (1988)

Fellatio has long been offered on the streets by prostitutes of both sexes:

She demands eight obols to give him a peck on his prick.

Hipponax of Ephesus (6th century BC)

As on a straw a Thracian man or Phrygian sucks his brew, forward she stooped, working away.

Archilochus, fragment (7th century BC)

Lesbia, the gifts of Bacchus you despise,
But pricks are drained by that fair mouth of thine.
In drinking water we'll pronounce thee wise,
Water is used for washing, but not wine.

Martial (1st century AD)

Never ask a man of the world: 'Fancy a blow-job?' Only little street girls express themselves like that. Instead, whisper softly in his ear: 'Would you care to use my mouth?'

Pierre Louys *Manuel de civilité pour les petites filles a l'usage des maison d'éducation* (1926)

The association of oral sex with both homosexuality and prostitution probably contributed to the stigma attached to the practice until relatively recently. There is now a general consensus that neither fellatio nor cunnilingus should be regarded as deviant or 'dirty' in any degree:

> *Theodore van de Velde's* Ideal Marriage *(1930), which ran through forty-two editions with sales of 700,000 copies in four years, explained in frank detail physiology, techniques of arousal and alternatives and variations. He stressed his concern to promote 'normal' monogamous marital harmony and to 'keep the Hell Gate of the Realm of Sexual Perversion firmly closed', though this did not exclude discussion of the previously 'perverse' cunnilingus and fellatio – the 'genital kiss' which he authorised as part of Love Play.*

Cate Haste *Rules of Desire* (1992)

> *It is true that in some cultures mouth-genital contacts have been condemned; but it is mistaken to regard fellatio and cunnilingus as deviant, since it is rare for either to replace intercourse except among homosexuals, and at least sixty per cent of males admit to the practice of one or other activity.*

Dr Anthony Storr *Sexual Deviation* (1964)

> *It wasn't many years ago that genital kisses, or rather the taboos on them, were a king pretext for divorce on grounds of perversity, cruelty and so on. We've come some way since then – now there are textbooks, and they figure in movies. Personal preferences and unpreferences apart, most people now know that they are one of the best things in sexual intimacy.*

Dr Alex Comfort *The Joy of Sex* (1972)

> *What more harm in a man's licking a woman's clitoris to give her pleasure, or of she sucking his cock for the same purpose, both taking pleasure in giving each other pleasure?*

Anon. *My Secret Life*, privately published novel (1890s)

Orgasms

But did thee feel the earth move?

Ernest Hemingway *For Whom the Bell Tolls* (1940)

Unlike its female counterpart, the male orgasm presents few mysteries. There can be little doubt as to what happens, when it happens, or why; the ejaculation of semen is an unmistakable event with an obvious biological purpose.

His cock, like that of a crop-gobbling donkey from Priene, overflowed.

Archilochus (6th century BC)

I cannot help asking whether we do not, in that very heat of extreme gratification when the generative fluid is ejected, feel that somewhat of our soul has gone out from us? And do we not experience a faintness and prostration along with a dimness of sight? This, then, must be the soul-producing seed, which arises from the outdrip of the soul, just as that fluid is the body-producing seed which proceeds from the drainage of the flesh.

In a single impact of both parties, the whole human frame is shaken and foams with semen, in which the damp humour of the body is joined to the hot substance of the soul.

Tertullian *A Treatise on the Soul* (2nd century)

In Chinese literature on sex the following two basic facts are stressed again and again. First, a man's semen is his most precious possession, the source not only of his health but of his very life, every emission of semen will diminish this vital force, unless compensated by the acquiring of an equivalent amount of yin essence from the woman. Second, the man should give the woman complete satisfaction every time he cohabitates with her, but he should allow himself to reach orgasm only on certain specified occasions.

R. H. Van Gulik *Sexual Life in Ancient China* (1961)

That girl was skilled at thrusting under the trees;
she gave me, we were brave, a blow for every blow,
and after my masculinity drops came in her.

Anon. 'Sexual Intercourse' (14th century)

Then off he came
And blusht for shame
Soe soone that he had endit.

Anon. 14th-century song, collected in *Loose Songs* (ed. Bishop Thomas Percy; late 18th century)

Stand, stately Tavie, out of the codpiece rise,
And dig a grave between thy mistress' thighs;
Swift stand, then stab 'till she replies,
Then gently weep, and after weeping die.
Stand, Tavie, and gain thy credit lost;
Or by this hand I'll never draw thee, but against a post.

Anon. 'Stand, Stately Tavie' (18th century)

It is I, you women, I make my way,
I am stern, acrid, large, undissuadable, but I love you,
I do not hurt you any more than is

necessary for you,
I pour the stuff to start sons and daughters fit for these States, I press with slow rude muscle,
I brace myself effectually, I listen to no entreaties,
I dare not withdraw till I deposit what has so long accumulated within me.

Walt Whitman 'Children of Adam' (1860)

In tumescence the organism is slowly wound up and force accumulates; in the act of detumescence the accumulated force is let go and by its liberation the sperm-bearing instrument is driven home.

The whole process of orgasm is exactly analogous to that by which a pile is driven into the earth by the raising and then the letting go of a heavy weight which falls on the head of the pile.

H. Havelock Ellis *The Mechanism of Detumescence* (1906)

For men, orgasm is widely and easily achieved; sexual activity without orgasm is deeply unsatisfying – presumably a reflection of the biological role that male orgasm plays in reproduction.

It is inconceivable that males who were not reaching orgasm would continue their marital coitus for any length of time.

Alfred Kinsey et al. *Sexual Behaviour in the Human Female* (1953)

The orgasm is the sugar coating with which the Creator (or Nature) has disguised the bitter pill of reproduction.

Paul A. Robinson *The Sexual Radicals* (1973)

93 per cent of the males interviewed claimed to have reached orgasm by the age of 15 through masturbation, heterosexual or homosexual activity.

For perhaps three quarters of all males, orgasm is reached within two minutes after the initiation of the sexual relation.

The evidence is now clear, that such arousal as petting provides may seriously disturb some individuals, leaving them in a more or less extended nervous state unless the activity has proceeded to orgasm.

Alfred Kinsey et al. *Sexual Behaviour in the Human Male* (1948)

However, in the 17th century, according to the teaching of the Church, orgasms were for one purpose only – and that purpose was not pleasure:

A person who feels a sexual climax coming on, save during marital intercourse, should lie still, taking care to avoid touching the genitals, should make the sign of the cross, accompanied by fervent prayers beseeching God not to allow him to slip into orgasmic pleasure.

Tomás Sánchez *De Sancto matrimonii sacramento disputationum* (1621)

And one opinion that is not mainstream:

In my experience, orgasm and ejaculation are not the same. In my experience there is a male orgasm separate and distinct from ejaculation, and these non-ejaculatory orgasms can be multiple.

John Stoltenberg *Refusing to be a Man* (1977)

The question of the female orgasm is far more controversial. At least there is some agreement about the nature of the experience.

When the sensations named for Aphrodite are mounting to their peak, a woman goes frantic with pleasure, she kisses with mouth wide open and thrashes about like a mad woman.

When a woman reaches the very goal of Aphrodite's action, she instinctively gasps with a burning delight and her gasp rises quickly to the lips with a love-breath, and there it meets a lost kiss, wandering about and looking for a way down. This kiss mingles with the love-breath and returns with it to strike the heart. The heart then is kissed, confused, throbbing.

Achilles Tatius *Leucippe and Cleitophon* (5th century)

When her climax came – and it appeared suddenly, like an accident – Jade trembled and made a high whinny, as if in distress. Then she was absolutely still, like a startled animal etched in the brightening beam of speeding headlights. Her mouth was open; it seemed as if she might drool but she closed her lips and lifted her chin, breathing out so heavily that her belly swelled and made her look pregnant for a moment.

Scott Spencer *Endless Love* (1980)

We have seen that the act of love requires of woman profound self-abandonment she bathes in a passive languor; with closed eyes anonymous, lost, she feels as if borne by waves, swept away in a storm, shrouded in darkness: darkness of the flesh, of the womb, of the grave. Annihilated, she becomes one with the Whole, her ego is abolished. But when the man moves from her, she finds herself back on earth, on a bed, in the light; she again has a name, a face: she is one vanquished, prey, object.

Simone de Beauvoir *The Second Sex* (1949)

The orgasm itself reminds me of a dam breaking. I can feel contractions inside me and a very liquid sensation. The best part is the continuing waves of build-up and release during multiple orgasms.

My vaginal and clitoral area gets absolutely hot and I seem to switch into a pelvic rhythm over which I have no conscious control; every contact with my clitoris at this point is a miniature orgasm which becomes more frequent until it is one huge muscle spasm!

First, tension builds in my body and head, my heart beats, then I strain against my lover, and then there is a second or two of absolute stillness, non-breathing, during which I know orgasm will come in the next second or two. Then waves, and I rock against my partner and cannot hold him tight enough. It's all over my body, but especially in my abdomen and gut. Afterwards, I feel suffused with warmth and love and absolute happiness.

Anon. women describing what they feel during orgasm, quoted by Shere Hite in *The Hite Report* (1976)

Whatever it is that happens to women at the climax of their lovemaking, it does not seem to have changed much over the last 15 centuries! However, not everyone agrees on exactly what is happening:

In the case of women, it is my contention that when during intercourse the vagina is rubbed and the womb is disturbed, an irritation is set up in the womb which produces pleasure and heat in the rest of the body...Once intercourse has begun, she experiences pleasure throughout the whole time, until the man ejaculates. If her desire for intercourse is excited, she emits before the man, and for the remainder of the time she does not feel pleasure to the same extent; but if she is not in a state of excitement, then her pleasure terminates along with that of the man.

Hippocrates *On the Generating Seed and the Nature of the Child* (4th century BC)

She burns and as it were, dries up the semen received by her from the male, and if by chance a child is conceived it is ill-formed and does not remain nine months in the mother's womb.

John Davenport *Curiositates Eroticae Physiologiae* (1875)

Orgiastic potency is defined as the capacity for complete discharge of all dammed-up sexual excitation through involuntary pleasurable contractions of the body.

Wilhelm Reich *Function of the Orgasm* (1942)

There were wives and husbands in the older generation, who did not even know that orgasm was possible for a female; or if they knew that it was possible, they did not comprehend that it could be desirable.

Alfred Kinsey et al. *Sexual Behaviour in the Human Female* (1953)

Is orgasm as necessary for women as it is for men in achieving sexual satisfaction?

It cannot be emphasized too often that orgasm cannot be taken as the sole criterion for determining the degree of satisfaction which a female may derive from sexual activity. Considerable pleasure may be found in sexual arousal which does not proceed to the point of orgasm, and in the social aspects of a sexual relationship. Whether or not she herself reaches orgasm, many a female finds satisfaction in knowing that her husband or other sexual partner has enjoyed the contact, and in realizing that she has contributed to the male's pleasure.

Alfred Kinsey et al. *Sexual Behaviour in the Human Female* (1953)

A woman may be emotionally satisfied to the full in the absence of any *orgasmic expression.*

Mary Jane Sherfey *A Theory of Female Sexuality* (1966)

Asked what aspect of sexual activity gave them the most pleasure, the majority preferred 'emotional intimacy, tenderness, closeness, sharing deep feelings with a loved one'. Orgasm came second.

Shere Hite *The Hite Report* (1976)

Children and most women can resort to crying as a means of easing the pain of disappointment, grief or unhappiness. Most men cannot do so – because, in a profound sense, they do not want to do so; they have learned that crying is 'unmanly'. Similarly, many women have learned that being sexually self-affirmative is 'unfeminine', hence, they are unable to discharge sexual tension through (coital) orgasm. Such women are now called anorgasmic (they used to be called frigid), but men who cannot weep are not called alachrymal. The former condition is thought to be a sexual dysfunction, but the latter is not considered to be a lachrymal dysfunction.

Thomas Szasz *Sex: Facts, Frauds and Follies* (1981)

Only approximately 30 per cent of the women in this study could orgasm regularly from intercourse.

Shere Hite *The Hite Report* (1976)

When should women have their orgasms and how many should they have?

Both parties should, in coitus, concentrate their full attention on one thing: the attainment of simultaneous orgasm.

Eustace Chesser *Love without Fear* (1939)

...she felt the soft bud of him within her stirring, and strange rhythms flushing up into her with a strange rhythmic growing motion, swelling and swelling till it filled all her cleaving consciousness, and then began again the unspeakable motion that was not really motion, but pure deepening whirlpools of sensation swirling deeper and deeper through all her tissue and consciousness, till she was one perfect concentric fluid of feeling, and she lay there crying in unconscious inarticulate cries...He sat down again on the brushwood and took Connie's hand in silence. She turned and looked at him. "We came off together that time," he said. She did not answer. "It's good when it's like that. Most folks live their lives through and they never know it," he said, speaking rather dreamily. "Don't people often come off together?" she asked with naïve curiosity. "A good many of them never. You can see by the raw look of them."

D. H. Lawrence *Lady Chatterley's Lover* (1928)

The modern erotic ideal: man and woman in loving sexual embrace experiencing simultaneous orgasm through genital intercourse. This is a psychiatric-sexual myth useful for fostering feelings of sexual inadequacy and personal inferiority. It is also a rich source of psychiatric 'patients'.

Thomas Szasz *The Second Sin* (1973)

More experienced and sensitive lovers enjoy their partner's climactic transports, which they are unable to do if they orgasm simultaneously.

Francis Stubbs *Evening Primroses* (1945)

When the man feels that he is about to emit semen he should always wait until the woman has reached orgasm.

Li Tung Hsuan *The Art of Love* (7th century)

The more quickly orgasm is attained, the more effective the performance is judged to be.

Alfred Kinsey et al. *Sexual Behaviour in the Human Female* (1953)

A woman will usually be satisfied with three to five orgasms.

Women are naturally multi-orgasmic; That is, if a woman is immediately stimulated following orgasm, she is likely to experience several orgasms in rapid succession. This is not an exceptional occurrence, but one of which most women are capable.

William Masters and Virginia Johnson *The Human Sexual Response* (1966)

Theoretically, a woman could go on having orgasms indefinitely, if physical exhaustion did not intervene.

Woman's inordinate orgasmic capacity did not evolve for monogamous, sedentary cultures.

Mary Jane Sherfey *A Theory of Female Sexuality* (1966)

The woman usually wills herself to be satisfied because she is simply unaware of the extent of her orgasmic capacity.

Mary Jane Sherfey *The Nature and Evolution of Female Sexuality* (1972).

Many women still faked orgasm in the belief that satisfying their partner was more important than their own satisfaction...

Cate Haste *Rules of Desire* (1992)

During this century there has been much discussion about whether or not there are two kinds of female orgasm – one brought about by the presence of a penis (or penis substitute) in the vagina:

It is nonsense to say that a woman feels nothing when a man is moving his penis inside her vagina: the orgasm is qualitatively different when the vagina can undulate around the penis instead of a vacancy.

Germaine Greer *The Female Eunuch* (1970)

and the other resulting from stimulation of the clitoris:

The facts of female anatomy and sexual response tell a different story. There is only one area for sexual climax although there are many areas for sexual arousal; that area is the clitoris. All orgasms are extensions of sensation from this area.

Anne Koedt *The Myth of the Vaginal Orgasm* (1970)

During my marriage I never once reached a climax during intercourse. The only way I could have one was for my husband to manipulate my clitoris.

Letter to *Forum* magazine quoted in *The Body Politic* (ed. Micheline Wandor; 1972)

There is still no sign of agreement on the matter:

Paul began to rely on manipulating her externally, on giving Ella clitoral orgasms. Very exciting. Yet there was always a part of her that resented it. Because she felt that the fact he wanted to, was an expression of his instinctive desire not to commit himself to her...A vaginal orgasm is emotion and nothing else, felt as emotion and expressed in sensations that are indistinguishable from emotion. The vaginal orgasm is a dissolving in a vague, dark generalised sensation like being swirled in a warm whirlpool. There are several different sorts of clitoral orgasms, and they are more powerful (that is a male word) than the vaginal orgasm. There can be a thousand thrills, sensations, etc., but there is only one real female orgasm and that is when a man, from the whole of his need and desire takes a woman and wants all

her response...But when she told him she had never experienced what she insisted on calling 'a real orgasm' to anything like the same depth before him, he involuntarily frowned, and remarked: "Do you know that there are eminent physiologists who say women have no physical basis for vaginal orgasm?"
"Then they don't know much, do they?"

Doris Lessing *The Golden Notebook* (1962)

The dichotomy of vaginal and clitoral orgasms is entirely false. Anatomically, all orgasms are centred in the clitoris, whether they result from direct manual pressure applied to the clitoris, indirect pressure resulting from the thrusting of the penis during intercourse, or generalized sexual stimulation of other erogenous zones like the breasts.

William Masters and Virginia Johnson *The Human Sexual Response* (1966)

Men have orgasms essentially by friction with the vagina, not the clitoral area, which is external and not able to cause friction the way penetration does. Women have thus been defined sexually in terms of what pleases men: our own biology has not been properly analyzed. Instead we are fed the myth of the liberated woman and her vaginal orgasm – an orgasm which in fact does not exist.

Anne Koedt *The Myth of the Vaginal Orgasm* (1970)

Just then, Dottie screamed faintly; it had gone all the way in. He put his hand over her mouth and then settled her legs around him and commenced to move it back and forth inside her. At first, it hurt so that she flinched at each stroke and tried to pull back, but this only seemed to make him more determined. Then, while she was still praying for it to be over, surprise of surprises, she started to like it a little. She got the idea, and her body began to move too in answer, as he pressed that *home in her slowly, over and over, and slowly drew it back, as if repeating a question. Her breath came quicker. Each lingering stroke, like a violin bow, made her palpitate for the next. Then, all of a sudden, she seemed to explode in a series of long, uncontrollable contractions that embarrassed her, like the hiccups, the moment they were over, for it was as if she had forgotten Dick as a person... She struggled against the excitement his tickling thumb was producing in her own external part; but as she felt him watching her, her eyes closed and her thighs spread open. He disengaged her hand, and she fell back on the bed, gasping. His thumb continued its play and she let herself yield to what it was doing, her whole attention concentrated on a tense pinpoint of sensation, which suddenly discharged itself in a nervous, fluttering spasm; her body arched and heaved and then lay still. When his hand returned to touch her, she struck it feebly away. 'Don't,' she moaned, rolling over on her stomach. This second climax, which she now recognized from the first one, though it was different, left her jumpy and disconcerted; it was something less thrilling and more like being tickled relentlessly or having to go to the bathroom.*

Mary McCarthy *The Group* (1963)

The recognition of clitoral orgasm would threaten the heterosexual institution. For it would indicate that sexual pleasure was obtainable from either men or *women, thus making heterosexuality not an absolute, but an option.*

Anne Koedt *The Myth of the Vaginal Orgasm* (1970)

This dichotomy of experience was summarized somewhat inconclusively by Cate Haste:

Masters and Johnson's Human Sexual Response *published in 1966 had exploded several myths about female sexuality, particularily the hierarchical distinction between the clitoral orgasm, designated since Freud 'immature', and the vaginal orgasm, designated 'mature' (proper) which had over the years gener-*

ated widespread anxiety among women about their sexual 'inadequacy, as well as sweeping generalisations about women's 'frigidity'. Masters and Johnson raised the status of the clitoris from being an aspect of foreplay to playing the central role by identifying it as 'the primary focus for sexual response in the human female's pelvis'. This conclusion had previously been drawn by Kinsey but had been largely ignored. They reiterated Kinsey's observations on the physiological similarities between men's and women's sexual responses and concluded that not only just a few, as Kinsey had observed, but the vast majority of women were capable of multiple orgasms.

Rules of Desire (1992)

See also IMPOTENCE AND FRIGIDITY

Kinsey's observation that male and female sexual responses were similar is interesting:

All orgasms appear to be physiologically similar quantities, whether they are derived from masturbatory, heterosexual, homosexual, or other sorts of activity. For most females and males, there appear to be basic physiologic needs which are satisfied by sexual orgasms, whatever the source.

Alfred Kinsey et al. *Sexual Behaviour in the Human Female* (1953)

There is no essential aspect of the orgasm of the adult which has not been observed in the orgasms which young children may have.

Alfred Kinsey et al. *Sexual Behaviour in the Human Male* (1946)

Sexology has ascertained that the clitoris and the penis are not biologically dissimilar in terms of arousal potential.

Kenneth Plummer 'The Making of the Modern Homosexual' in *Liberating Lesbian Research* (1981)

However:

The clitoris is unique in that it is the only organ in human anatomy whose purpose is exclusively that of erotic excitation and release.

William Masters and Virginia Johnson *The Human Sexual Response* (1966)

An interesting observation in the absence of an explanation of the biological role of the female orgasm (whether or not it occurs seems not to alter the chances of conception).

The greater openness about the female orgasm that has been a feature of recent years has undoubtedly led many women to expect more from their sex lives.

The complete mutual satisfaction, physical and psychic, of mother and child, in the transfer from one to another of a precise organicized fluid, is the one true physiological analogy of the relationship of a man and a woman at the climax of the sexual act.

H. Havelock Ellis *Analysis of the Sexual Impulse* (1903)

The apex of raptures sweeps into its tides the whole essence of the man and woman, vaporizes their consciousness so that it fills the whole of cosmic space.

Dr Marie Stopes *Married Love* (1918)

Women who have taken it for granted that the sexual satisfaction was unimportant are now reading about women having multiple orgasms. Many men realise they've *been ripped off by being programmed to deny their expressive aspects. It becomes a possibility to throw out some of the old sex roles and change drastically.*

Sophie Freud Loewenstein *New York Times* (28 Nov. 1972)

I was sleeping with men and not coming. I was allowing them to be the ones who knew about lovemaking and running the show. And I just kind of joined in.

Anon., quoted by Anna Coote and Beatrix Campbell in *Sweet Freedom* (1982)

Although the frequency of marital coitus was declining...the regularity of her orgasm in marital intercourse was rising. This increase in orgiastic reliability and overall sexual satisfaction eventually offset the forces that caused the initial drop in coital activity.

Morton Hunt *Sexual Behaviour in the 1970s* (1974)

The women's movement is merely the latest attempt to fulfil the objectives of orgasm, by which a man and woman cease to be known as such and instead become full persons.

Declan Kiberd *Men and Feminism in Modern Literature* (1985)

It seems, however, that the modern obsession with orgasms, male and female, may only be creating new burdens and anxieties.

At the center of that religion of marriage was a cult every bit as hallowed as that of the Virgin: the cult of the orgasm, mutual and simultaneous. It descended to the young people of my generation from both Lawrence and Freud as the Inner Mystery, something they all aspired to, a sign of grace. Because of it I had impossible expectations of my marriage, my sex life, myself. I was an absolutist of the orgasm before I had had enough experience to ensure even sexual competence.

Al Alvarez *Life after Marriage* (1982)

She not only has to prove him a man by making him experience orgasm; she must also prove her femininity by the same experience, because otherwise she must fear she is frigid. Sexual intercourse cannot often stand up to such complex emotional demands of proving so many things in addition to being enjoyable.

Bruno Bettelheim *The Problem of Generations* (1962)

One medical expert reported men were seeing their partner's orgasm as a reflection of their virility; if women failed, men felt inadequate. Women who failed might also feel inadequate, a new word for frigid. If women succeeded, it was a tribute to male technique.

Cate Haste *Rules of Desire* (1992)

The orgasm has replaced the Cross as the focus of longing and the image of fulfilment.

Malcolm Muggeridge *Tread Softly For You Tread On My Jokes* (1966)

The cult of the Orgasm succeeded the cult of Mammon as the basic passion of American life.

Daniel Bell *The Cultural Contradictions of Capitalism* (1978)

The new opiate of the people, like all religions, has its ritual observance. The discipline imposed is the discipline of the orgasm, not just any orgasm, but the perfect orgasm, regular, spontaneous, potent and reliable.

Germaine Greer *Sex and Destiny* (1984)

Orgies

In the ancient world orgiastic behaviour often had a religious significance, being associated with fertility rites and the cults of particular gods or goddesses. This is reflected in the derivation of the word 'orgy' – from a Greek word meaning 'nocturnal festival'. Greek and Roman mystery religions often made use of frenzied dancing, drinking, and sexual activity to induce a mood of communal hysteria:

> *The rites of the Good Goddess! Shrieking flutes excite the women's loins, wine and trumpet madden them, whirling and shrieking, rapt by Priapus. Then, then, their hearts are burning with lust, their voices stammer with it, their wine gushes in torrents down their soaking thighs. Their itching cannot bear delay: this is sheer Woman, shrieking and crying everywhere in the hall, 'It is time, let in the men!'...And if no man can be found, they content themselves with an ass.*
>
> Juvenal *Satires* (2nd century)

> *The orgy is not associated with the dignity of religion, extracting from the underlying violence something calm and majestic compatible with profane order; its potency is seen in its ill-aimed aspects, bringing frenzy in its wake and a vertiginous loss of consciousness. The total personality is involved, reeling blindly towards annihilation, and this is the decisive moment of religious feeling...*
>
> *In the orgy the celebration progresses with the overwhelming force that usually brushes all bonds aside. In itself the feast is a denial of the limits set on life by work, but the orgy turns everything upside-down. It is not by chance that the social order used to be turned topsy-turvy during the Saturnalia, the master serving the slave, the slave lolling on the master's bed. These excesses derive their most acute significance from the ancient connection between sensual pleasure and religious exaltation.*
>
> Georges Bataille *Eroticism* (1987)

The mysteries of the wine god Bacchus (Dionysius), originally for women only, seem to have become orgies in the modern sense sometime after they reached Rome and men were admitted:

> *After the rites had become open to everybody, so that men attended as well as women, and their licentiousness increased with the darkness of night, there was no shameful or criminal deed from which they shrank. The men were guilty of more immoral acts among themselves than the women. Those who struggled against dishonour or were slow to inflict it on others, were slaughtered in sacrifice like brute beasts. The holiest article of their faith was to think nothing a crime.*
>
> Livy *History of Rome* (1st century AD)

The Bacchic rites acquired such an unsavoury reputation that the Roman Senate was moved to prohibit them in 186 BC. During the Imperial era, however, hedonism and excess of all kinds were allowed to flourish:

> *The Roman idea of love was purely sexual. Lust was the rule for everything: sex, food, or violence. Orgies and feasts lasted*

for days. There was a limit on how much sex one could participate in, but there was no end to the eating orgies.

Sander J. Breiner *Slaughter of the Innocents* (1990)

Tiberius on retiring to Capreae made himself a private sporting house, where sexual extravagancies were practised for his secret pleasure. Bevies of girls and young men, whom he had collected from all over the Empire as adepts in unnatural practices, and known as spinfriae, *would copulate before him in groups of three, to excite his waning passions…*

Nero so prostituted his own chastity, that after defiling almost every part of his body, he at last devised a kind a game in which, covered with the skin of some wild animal, he was let loose from a cage and attacked the private parts of men and women, who were bound to stakes…

Suetonius *Lives of the Twelve Caesars* (c. 100 AD)

Indeed, Rome seems to have a special association with orgies – from the days of Nero to those of the Borgias and Fellini's *La Dolce Vita*. The Borgias were particularly enthusiastic party-goers:

Dear son,
We have heard that Your Worthiness, forgetful of the high office with which you are invested, was present from the 17th to the 24th hour, 4 days ago, in the garden of Giovanni de Bichis, where there were several women of Siena, women wholly given over to worldly vanities. We have heard that a dance was indulged in with all wantonness; none of the allurements of love were lacking, and you conducted yourself in a wholly worldly manner. Shame forbids mention of all that took place…In order that your lust might be all the more unrestrained, the husbands, fathers, brothers, and kinsmen of the young women and girls were not invited to be present. You and a few servants were the leaders and inspirers of this orgy.

Pope Pius II, letter to his son Rodrigo Borgia, later Pope Alexander VI (11 June 1460)

On the evening of 30th October 1501 there was a feast in the rooms of the Duke of Valentinois [Cezare Borgia] *in the Papal Palace. 50 prostitutes of the kind known as courtesans and who are not of the common people, were present. After the meal they danced with the servants and the others who were present. At first they wore their dresses, then they stripped themselves completely naked. The meal over, the lighted candles which were on the table, were set out on the floor, and chestnuts were thrown down for the naked courtesans to pick up, crawling on hands and knees between the candlesticks. The Pope, the Duke, and Lucrezia his sister were present watching. Finally a collection of silk cloaks, of hose, of brooches, and of other things was displayed, and promised to those who had connexion with the greatest number of prostitutes. This took place in public, the spectators, who acted as judges, gave the prizes to those who were judged the victors.*

John Burchard, secretary to Pope Alexander VI, *Diary* (Oct. 1501)

Fellini portrayed a modern Rome preoccupied with decadent parties:

La Dolce Vita *(1959) Federico Fellini's exposé of 'the sweet life', a sprawling persuasive, orgiastic movie assumed by many to have contributed to a decline in standards because it reported without condemning .*

Leslie Halliwell *Filmgoer's Companion* (1979)

But, of course, Romans, ancient or modern, have no monopoly on such behaviour. Orgies of one kind or another have occurred in most cultures and periods, poor taste being one of the most universal of human characteristics:

When women enter the banquet-hall, at first their dress is modest: then they each take off their outer garments. Finally they throw off the most intimate coverings of their bodies. Nor is this an abomination of prostitutes, but the practice of matrons and girls who consider the degradation of their exposed person as a mark of courtesy.

Quintus Curtius Rufus *The History of Alexander the Great* (1st century AD)

There is such a renninge, leapinge, and flynginge amongst them, and then there is such a lyftinge up and discouering of damesels clothes and of other wemens apparell that a man might thynk all these dauncers had cast all shame behinde them and were become stark madde and out of their wyttes and that they were sworn to the the devels daunce. And that noyse and rombling endureth euen until supper.

Heinrich Bullinger *The Christian State of Matrimonye* (15th century)

Orgies are common in Japanese and Chinese art, and were common enough in the traditional Japanese pattern of life to have given rise to a game called 'Crossing the Valley.' The girls lay down on the floor and the boys had to do them all in turn, from one end of the room to the other. The winner was the boy who 'crossed the valley' without coming...

The American petting party is a kind of catharized or yogi-ized orgy for adolescents, based on the ritual retention of semen.

Wayland Young *Eros Denied* (1964)

If all the young ladies who attended the Yale promenade dance were laid end to end, no one would be the least surprised.

Dorothy Parker, quoted by Alexander Woollcott in *While Rome Burns* (1934)

Of course, one motive for participating in an orgy might be intellectual curiosity. It is said that Voltaire, having attended an orgy for the first time, turned down an invitation to a second one on the following night, commenting:

Once: a philosopher; twice: a pervert!

Voltaire's near contemporary, the Marquise de Sade, had no such inhibitions about combining philosophy with perversion – in either his life or his writings:

"Come on," said Raphael, as his prodigious desires seemed to have reached the point of no return, "it's time to sacrifice the victim; each of us must prepare to submit her to his favourite enjoyments." And the vile man, having put me on the sofa, in the most opportune position for his deplorable pleasures, had me held by Antonin and Clément...Raphael – Italian, a monk and depraved – satisfied himself insultingly, without my ceasing to be a virgin...Clément came forward, inflamed by the sight of his Superior's infamy, and even more by what he'd done while watching...He got me down on my knees, and getting tight up against me in this position, practised his false passions in a place which stopped me complaining of its irregularity while the sacrifice was going on. Jérôme followed. His temple was the same as that of Raphael, but he didn't get to the inner sanctuary and was content to stay at the vestibule..."What a good start!" Antonin said as he grabbed me. "Come here, my chicken, come and let me revenge the irregularities of my brothers and pluck the first fruits that their excesses have left me"...the normal pain of losing a virginity was the least thing I had to bear in this dangerous attack. But it was at the moment of orgasm that Antonin finished with such ferocious cries...that I believed for that moment that I was the prey of a savage animal who could only be satisfied by devouring me. When these horrors were completed, I fell back on the altar of my sacrifice, not knowing where I was and almost unconscious.

Marquis de Sade *Justine, or the Misfortunes of Virtue* (1791)

While anonymous group sex may be an attractive theme for fantasy, it is probable that any sensitive person would find the reality awkward, exhausting, and depressing. In the 1960s orgies were said to be the rage in the world of Christine

Keeler and Stephen Ward – but even they did not seem to be too enthusiastic:

Stephen was going to the occasional orgy, but he was now rather bored with them. He always asked if I wanted to go along, but I refused. They didn't turn me on. One night though, when Mandy was with me at the flat, we agreed to pick him up after the party...The guests were bankers, brokers and professionals from Harley Street, plus a smattering of artists, for luck. The girls were young and very sexy. There was only one rule: never, on any account, have anything to do with another person privately. If a couple disappeared into a corner, they were quickly flushed out and jeered at. It wasn't sporting. Stephen never joined in. He preferred watching or holding court in a corner, talking with people who had just finished themselves off.

Christine Keeler *Scandal* (1989)

Orgies are for sexual athletes.

Quentin Crisp (1975)

...on Fire Island...the atmosphere is sick, sick, sick. Never in my life have I seen such concentrated, abandoned homosexuality. It is fantastic and difficult to believe...Thousands of queer young men of all shapes and sizes camping about blatantly and carrying on – in my opinion – appallingly...I have always been of the opinion that a large group of queer men was unattractive. In Fire Island it is more than unattractive, it's macabre, sinister, irritating and somehow tragic.

Noël Coward *Diaries* (1982)

A few closing opinions to reflect the ambiguity of human feelings on the subject:

Home is heaven and orgies are vile
But you need an orgy, once in a while.

Ogden Nash *Home, 99.44100% Sweet Home* (1940)

An orgy looks particularly alluring seen through the mists of righteous indignation.

Malcolm Muggeridge *The Most of Malcolm Muggeridge*, 'Dolce Vita in a Cold Climate' (1966)

If God had meant us to have group sex, I guess he'd have given us all more organs.

Malcolm Bradbury *Who Do You Think You Are?*, 'A Very Hospitable Person' (1976)

Perversion

Erotic is when you do something sensitive and imaginative with a feather. Kinky is when you use the whole chicken.

John Collee *Observer* (8 Nov. 1992)

Attempts to define what is 'normal' or 'abnormal' in sexual behaviour are notoriously self-defeating. Such definitions often turn out to be circular:

By normal sex life, we mean the forms of sex that commonly occur in healthy natural people, and we group in abnormal sex all forms of sex that occur only rarely, and in their form deviate from ordinary forms in essential points.

J. Fabricius-Møller *Sexual Life* (1944)

or to be based on little more than the social conventions of a particular place and time:

The man who avoids women and the woman who seeks out men are abnormal.

Richard von Krafft-Ebing *Psychopathia Sexualis* (1886)

Is the criterion of normality to be statistical, biological, or moral? These categories often seem to become confused:

The elements of a comprehensive definition of sexual perversion should include sexual activity or fantasy directed towards orgasm other than genital intercourse with a willing partner of the opposite sex and of similar maturity, and contrary to the generally accepted norm of sexual behaviour in the community.

P. D. Scott *The Pathology and Treatment of Sexual Deviation* (1964)

Yet surveys indicate that most adults enjoy sexual fantasies of precisely this kind (see SEXUAL FANTASIES) – are they all to be labelled 'abnormal'? Similarly, any attempt to define sexual normality purely in terms of the reproductive goal will lead to the conclusion that most of us are perverts:

No healthy person, it appears, can fail to make some addition that might be called perverse to the normal sexual aim; and the universality of this finding is in itself enough to show how inappropriate it is to use the word perversion as a term of reproach.

Sigmund Freud *Three Essays on the Theory of Sexuality* (1905)

Another difficulty arises from the fact that much 'normal' sexual behaviour includes elements that – taken in isolation – might be seen as 'perverted':

The borderline between normal and abnormal is by no means sharp, and there are all kinds of intermediate stages.

J. Fabricius-Møller *Sexual Life* (1944)

Where, for instance, does one draw the line between:

a lover's pinch that hurts and is desired

William Shakespeare *Antony and Cleopatra* (1606)

and more extreme sadomasochistic practices?

The pleasure-pain syndrome is so characteristic of ordinary love-making that the boundary across which such activity becomes a perversion is not easy to draw.

G. Hughes *Consent in Sexual Offences* (1962)

Similarly, at what point does the lover's fascination with specific parts of the beloved's body, items of clothing, or other associated objects become fetishism? Phyllis Greenacre both states the problem and suggests the answer:

Perhaps the most frequent normal fetishistic phenomenon of adulthood is the love-token, or memento, which enhances the courtship love-play and may find its place as a preferred, but not a necessary, contribution to the foreplay of intercourse.

Fetishism as a perversion may be described in phenomenological terms, as the obligatory *use of some non-genital object as a part of the sexual act, without which culmination cannot be achieved.*

Fetishism (1964)

Perhaps there is a key element in any definition of perversion:

One factor which would appear to characterize the pervert...is that he has no choice; his sexuality is fundamentally compulsive.

J. McDougall *Primal Scene and Sexual Perversion* (1972)

The compulsive behaviour may be either an adjunct to or a substitute for ordinary intercourse:

Perverse behaviour usually occurred in two distinct phases; the specific perverse activity, followed by apparently normal intercourse in which the person's potency was augmented by the antecedent perverse behaviour.

M. Oston *Sexual Deviation: a Psycho-analytical Approach* (1974)

Although women may suffer from sexual compulsions, the criminal or antisocial forms of abnormality are almost entirely limited to men:

In reality, despite the daydreams of many men, females rarely force sexual intercourse on males.

C. H. McCaghy *Deviant Behaviour* (1976)

Voyeurism also occurs only in men. There are no reports of women seeking gratification of their sexual impulses by, for example, roaming around military bases and spying on soldiers.

Preben Hertoft *Psychosexual Problems* (1976)

See also EXHIBITIONISM

Various attempts have been made to find the cause or causes of sexual abnormality. At one time it was thought that perversion could be inherited:

Perverse instincts which injure no-one when carried into practice (fetishism, for example), are ethically indifferent and harmless, in that their possessors, generally speaking, do not multiply. It is, however, immoral for such persons to marry. Anyone who suffers from an hereditary perversion of the sex instinct should avoid marriage and all procreation of children.

Auguste Forel *Sexual Ethics* (1908)

Psychoanalysts have generally sought explanations in early childhood:

It is impossible to begin to understand sexual perversions without a knowledge of infantile sexuality, of its peculiar features, its development and vicissitudes and of the transformations which it normally goes through at puberty before emerging as adult sexuality.

Ismond Rosen *The General Psychoanalytical Theory of Perversion* (1964)

There is a tendency to blame the mother:

In the child destined to a perverse solution of sexual desire the mother's unconscious plays a vital role. One is tempted to surmise that the mother of the future pervert herself denies sexual reality and denigrates the father's phallic function. It is possible that she gives the child in addition the feeling that he or she is a phallic substitute.

J. McDougall *Primal Scene and Sexual Perversion* (1972)

Attempts to explain individual disorders range from the obviously sensible:

The paedophiliac is usually shy and timid and may show a wide range of psychopathological behaviour...Fear has prevented the development of adult heterosexuality and they tend to seek comfort and sexual gratification with children.

D. J. Power *Sexual Deviation and Crime* (1976)

to the extremely unlikely:

Quite by accident I recently hit on what I hope is the ultimate secret of foot fetishism. In the foot it has become permissible to worship the long lost and ardently longed-for woman's penis of the primordial age of infancy. Evidently some people search as passionately for this precious object as the pious English do for the lost ten tribes of Israel.

Sigmund Freud, in a letter to Carl Jung (21 Nov. 1909)

The moral implications of sexual abnormality are a matter of much debate. Some radical thinkers see the pervert as a heroic figure, who elevates sex from a blind biological urge into a truly human and imaginative activity:

The taboo within us against sexual liberty is general and universal; the particular prohibitions are variable aspects of it.

Georges Bataille *Eroticism* (1987)

A common view today is that consensual acts, however extreme or bizarre, are necessarily morally neutral. Others find this assumption overly bland. To many, such practices as coprophilia, necrophilia, bestiality, or serious sadomasochism make a travesty of love and lovemaking:

The delight in perversions is caused by the destruction, humiliation, desecration, the deformation *of the perverse individual himself and of his partner.*

E. Straus *Geschehnis und Erlebrus* (1930)

The sadist, like the necrophiliac, the paedophile, and the rapist, can accept the other only in terms that are dictated by himself...The other's body is the means to accomplish a private ceremony.

Roger Scruton *Sexual Desire: A Philosophical Investigation* (1986)

See also MORALITY

For some, too, the taking of pleasure in the infliction of pain is *always* wrong and dangerous:

The wish to hurt, the momentary intoxication with pain, is the loophole through which the pervert climbs into the minds of ordinary people.

Jacob Bronowski *The Face of Violence* (1954)

The greatest achievement of Sade is undoubtedly to demonstrate that just because an idea is original, revolutionary, outrageous, avant-garde or frowned upon, doesn't mean it contains anything of merit.

Alexander Baron *The Wickedest Woman in the World* (1991)

The sadist may be utterly demonic in his actions, so may use considerable violence, even to the extent that his victim's death may result; this is called sexual murder.

J. Fabricius-Møller *Sexual Life* (1944)

Sadism per se *is not a mental disorder within the meaning of the Mental Health Act 1959 and does not legally excuse or mitigate murder or other serious crimes against the person. It may be an expression of psychopathic disorder, psychosis, subnormality or organic brain disease.*

D. J. Power *Sexual Deviation and Crime* (1976)

See also SADISM AND MASOCHISM

One of the rarest and most extreme forms of sexual abnormality is vampirism:

The syndrome consists of a compulsive interest in blood, confusion about personal identity and an abnormal interest in death – often manifested by necrophilia or necrophagia (pleasure derived from the eating of parts of dead bodies)...
The vampire is the freest of all characters, doing just what he or she pleases. With the combination of necrophilia, necrophagia, serial killing, blood, sex, death and cannibalism, every possible taboo is violated.

Raj Persand 'Blood-lust in the Clinic' *Independent* (2 Feb. 1993)

Finally, a short list of clinical terms for some of the lesser known sexual disorders:

acrotomophilia — *sexual pleasure from imagining that one's partner is an amputee*
apotemnophilia — *sexual pleasure from imagining oneself as an amputee*
asphyxiophilia — *sexual pleasure from the idea of strangulation*
autoassassinatophilia — *sexual pleasure from staging or imagining one's own murder*
coprophilia — *sexual pleasure from faeces or their evacuation*
gerontophilia — *sexual attraction to a much older partner*
kleptophilia — *sexual pleasure from stealing*
klismaphilia — *sexual pleasure from being given an enema*
homocidophilia — *sexual pleasure from the idea of murdering one's partner*
mysophilia — *sexual pleasure from soiled underwear*
narratophilia — *sexual pleasure from erotic narratives*

Pornography and Erotica

What is pornography?

Pornography is a more civilized version of rape. That is to say, it is an appeal to the masculine desire to conquer and penetrate without personal involvement.

Colin Wilson 'Literature and Pornography' in *The Sexual Dimension in Literature* (ed. Alan Bold; 1982)

Pornography is the theory, and rape is the practice.

Robin Morgan *Going Too Far: the Personal Chronicle of a Feminist* (1978)

Pornography is the attempt to insult sex, to do dirt on it.

D. H. Lawrence 'Pornography and Obscenity' (1929)

Pornography is a social problem. It is a commodity brought into existence by certain characteristics of a highly developed civilisation.

Sir Herbert Read in *Does Pornography Matter?* (1961)

Pornography includes all forms of visual and verbal humiliation of women for the sexual titillation of men, from page 3 in the Sun *to strip tease and flagellation movies, plus the exploitation and humiliation of women for economic gain, e.g. advertising, entertainment, etc.*

London Rape Action Group *Women against Violence against Women* (1985)

Pornography is a serious problem, but it does not exist in isolation. The pornographic mind expresses itself wherever men assume the right to buy women, or control their lives, wherever women are subordinated to men...

Pornography is big business and exists to make money – some £500 million a year in the United Kingdom and $10 billion in the United States.

Anne Borrowdale *Christian Attitudes to Women, Men and Sex* (1991)

Pornography is more than a nudey magazine, it is a prevailing atmosphere of sexual licence.

Jerry Falwell *Listen, America* (1980)

[Pornography] *is raw sex stripped of all beauty and poetry.* [Pornographers'] *purpose is to treat the sexual act as no more than the gratification of animal passions, their object is to stimulate a prurient desire for the sex without love that is lust.*

James Jackson Kilpatrick *The Smut Peddlers* (1960)

...pornography is a lonely business. It is the sex of the solitary.

Leslie Paul *Eros Discovered: Restoring Sex to Humanity* (1970)

Pornography is indefinable, and as irrepressible as prostitution.

Charles Skilton *Pornography and Society* (1972)

Don't be daft. You don't get any pornography on there, not on the telly. Get filth, that's all. The only place you get pornography is in yer Sunday papers.

Johnny Speight *Till Death Do Us Part*, BBC TV series (1960s–80s)

The word itself is a 19th-century coinage from the Greek, meaning 'a description of prostitutes or prostitution':

In the mind of the scholar responsible for the word in the big Oxford Dictionary *there seems to have been present a suspicion that it carried the idea of* inciting *to unchaste and lewd behaviour, for he quotes* Webster *as offering the murals at Pompeii, in rooms designed for the Bacchanalian orgies, as examples of pornography.*

Dom Denys Rutledge in *Does Pornography Matter?* (1961)

Some writers attempt to draw a distinction between pornography (bad) and erotica (good, or at least acceptable):

The two sorts of images are as different as love is from rape, as dignity is from humiliation, as partnership is from slavery, as pleasure is from pain.

Gloria Steinem *Erotica vs Pornography* (1975)

Porn and erotica are very different subjects. In pornography, there is no love and it transforms the other person into an object. One person is always exerting power over the other. In erotica, it is both people looking for something, for pleasure.

Benoîte Groult, interviewed on the French TV programme *Apostrophe*, after the publication of *Salt on Our Skin* (1991)

...erotica and porn are like sex: women are more turned on by the foreplay and titillation; men prefer the hard stuff.

Janine di Giovanni *Sunday Times* (30 Aug. 1992)

Attempts to define pornography are further confused by the legal concept of obscenity. Some legal views:

I think the test of obscenity is this, whether the tendency of the matter charged as obscene is to deprave and corrupt those whose minds are open to such immoral influences, and into whose hands a publication of this sort may fall.

Sir Alexander Cockburn, Lord Chief Justice, in R. v Hiclin (1868)

...the word 'obscene' be allowed to indicate the present critical point in the compromise between candor and shame at which the community may have arrived here and now.

Judge Learned Hand, in US v Kennerly (1913)

In order for you to find a book to be obscene you must find that its predominant theme is an appeal to prurient sexual interests and desire which goes substantially beyond the standards tolerated by the community as a whole in these present times.

Judge Bryan, in US v Gilbert Fox, Vixen Press, et al. (1959)

The essence of pornography I take to be the deliberate excitation of sexual feelings; but a book can be obscene, it is said, without any such deliberate purpose.

Lord Birkett Q.C. in *Does Pornography Matter?* (1961)

For others, too, pornography and obscenity are by no means synonymous:

Pornography is the art which attracts you towards sex; obscenity the nauseous substitute for sex which repels you from the total experience. The former moves you toward sex, the latter from it.

Ronald Duncan, introduction to *Selected Lyrics and Satires of John, second Earl of Rochester* (1948)

Obscene is not the picture of a naked woman exposed but that of a fully clad general who exposes his medals won in a war of aggression.

Herbert Marcuse *An Essay on Literature* (1969)

For the US lawyer and politician Theodore Schroeder:

Obscenity is not ever the quality of a book or picture, but always and ever only the quality of the viewing mind.

Constructive Obscenity (1907)

The emotionally intense judgements against so-called 'obscene' objects are re-

ally a confession of an extravagant interest in sex.

The Nudist, 'A Psychological Challenge to Prudery' (March 1937)

Do either pornography or erotica do any harm?

I don't think pornography is very harmful, but it is terribly, terribly boring.

Noël Coward 'Sayings of the Week' *Observer* (24 Sept. 1972)

Sex is becoming a strangely joyless national compulsion. The sex-glutted novels have become increasingly explicit and increasingly dull. The endless flow of manuals describing new sex techniques hint at an endless lack of excitement.

Betty Friedan *The Feminine Mystique* (1963)

In the US, a Presidential Commission on Obscenity and Pornography reported in 1970 that pornography was unlikely to be harmful. It even suggested:

Although somewhat far-fetched, it seems possible that graded exposure [to pornography] *may immunize in somewhat the same fashion that exposure to bacteria and viruses builds resistance.*

The President was not amused:

The Commission contends that the proliferation of filthy books and plays has no lasting effects on a man's character. If that were true, it must also be true that great books, great paintings and great plays have no ennobling effects on a man's conduct. Centuries of civilization and ten minutes of common sense tell us otherwise.

Richard Nixon (1970)

The relationship between porn and criminality had been a repeated theme of a former director of the FBI:

The increase in the number of sex crimes is due precisely to sex literature madly presented in certain magazines. Filthy literature is a great moral wrecker. It is creating criminals faster than jails can be built.

J. Edgar Hoover, in a speech (1951)

I say that we can no longer afford to wait for an answer. What we do know is that in an overwhelmingly large number of cases sex crime is associated with pornography. We know that sex criminals read it, are clearly influenced by it. I believe pornography is a major cause of sex violence. I believe that if we can eliminate the distribution of such items among impressionable school age children, we shall greatly reduce our frightening crime rate.

J. Edgar Hoover, in a speech (1959)

Investigations into the alleged link between pornography and sex crimes have produced conflicting findings:

About one third of the control group and one half of the prison group reported having personally owned pornography...Between these two proportions lie those of the majority of sex offenders. Summing up the evidence, it would appear that the possession of pornography does not differentiate sex offenders from non-sex offenders.

Institute of Sex Research *Sex-Offenders, an Analysis of Types* (1965)

The weight of evidence is accumulating that intensive exposure to soft-core pornography desensitizes men's attitude to rape, increases sexual callousness and shifts their preferences towards hard-core pornography...

Exposure to violent pornography increases men's acceptance of rape myths and of violence against women.

M. Baxter 'Flesh and Blood' *New Scientist* (5 May 1990)

...that we get hung up on cold clinical arguments about what proof *there is that pornography affects behaviour is a measure of how coldly indifferent we have become.*

Mary Whitehouse *Whatever Happened to Sex?* (1977)

Others are convinced that pornography has no evil effects:

> *No one ever died from an overdose of pornography.*
>
> William Margold, quoted by Sam Frank in *Sex in the Movies* (1986)

> *The fact remains that, no matter how disturbing violent fantasies are, as long as they stay within the world of pornography they are still only fantasies. The man masturbating in a theater showing a snuff film is still only watching a movie, not actually raping and murdering.*
>
> Dierdre English *Mother Jones* (Apr. 1980)

> *It has always been argued by censorious groups that all porn corrupts and absolute porn corrupts absolutely. I doubt that if only because the great erotic bibliographers and others seem psychologically cleansed by constant immersion in forbidden literature...*
>
> Alan Bold, introduction to *The Sexual Dimension in Literature* (1982)

> *To claim an important effect from erotica, it really is necessary to demonstrate something over and above that which could be produced by mere fantasy.*
>
> H. J. Eysenck *Sex, Violence, and the Media* (1978)

> *This belief in the inciting effects of pornography tells us something about the minds of legislators and the respectable people who support them; for them, apparently, illicit sexual indulgence is a temptation so near the surface that it will erupt into action if the possibility is ever put into people's minds.*
>
> Geoffrey Gorer in *Does Pornography Matter?* (1961)

> *Because the erotic preferences usually reveal themselves at puberty, it is often assumed that they were instilled by a first sexual experience at that time or caught from exposure to erotic pictures, books or films, an assumption that is responsible for much of today's judicial panic about pornography.*
>
> J. Money and P. Tucker *Sexual Signatures* (1977)

> *The belief that any sexy books, pictures or plays ever hold or emit any force for evil is one hundred per cent illusional.*
>
> Theodore Schroeder *Puritanic Sex Censorship* (1947)

> *In the same way aspirin eases a headache, and penicillin battles the 'flu, a dose of pornography can work medicinal magic on sufferers of sexual stress.*
>
> Dr Jay Mann, in a Florida courtroom (1977)

Whether or not pornography incites men to crime, it does, in the opinion of most feminists, degrade women. In the first place, a diet of unrestrained fantasy can give men harmfully false ideas about both male and female sexuality:

> *Pornography teaches men that they have, and deserve to have, sexual power over women and that it is masculine and glamorous to exercise and abuse that power.*
>
> Paula J. Caplan *The Myth of Women's Masochism* (1984)

> *New cultural norms are created by pornography, norms which say women can only find pleasure when they are tortured, beaten, raped or when they have objects thrust into their bodies.*
>
> Elfriede Jelinek, interviewed in the *Guardian* (15 Oct. 1992)

> *Surveying some of the victims of battery, I have encountered women who openly confess that their sex lives changed considerably once their husbands got into pornography. The pornography, often from magazines, gave their spouses all kinds of ideas about what was sexy, and made their spouses wonder why their wives were not being sexy in the way the pornographic models were sexy. Many of these women report being forced to replicate sexual acts in the pornography.*
>
> Susan Cole *Combating the Practice of Pornography* (1984)

A happily married man, perhaps:

> *...becomes seriously concerned with whether he is obtaining the necessary gratification of his sex desires from his normally endowed and inclined wife.*
>
> Dr M. A. Tarumianz, in a Delaware trial (1952)

> *All over this country a new campaign of terrorism and vilification is being waged against us. Fascist propaganda celebrating sexual violence against women is sweeping this land. Pornography is the propaganda of sexual terrorism.*
>
> Andrea Dworkin *New York Times* (4 Dec. 1978)

And secondly, it is alleged, displays of the pudenda of naked girls demean the whole sex by reducing women to the status of objects:

> *Consider also our spirits that break a little each time we see ourselves in chains or full labial display for the conquering male viewer, bruised or on our knees screaming a real or pretended pain to delight the sadist, pretending to enjoy what we don't enjoy, to be blind to the images of our sisters that really haunt us – humilated often enough ourselves by the truly obscene idea that sex and the domination of women must be combined.*
>
> Gloria Steinem *Erotica and Pornography* (1973)

> *She is the pin-up, the centerfold, the poster, the postcard, the dirty picture, naked, half-dressed, laid out, legs spread, breast or ass protruding. She is the thing she is supposed to be: the thing that makes him erect...*
>
> *Women do not believe that men believe what pornography says about women. But they do. From the worst to the best of them, they do.*
>
> Andrea Dworkin *Pornography: Men Possessing Women* (1981)

> *As the racket* [pornography] *grows a steady stream of teen-age girls must be attracted into nude modeling, perversion and prostitution. Boys must be tempted into the sordid business of serving as sex partners, photographers, film processors, and salesmen.*
>
> James Jackson Kilpatrick *The Smut Peddlers* (1960)

That there are fewer male equivalents of girlie magazines may suggest that women tend to be turned on by visual stimuli less than men. However, there is no doubt that some women enjoy porn:

> *For women, as for men, it can also be a source of erotic pleasure. For a woman to enjoy pornography is less to collaborate in her oppression than to defy it, to insist on an aspect of her sexuality that has been defined as a male preserve.*
>
> Ellen Willis *Village Voice* (12 Nov. 1974)

> *What changed our sex life was that a bunch of us girls starting reading books and passing them around. Everything from how-to-do-it sex books to real porno paperbacks. Some of the men said that the stuff was garbage, but I can tell you that my husband was always ready to try out anything. Some of it was great, some was awful, and some was just funny, like the honey business.*
>
> Anon. waitress, quoted by Morton Hunt in *Sexual Behaviour in the 1970s* (1974)

In 1992 Virgin Publishing set up a new imprint specifically to provide erotic writing for women; its booklet of advice for would-be authors states:

> *Setting up an erotica imprint for women is a step in the right direction of freedom and sexual equality. Sex is surely a good thing. People like doing it. They like reading about it.*
>
> *Don't be tempted to write a literary masterpiece. Our readers want a sexy story...more plot means less room for sex.*
>
> *While heterosexual men are not interested in sexual descriptions of their own gender, women are – we think – turned on by descriptions of women being turned on...*
>
> Peter Darvill-Evans (1992)

What, though, of the women who appear in pornographic material? Although some may be turned on by the thought of being the focus of so many men's fantasies, in most cases the inducement is straightforwardly financial:

Nobody made me pose topless. I wasn't being exploited by the press, I was exploiting them. Anyway, if Glenda Jackson can show her boobs and call it art, why can't I?

Samantha Fox, interviewed in *The Times* (5 Dec. 1992)

Most of the girls I have met in this business do it for the money. They don't care how dirty the jobs are they do, just that they get good money for it.

Brigitte, pornography actress, quoted by David Hebditch and Nick Anning *Porn Gold* (1988)

Alternatively, coercion of one kind or another may be involved. The case of Linda Marchiano ('Linda Lovelace') is now well known:

After her leading role in Deep Throat, *Linda Lovelace became the industry's first major star, her name constantly on the lips of dinner guests at early 1970s cocktail parties. But Lovelace was to leave the industry and campaign vigorously against pornography. She is on record as insisting that she was forced to perform in the movie, a gun being held – literally – to her head while she performed the act of fellation. Those involved in the production have strongly denied that she was in any way unwilling.*

David Hebditch and Nick Anning *Porn Gold* (1988)

Linda Marchiano gives a particularly disturbing account of how one woman was coerced into pornography. But women's sexual portrayals or nude photographs can end up in pornography – or even simply on public display – in a number of ways. Pictures are taken surreptitiously, or a woman consents to being photographed by her husband or boyfriend and the photographs end up without her consent in the public view, or the photographs are made through physical abuse and intimidation, and the woman loses control of them.

Lauren Robel *Pornography and Existing Law: What the Law Can Do* (1989)

3 per cent [of respondents to a *Cosmopolitan* survey] *had participated in making pornography. Of these three-quarters were models, actors, or strippers; a third were forced to participate in pornography by father, brother or partner; a third did it for the money; a quarter felt bad about it at the time, and half felt bad about it in retrospect.*

Cosmopolitan (Mar. 1990), quoted by Catherine Itzen in *Pornography* (1992)

Clearly, the issue of pornography is one that leaves many liberal thinkers in a quandary. Much as they dislike the commercial exploitation of sex, they find censorship an even greater evil:

Censorship is more depraving and corrupting than anything pornography can produce.

Tony Smythe, chairman of the National Council for Civil Liberties, 'Sayings of the Week' *Observer* (18 Sept. 1972)

The pornographic imagination says something worth listening to, albeit in a degraded and often unrecognizable form.

Susan Sontag *The Pornographic Imagination* (1966)

The only way to 'eradicate' pornography is to eradicate the need for it and this cannot be done by banning it or driving it underground.

Martin Tomkinson *The Pornbrokers* (1982)

Opponents of censorship point out that pornography has often flourished in sexually repressive cultures:

The serpent of shame entered the garden of sex some years after the reign of Good Queen Bess and pornography hasn't been the same since. For the first time in literary history there came into being a direct censorship of the obscene. Immediately thereafter a new type of salacious literature appeared, aimed solely at the sexual arousal or tickling of the reader. Laughter and beauty and joy departed from this pornography.

David Loth *The Erotic in Literature* (1962)

The two variations on normal sexual intercourse most commonly referred to were female masturbation with dildoes and anal penetration. But it seems not unlikely that the harping on the latter may have been partly due to the poverty of imagination of the poets, and to the accident that the word 'tarse' (penis) happens to rhyme with 'arse'.

Lawrence Stone *The Family, Sex, and Marriage in England 1500–1800* (1977)

By the 19th century, even Shakespeare was too bawdy for some:

Bare-faced obscenities, low vulgarities and nauseous vice so frequently figure and pollute his pages that we cannot but regret the luckless hour he became a writer for the stage.

John Styles *An Essay on the Character, Immoral and Antichristian Tendency of the Stage* (1806)

And yet pornography proliferated as never before:

The prevalence and the very nature of Victorian pornography is directly the result of the Victorian fear of sex and sense of shame at all things sexual.

D. F. Barber *Pornography and Society* (1972)

The Victorian pornographic novel represents the fantasy of the Victorian male: all men are sexual athletes, all women flow with the juices of love. Jealousy and possessiveness have little part to play in this fantasy, for here, everything is for the best in the best of all possible worlds...

If the Victorian novel attempts to represent the whole range of human experience, the pornographic variety presupposes a world where all human experience is concerned exclusively with sex...The range of sexual activities in this genre is wide, from incest to male and female homosexuality, but the most frequently found are rape and flaggelation. This in itself is revealing of a sexually repressed and totally male-dominated society.

Peter Webb 'Victorian Erotica' in *The Sexual Dimension in Literature* (ed. Alan Bold; 1982)

As literacy spreads, the anxiety of paterfamilias for the chastity of his wife and daughters, or the morals of his servants, finds expression in the growing belief that erotic literature is always and necessarily corrupt.

Donald Thomas *A Long Time Burning* (1969)

Words echoing those of the Treasury counsel to whom fell the task of leading the prosecution in the 1960 trial of D. H. Lawrence's *Lady Chatterley's Lover* (1928):

Would you allow your wife or your servant to read this book?

Mervyn Griffith-Jones

The jury unanimously said they would. Though one wag remarked:

More to the point, would you allow your gamekeeper to read it?

This trial proved to be a watershed.

Sexual intercourse began
In Nineteen sixty-three
(Which was rather late for me) –
Between the end of the Chatterley *ban*
And the Beatles' first LP.

Philip Larkin 'Annus Mirabilis' (1974)

Before the Chatterley trial it was roughly true that:

A man may vote as he wishes, believe what he likes, but he must not be sexually aroused by printed matter.

D. F. Barber *Pornography and Society* (1972)

However, since then virtually anything can be published in the UK as long as it does not contain material that tends to 'deprave or corrupt' under the terms of the Obscene Publications Acts (1959 or 1964). The trouble with such definitions is that no two people react identically to the same stimuli. D. H. Lawrence himself, for example was disgusted by dirty postcards:

Take the very lowest instance, the picture postcard sold underhand, by the underworld, in most cities. What I have seen of them have been of an ugliness to make you cry. The insult to the human body, the insult to a vital human relationship! Ugly and cheap they make the human nudity, ugly and degraded they make the sexual act, trivial cheap and nasty...

'Pornography and Obscenity' (1929)

No one knows what goes on inside people looking at the same pornographic film: one might be in the process of self-education; a second one is thinking about something else; a third is contemplating beauty; a fourth is working himself up to an orgasm.

André Guindon *The Sexual Language* (1976)

While many now regard erotica and soft porn as generally harmless (and in some cases beneficial), pornography that incites or encourages violence raises more worrying issues:

Magazines devoted to sado-masochism are the best-selling of all pornographic periodicals.

Dr Thomas Stuttaford *The Times* (3 Dec. 1992)

The other class of pornography that most people would consider totally unacceptable under any circumstances is that which involves children:

It is important to realize that child pornography can only be reproduced through the victimization of a child, and that the photograph or film is in fact a permanent record of the sexual abuse of a child. The taking of the photograph is in itself an act of child molestation or sexual abuse.

Obscene Publications Squad (1988)

The pictures, films and tapes range from revealing stills of naked children, through more explicit shots of their genitalia thumbed apart, to the recording of oral, anal and vaginal abuse and intercourse.

Commonly the children are required to have sex with other youngsters as well as adults (both male and female). Frequently they are made to urinate on each other or their abusers. Almost invariably their faces, chests or genitalia are coated in semen when the adult men ejaculate over them. Occasionally they are photographed having sex with an animal.

Tim Tate *Child Pornography: an Investigation* (1990)

Children used in pornography seem to come from every class, religion, family and background. A majority are exploited by someone who knows them by virtue of his or her occupation or through a neighbourhood community or family relationship.

Many are too young to know what has happened; others are powerless to refuse the demand of an authority figure; some seem to engage in the conduct 'voluntarily', usually in order to obtain desperately needed adult affection.

Final Report of the Attorney General's Commission on Pornography (1986)

It is important for the law enforcement officer to realize that most of the children in pre-pubescent child pornography were not abducted into sexual slavery. They were seduced into posing for these pictures or videos by a paedophile they probably knew. They were never missing children. In some cases their own parents took the pictures or made them available for others to take the pictures. Children in pubescent child pornography, however, are more likely to be missing children – especially runaways being exploited by morally indiscriminate pimps or profiteers.

Kenneth Lanning *Child Molesters: A Behavioral Analysis for Law-enforcement Officers Investigating Cases of Child Sexual Exploitation* (1986)

See also CHILD ABUSE

Perhaps, again, the last words should go to the cynics:

In almost every human society, pornography and exhibitionism are reckoned as offences, except when, as not infrequently occurs, they form part of a religious ceremony.

Bertrand Russell *Why I am Not a Christian* (1957)

Its avowed purpose is to excite sexual desire, which, I should have thought, is unnecessary in the case of the young, inconvenient in the case of the middle aged, and unseemly in the old.

Malcolm Muggeridge *Tread Softly For You Tread On My Jokes* (1966)

Postscript: for anyone wondering what happens to discarded pornography, the 1993 edition of the AA's hotel guide has an answer:

...pornographic magazines are the fifth most frequently discarded item in hotels.

Guardian (25 Nov. 1992)

Promiscuity

Human beings can be motivated by the appropriate stimulus to copulate at any time of the year, month, or day, from the onset of puberty until they die. In the absence of any restraints, promiscuity might therefore seem to be a consequence of human nature:

I have made love to 10,000 women since I was 13½. It wasn't in any way a vice. I've no sexual vices. But I needed to communicate.

Georges Simenon, interview in *L'Express* (21 Feb. 1977)

Adulterers and customers of whores
And cunning takers of virginities
Caper from bed to bed, but not because
The flesh is pricked to infidelities.

The body is content with homely fare;
It is the avid, curious mind that craves
New pungent sauce and strips the larder bare,
The palate and not the hunger that enslaves.

John Press 'Womanisers' (20th century)

The promiscuous lover displays the human virtue of expectation, stranger even than the Christian virtue of hope. There is always, round the corner, something better. Or at any rate there is something just as good. This is optimism, a quality not to be derided. Promiscuity can sometimes be regarded as the simple wish to relate closely and warmly to as many people as practicable.

Francis Bennion *The Sex Code* (1991)

It is not, of course, only men who can be promiscuous:

There are some women, though not all of them, who are indiscriminate slaves to lust, like animals they rut without discretion.

Origen *In Genesim homeliae* (3rd century). He allegedly castrated himself to preserve his chastity

She often 'layed her down in the highway between Axbridge and Crosse, and called to all persons passing, by spreading her legs abroad, saying: "Come play with my cunt and make my husband a cuckold."'

G. R. Quaife *Wanton Wenches and Wayward Wives: Peasants and Illicit Sex in Early Seventeenth-Century England*

The Professor of Gynaecology began his course of lectures as follows: Gentlemen, woman is an animal that micturates once a day, defecates once a week, menstruates once a month, parturates once a year and copulates whenever she has the opportunity.

W. Somerset Maugham *A Writer's Notebook* (1949)

Behold yond simpering dame,
Whose face between her forks presages snow;
That minces virtue, and does shake the head
To hear of pleasure's name;
The fitchew, nor the soiled horse, goes to't
With a more riotous appetite.
Down from the waist they are Centaurs,
Though women all above:

But to the girdle do the gods inherit,
Beneath is all the fiends';
There's hell, there's darkness, there's the sulphurous pit,
Burning, scalding, stench, consumption; fie, fie, fie!

William Shakespeare *King Lear* (1605)

Indeed, promiscuous behaviour in women is a staple theme of bawdy poems, songs, and epigrams:

How often Cleveland, hast thou here been found
By a lascivious herd encompass'd round?
How often have you hence retir'd, and lain
A leash of stallions breathless on the plain?
Then back return'd; another leash enjoy'd,
Another after that, when those were cloy'd;
And so elsewhere, and here, half your life employ'd.

Robert Gould, on the Duchess of Cleveland, 'The Play-House, a Satyr' (late 17th century)

Under her beauteous bosom there did lie
A belly as smooth as any ivory.
Yet nature to declare her various art
Had plac'd a tuft in one convenient part;
No park with smoothest lawn or highest wood
Could e'er compare with this admir'd abode.
Here all the youth of England did repair
To take their pleasure and to ease their care.

Charles Sackville, 6th Earl of Dorset 'Duel of the Crabs' (1701)

An' heard ye o the coat o arms
The Lyon brought our lady, O?
The crest was couchant sable cunt
The motto ready, ready, O,
Green grow the rashes, O
Green grow the rashes, O,
The lassies they hae wimble-bores,
The widows they hae gashes, O.

Robert Burns 'Green Grow the Rashes, O' (1780s)

Lady Capricorn, he understood, was still keeping open bed.

Aldous Huxley (1923)

Some have taken the Mae West approach – disarming criticism by their brazen wit:

I'm glad you like my Catherine. I like her too. She ruled thirty million people and had three thousand lovers. I do the best I can in two hours.

In a speech from the stage after her performance in *Catherine the Great*

I'm tired, send one of them home.

On being told that ten men were waiting to meet her in her dressing room

Good girls go to heaven.
Bad girls go everywhere.

Helen Gurley Brown *Sex and the Single Girl* (1963)

Biologically, however, there are restraints to female promiscuity – sometimes as a result of pregnancy, but more often to prevent unwanted pregnancies. Moreover, in some cultures, notably Judaeo-Christian societies, restraints on both male and female promiscuity have been imposed by the tradition of monogamy. However,

For a male and female to live continuously together is...biologically speaking, an extremely unnatural condition.

Robert Briffault *The Sin of Sex* (1931)

These monogamous restraints are often supported by religious sanctions; in some cases, particularly in Christian teaching, almost any form of sexual activity not specifically aimed at procreation is tainted by the concept of sin. Such pre-permissive attitudes are summed up in the words of the Roman Catholic Lord Longford:

No sex without responsibility.

Observer (3 May 1954)

See also CHASTITY AND CELIBACY

However, restraints related to unwanted babies and religious teaching have for many people lost their cogency in a secular age in which effective contraceptives are freely available. Modern restraints on promiscuity are not imposed from outside on the individual, rather they result from his or her own inclinations and disinclinations. Too much sex, or sex without LOVE, may for some people be worse than no sex at all:

It's all this cold-hearted fucking that is death and idiocy.

D. H. Lawrence *Lady Chatterley's Lover* (1926)

and from the same author:

You mustn't think I advocate perpetual sex. Far from it. Nothing nauseates me more than promiscuous sex in and out of season.

Letter to Lady Ottoline Morrell (22 Dec. 1928), referring to *Lady Chatterley's Lover*

To suppose that all women, as soon as they repudiate coercion, will adopt promiscuity is as fantastic as to suppose that but for the police they will attend the Ascot Races stark naked.

Robert Briffault *The Sin of Sex* (1931)

Everything can be overdone and sex is no exception:

Sex is the tabasco sauce which an adolescent national palate sprinkles on every course in the menu.

Mary Day Winn *Adam's Rib* (1931)

Those who are forever having intercourse with women, or drinking, or listening to music – though these are the strongest and deepest-rooted of all the lusts – do not enjoy these indulgences so much as men who do not incessantly gratify them; for these passions become for them exactly the same as any other passion – that is to say, they become commonplace and habitual.

Rhazes *The Spiritual Physick* (c. 10th century)

According to the 12th-century Jewish philosopher Maimonides too much sex may not only be boring. For men it can be quite disastrous:

Effusion of semen represents the strength of the body and its life… whenever it is emitted to excess, the body becomes consumed, its strength terminates and its life perishes…he who immerses himself in sexual intercourse will be assailed by premature ageing, his strength will wane, his eyes will weaken, and a bad odour will emit from his mouth and his armpits, his teeth will fall out and many other maladies will afflict him.

Mishreh Torah

For women, the traditional wisdom has often linked promiscuity with infertility, illness, or neurotic behaviour. This association of ideas has not been entirely banished by medical science:

Scientists on IVF [in vitro fertilization] *programmes often describe the women they treat as 'non-achievers' and 'failures' with 'defective' bodies…. Many are punitive, and blame women's infertility on supposed infections contracted from sexual promiscuity or on earlier abortions…*

Celia Kitzinger *New Internationalist* (Mar. 1991)

Psychiatrists, too, have little time for the libertine:

…promiscuity is based upon the neurotic inability to find or to form an adult relationship.

Dr G. B. Barker (1969)

Very often if the masculine character traits *of a man are weakened because emotionally he has remained a child, he will try to compensate for this lack by the exclusive emphasis on his male role in* sex. *The result is the Don Juan, who needs to prove his male prowess in sex because he is unsure of his masculinity in a characterological sense.*

Erich Fromm Barker *The Art of Loving* (1957)

Although other traditions (especially the Chinese) take a more positive view of male promiscuity:

The more women with whom a man has intercourse, the greater will be the benefit he derives from the act.

Ko Hung *Nei p'ien* (c. 300)

When the common people hear that the Yellow Emperor ascended heaven because he had sexual intercourse with twelve hundred women, they think this was the only *reason why he achieved longevity. It is true that he had intercourse with twelve hundred women, but this was not the sole cause of his success.*

Ko Hung *Nei p'ien* (c. 300)

If a man continually changes the women with whom he has intercourse, the benefit will be great. If in one night he can have intercourse with more than ten women it is best.

Yü-fang-pi-chüch *I-hsin-fang* (c. 600)

His lust leaves no virgin to her lover, neither the warrior's daughter nor the wife of the nobleman.

Epic of Gilgamesh (c. 2000 BC)

Among the other honours and rewards our young men can win for distinguished service in war and in other activities, will be more frequent opportunities to sleep with women.

Plato *Republic* (4th century BC)

The idea that promiscuity was a positive good for both sexes did not really emerge until the 'sexual revolution' of the 1960s:

Making love is good in itself, and the more it happens in any way possible or conceivable between as many people as possible, the better.

David Cooper *The Death of the Family* (1970)

For the hippies, sex is not a matter of great debate, because as far as they are concerned the sexual revolution is accomplished. There are no hippies who believe in chastity, or look askance at marital infidelity, or see even marriage itself as a virtue. Physical love is a delight, to be chewed upon as often and as freely as a handful of sesame seeds.

Newsweek (6 Feb. 1967)

Girls say yes to guys who say no.

US Draft Resistance Slogan (late 1960s), quoted in Hole and Levine *The Rebirth of Feminism*

This view was also shared by some homosexuals:

Later on I walked him to King's Cross where he caught a bus home. On the way we talked about sex. "You must do whatever you like," I said, "as long as you enjoy it and don't hurt anyone else, that's all that matters." "I'm basically guilty about being a homosexual you see," he said. "Then you shouldn't be," I said. "Get yourself fucked if you want to. Get yourself anything you like. Reject all the values of society. And enjoy sex. When you're dead you'll regret not having fun with your genital organs."

Joe Orton, diary entry for July 1967, published in *The Orton Diaries* (1986)

To some extent, the sexual revolution amongst women was a consequence of the advent of the contraceptive pill – although some argue that the correlation is less simple than is often suggested:

Does the convenient contraceptive promote promiscuity? In some cases, no doubt it does, as did the automobile, the drive-in movie, and the motel. But the consensus is that a girl who is promiscuous on the pill would have been promiscuous without it.

New York Saturday Evening Post (15 Jan. 1966)

The contraceptive pill influenced the steady loosening of constraints, although it was probably not the only factor and its most dramatic impact on behaviour was in the early 1970s.... On the market since 1961, its use spread rapidly among married women.... It was not so easily available to single women until the Family Planning Act 1967 enabled local authorities to set up or support family planning clinics.... Some Family Planning Association clinics continued until 1969 to provide advice and facilities only to married couples, and to engaged couples if they had a note from the vicar. Only 9 per cent of all single women in the 1970 Bone survey had ever used the pill.

Cate Haste *Rules of Desire* (1992)

Did the sexual revolution and the abandonment of restraints make for greater happiness?

> *There was a lot of fucking going on. It was paradise for men in their late twenties: all these willing girls. But the trouble with the willing girls was that a lot of the time they were willing not because they particularly fancied the people concerned but because they felt they ought to. There was a huge pressure to conform to non-conformity...There was a lot of misery. Relationship miseries: ghastly, ghastly jealousy, although there was supposed to be no jealousy, no possessiveness. What it meant was that men fucked around. You'd cry a lot, and you would scream sometimes, and the man would say, "Don't bring me down – don't lay your bummers on me...don't hassle me, don't crowd my space." There were multiple relationships but usually in a very confused way; usually the man wanted it.*

Nicola Lane, quoted in Jonathan Green *Days in the Life* (1988)

Women also remained quick to condemn their more promiscuous sisters – as Germaine Greer points out:

> *Girls who pride themselves or their monogamous instincts have no hesitation in using the whole battery of sex-loathing terms for women who do not.*

The Female Eunuch (1970)

Although in the same book, Germaine Greer expresses her own somewhat ambivalent opinions:

> *...nobody feels embarrassed about admitting disgust attendant on promiscuity, although it might be argued that if sex is a good thing it ought not to become disgusting if done often, or with different people.*
>
> *For all the pseudo-sophistication of twentieth-century sex theory, it is still assumed that a man should make love as if his principal intention was to people the wilderness.*

However, it is probably a mistake to judge the sexual mores of any era by its rhetoric or by the lifestyles of the conspicuous few. For example, the 19th-century may have a reputation for sexual repression, yet:

> *The Victorians found time, as men and women have found time since the Creation, for much sexual promiscuity; a dead baby in the street was as common a sight then as an abandoned car is now.*

C. H. Rolph *Books in the Dock* (1969)

Appearances can be misleading – for eras as for individuals:

> *Nine adulteries, 12 liaisons, 64 fornications and something approaching a rape*
> *Rest nightly upon the soul of our delicate friend Florialis,*
> *And yet the man is so quiet and reserved in demeanour*
> *That he passes for both bloodless and sexless.*
> *Bastidides, on the contrary, who both talks and writes of nothing save copulation,*
> *Has become the father of twins,*
> *But he accompanied this feat at some cost;*
> *He had to be four times cuckolded.*

Ezra Pound 'The Temperaments' (20th century)

In the end, the sexual behaviour of individuals – men and women, heterosexual or homosexual – is determined by the equilibrium they achieve between their desires and the restraints that apply to them. Attitudes to monogamy, personal loyalty, the availability of contraceptives, and the threat of sexually transmitted diseases are the main factors that each person has to consider in deciding whether or not a particular occasion should become a sexual event. Perhaps it is the last of these factors, since the late 1980s and the arrival of AIDS, that now chiefly governs these decisions:

> *Before you take a girl to bed these days you have to have a medical discussion about the plague. So I don't bother much.*

Jack Nicholson 'Quote Unquote' *Independent* (27 Feb. 1993)

And, finally, two unlikely bedfellows in total agreement:

The strongest possible piece of advice I would give to any young woman is: Don't screw around, and don't smoke.

Edwina Currie 'Sayings of the Week', *Observer* (3 Apr. 1988)

The sexual restraint of chastity is the only safe and virtuous way to put an end to the tragic plague of Aids.

Pope John Paul II 'Quote Unquote' *Independent* (13 Feb. 1993)

See also SEXUALLY TRANSMITTED DISEASES

Prostitution

Prostitution is as old as civilization. Commercial sex has survived even the most draconian and repressive attempts to eradicate it.

Ruth Morgan Thomas *AIDS Risks, Alcohol, Drugs and the Sex Industry: a Scottish Study* (1990)

Why do women become prostitutes?

It is a silly question to ask a prostitute why she does it...These are the highest-paid 'professional' women in America.

Gail Sheehy *Hustling* (1971)

They're whores, and that's not a term of abuse. It's a good honest biblical word for an honourable profession of ancient lineage. They make love with men for a living and don't you ever think badly of them for that. Any woman worthy of the name would do the same if her children were hungry.

Allegra Taylor *Prostitution: What's Love got to Do with It?* (1991)

Necessity never makes prostitution the business of men's lives; though numberless are the women who are thus rendered systematically vicious. This, however, arises, in a great degree from the state of idleness in which women are educated, who are always taught to look up to man for a maintenance, and to consider their persons as the proper return for his exertions to support them.

Mary Wollstonecraft *A Vindication of the Rights of Women* (1792)

...prostitution is caused, not by female depravity and male licentiousness, but simply by underpaying, undervaluing, and overworking women so shamefully that the poorest of them are forced to resort to prostitution to keep body and soul together.

George Bernard Shaw, Preface to *Mrs Warren's Profession* (1894)

Whether our reformers admit it or not, the economic and social inferiority of women is responsible for prostitution.

Emma Goldman *Anarchism and Other Essays* 'The Tragedy of Women's Emancipation' (1911)

...prostitution is the logical consequence of the feminine attitude. In so far as she is attractive, a woman is a prey to men's desire. Unless she refuses completely because she is determined to remain chaste, the question is at what price and under what circumstances will she yield. But if the conditions are fulfilled she always offers herself as an object. Prostitution proper only brings in a commercial element.

Georges Bataille *Death and Sensuality* (1969)

The same reasons were given over 2000 years ago:

At first
Modest and thriftily, tho' poor, she liv'd,
With her own hands a homely livelihood
Scarce earning from the distaff and the loom.
But when a lover came with promis'd gold,
Another, and another, as the mind

Falls easily from labour to delight,
She took their offers, and set up the trade

Terence *Andria* (166 BC)

Clearly, money is a very basic reason – and it certainly can be a well-paid profession:

There is something utterly nauseating about a system of society which pays a harlot 25 times as much as it pays its Prime Minister, 250 times as much as it pays its Members of Parliament, and 500 times as much as it pays some of its ministers of religion.

Harold Wilson, referring to Christine Keeler in a speech in the House of Commons (June 1963)

The money you can earn is mind-blowing. In one month working in an escort agency I earned £5,000 – enough to support myself through a year at university. I can't see why people are so shocked at the idea of students working in the sex industry...it takes up very little time and is a very high earner.

Jane, philosophy student at London University, quoted in the *Sunday Times* (11 Apr. 1993)

There are, however, a number of non-economic views:

Prostitution is not so much of a temptation which ensnares morally collapsed girls as it is a job opportunity and a scheme of life for low resource girls.

Walter C. Reckless *A Sociologist Looks at Prostitution* (1943)

It is the appeal of civilization, though not of what is finest and best in civilization, which more than any other motive, calls women to the career of a prostitute.

H. Havelock Ellis *Studies in the Psychology of Sex* (1937)

The fact that in several cases both the mother and maternal grandmother were harlots, permits us to conclude that the total mental personality which especially predisposes to prostitution is frequently hereditary.

Tage Kemp *Prostitution: An Investigation of its Causes* (1936)

The working-class prostitute [in the 19th century] *was regarded as suffering from an overproduction of male hormones and sometimes from chromosomatic imbalance.*

Susan Edwards *Female Sexuality and the Law* (1981)

Prostitution gives her an opportunity to meet people. It provides fresh air and wholesome exercise, and it keeps her out of trouble.

Joseph Heller *Catch-22* (1961)

Ms St Clair claims she loves her work. "I'm an extrovert nymphomaniac," she says. "It's perfect for me." Her pleasures are "sleeping, eating, counting money and sex – in that order"...She insists that she has turned down scores of offers of marriage – "Why buy a book when you can join a library?"

Lindi St Clair, quoted in the *Independent* (25 Apr. 1992)

This miscellany of views seems to evade the central horror of the teenager who, having been abused as a child or fallen into drug abuse, runs away from home – to London or another big city. The pimps are there waiting – they feed her, house her, provide her with drugs, and usually seduce her before sending her out onto the streets:

I watched in fascination as she [tore the syringe from her arm] *...and asked, naively, if she had seen a doctor. Shc said it was too late, that she was forced to pick up 'fat, disgusting scum' to feed her habit.*

Paula McGinley 'The night I Met a Prostitute in My Back Yard' *Independent* (4 Dec. 1992)

It seems to me that young women, whatever their mode of life, are entitled to be protected. If this young girl was feeding her drug addiction with the proceeds of prostitution, it simply lends force to the lobby which seeks to provide legalized brothels which can be properly and medically supervised.

James Hipwell, coroner at the inquest on a murdered teenage prostitute, quoted in *The Times* (27 Nov. 1992)

However, not all prostitution is carried on at this pitiful level:

This prostitute society has its own class structure with varying standards of behaviour, the same qualities making for success in this as in any other professional sphere.

C. H. Rolph *Women of the Streets* (1955)

For example, there is the middle-class girl with low self-esteem and high aspirations. She works in the best hotels in town, for an escort agency. Well-dressed and well-spoken, she charges according to the hotel to which she is called. She will do anything, no matter how kinky, as long as it doesn't hurt; she gets her kicks from being admired and the high fees she commands, not from the sex, which leaves her totally unmoved, though she is likely to have a separate sex life 'for her'. Some students who have turned to prostitution to support themselves even find they quite like it:

My regular clients knew I was a student and I don't think any of them were shocked. They enjoyed the fact that I was well educated. I quite liked a few of them and genuinely enjoyed having sex with them.

Jane, philosophy student at London University, quoted in the *Sunday Times* (11 Apr. 1993)

Such girls are quite likely to support Tomorrow, the English Collective of Prostitutes, who encourage

...public acceptance of their existence as part of the local welfare economy. What they want is recognition of prostitutes as small traders engaged in a form of social therapy, not ostracism and moral apartheid.

The Times (9 Nov. 1992)

Tomorrow's slogans include:

No one screws more prostitutes than the Government. In 1990 prostitutes were fined £½ million.

Practising safe sex can get you arrested.

Prostitutes are arrested for carrying condoms.

What do you call men who take money from prostitutes? Magistrates.

Independent (11 Nov. 1992)

One of the occupational hazards of prostitution is catching a sexually transmitted disease (STD):

AIDS is not the first incurable, fatal sexually transmitted disease. Syphilis once had a very similar position to the one that is occupied by AIDS today. Past experience suggests that neither the threat of disease nor the risks of stigma, abuse, imprisonment, or violence have deterred people from working as prostitutes. The sex industry is extensive. Moreover, those who sell sexual services are vastly outnumbered by those who buy such services.

Ruth Morgan Thomas *AIDS Risks, Alcohol, Drugs and the Sex Industry; a Scottish Study* (1990)

Prostitution has been defined as the exchange of sexual services for money or things of monetary value, such as drugs. One of the things of no monetary value that can be exchanged between a prostitute and a client is a sexually transmitted disease.

Martin A. Plant *AIDS, Drugs and Prostitution* (1990)

In Vienna during the 1830s and 1840s, public hospitals annually admitted between 6000 and 7000 prostitutes suffering from venereal disease. In 1856, London hospitals admitted over 30,000 cases, and in Paris most prostitutes sent to prison had the 'clap'. Whole armies became infected – the Garde Impériale lost 20,000 duty days in only three months during 1865. It was estimated that, in Copenhagen one in three citizens contracted some form of venereal disease.

Roy Eskapa *Bizarre Sex* (1987)

Women who solicit soldiers for immoral purposes are usually disease spreaders and friends of the enemy.

Keeping Fit to Fight, pamphlet issued to US troops (1917)

I picked up a girl in the Strand; went into a court with intention to enjoy her in armour. But she had none. I toyed with her. She wondered at my size, and said if I ever took a girl's maidenhead, I would make her squeak. I gave her a shilling and had enough command of myself to go without touching her. I afterwards trembled at the danger I had escaped.

James Boswell *Boswell's London Journal* (1761)

It is ironic that AIDS should appear only a few decades after the main STDs had succumbed to antibiotics. AIDS is a frightening disease with a prognosis quite as dire as untreated syphilis:

In the context of HIV and other sexually transmitted diseases, it is important to remember that in any new relationship each partner will potentially inherit the sexual past history of the other.

Roger Gaitley and Philip Seed *HIV and AIDS* (1989)

See also SEXUALLY TRANSMITTED DISEASES

However, as any high-class prostitute will tell you, the risk of either catching or transmitting an STD is lower for prostitutes than it is for girls who regularly go in for one-night stands. Many prostitutes insist on 'safe sex', and even in their private lives make their men use condoms, which is not so of many happy-go-lucky young women. 'Specials', without condoms, are no longer on the menu:

The rate of venereal disease among prostitutes is lower than among high school students because they're professionals and it would be bad for business to do otherwise.

Dr Jennifer Jones, speech given at the Hookers' Convention, San Francisco (1975)

Statistically...you have more chance of contracting Aids from a Catholic priest than from a prostitute.

Nina Lopez-Jones, spokeswoman for Tomorrow, quoted in the *Independent on Sunday* (13 Sept. 1992)

Large numbers of prostitutes have been monitored for HIV and Aids at clinics in London and New York. Unless they are drug users they rarely become HIV-positive; and some London hospitals have reported no cases of Aids in prostitutes...except when they were illicit drug-users.

Neville Hodgkinson 'Moving in a positive direction' *Sunday Times* (11 Apr. 1993)

Given the temptation of good money, can any girl willing to take the health risk become a prostitute? Or does it need special training?

Any idiot can learn to make love well enough to please most men. All you have to do is lie there, wiggle a little, sigh and moan, pant, and generally act as if it's about the greatest thing that ever happened to you. Maybe you cut loose with a torrent of oaths every now and then, and you bite him and scratch him if you see he goes for that. And if it's not too implausible, you beg him not to hurt you with that enormous *thing he's got. What imbecile can't learn to do these things?*

German prostitute, quoted by Robert E. L. Masters in *The Hidden World of Erotica* (1973)

There is not so much difference between the hooker and the non-hooker as one might expect.

Ellen Strong *The Hooker* (1970)

Here are comments from three anonymous London prostitutes:

There's some of them lies still as stones, they think it's more lady-like or something. But I say they don't know which side their bread's buttered on. Listen, if you lie still the bloke may take half the night sweating away. But if you bash it about a bit he'll come all the quicker and get out and away and leave you in peace. Stupid to spin it out longer than you need, isn't it?

When I'm with a client I always put the rubber on him very gently, you know, stroking him and spinning it out as long as I can. 'You ought to have been a nurse', they say. That's always what it makes them think of. And then with a bit of luck they come before they even get into me. When they do I look ever so lov-

ing and gentle and say 'Traitor!' Well, I'm not paid just to be a bag, am I?

One time there was a client took me back to his place. I had to tie him up. All the girls have to know how to tie a bloke to a chair properly. I did him really well, couldn't move an inch. Then I had to strap his prick up to his belly with elastoplast. I was feeling angry, I suppose, because there was some elastoplast over and I put one piece across his mouth and another across his eyes. 'There's for you, you bastard,' I thought, 'You asked to be strapped up, and you gets strapped up.' He'd told me earlier he had a cleaner come in every second morning. I hope she did, that's all I can say. That was two months ago.

Wayland Young *Eros Denied* (1964)

one from a fictional New Yorker:

After I became a prostitute, I had to deal with penises of every imaginable shape and size. Some large, others quite shrivelled and pendulous of testicle. Some blue-veined and reeking of Stilton, some miserly. Some crabbed, enchanted, dusted with pearls like the great minarets of the Taj Mahal, jesting penises, ringed as the tail of a raccoon, fervent, crested, impossible to live with, marigold-scented. More and more I became grateful I didn't have to own one of these appendages.

Tama Janowitz *Slaves of New York* (1986)

And one from a London housewife, following her acquittal on a charge of controlling prostitutes in a sex-for-luncheon vouchers case:

I know it does make people happy but to me it is just like having a cup of tea.

Cynthia Payne (8 Nov. 1987)

Whatever view one takes of prostitutes – it takes two to tango:

There is no escape from the conclusion that, while woman's want of bread induces her to pursue this vice, man's love of vice itself leads him there.

Susan Anthony, public lecture on social purity (1895)

Inevitably, prostitution has flourished in societies that have demanded strict chastity from 'respectable' women, thus denying young men any other sexual outlet:

Prostitution sacrifices a segment of the female population in order to preserve the 'purity' of the rest.

Abram Kardiner *Sex or Morality* (1955)

When a very famous man had once visited a brothel, he said: praised be to eternity the sensible opinion of the old Cato. As soon as desire brings the blood in the veins of a young man to boiling heat, it is right and just that they should go this way and not seduce respectable married women.

Horace *Satires* (c. 35 BC)

Remove prostitutes from human affairs and you will pollute all things with lust.

St Augustine *De ordine* (5th century)

Prostitution is like the filth in the sea or the sewer in a palace. Take away the sewer, and you will fill the palace with pollution. Take away prostitutes from the world, and you will fill it with sodomy.

St Thomas Aquinas *Opuscula* (13th century)

Middle class [Victorian] *men tended to have recourse to prostitutes or semi-prostitutes – servants or lower-class factory workers – because sexual intercourse, when enjoyed, was essentially a conspiracy to do something wicked, and was therefore unsuited to 'respectable' people.*

Glen Petrie *A Singular Iniquity* (1971)

It is easy to forget how limited the sexual opportunities were for middle-class young men in the 1860s, largely because of the strictness with which girls or young women of their own class were watched or chaperoned. In the lower classes, where appearances, or even conventional morality and respectability, were far less important, the men were freer to act out their natural impulses, and for men of the upper classes, with many available young girls acting as servants in their houses or as workers on their estates, there was also a greater opportunity for sexual expression. Since almost the only other alternative was the sleazy world of prostitution, it is not surprising if neither Hopkins nor the majority of his scrupulous friends ever slept with a woman.

Robert Bernard Martin *Gerard Manley Hopkins: A Very Private Life* (1991)

We must go walk the streets, my sisters,
love is our shameful trade,
Never complain though the hours be long
and our work so poorly paid,
Fate has decreed that we serve men's
need and forfeit our worthless life,
All to defend the family home and protect
the virtuous wife.

Auguste Barbier *Lazare* (1837)

Prostitution is a blight on the human race...for if you men did not impose chastity on women as a necessary virtue while refusing to practise it yourselves, they would not be rejected by society for yielding to the sentiments of their hearts, nor would seduced, deceived and abandoned girls be forced into prostitution.

Flora Tristan *The London Journal of Flora Tristan* (1842)

Ignorant laws, ignorant prejudices, ignorant codes of morals, condemn one portion of the female sex to vicious excess, another to as vicious restraint, and generally the whole of the male sex to debasing licentiousness, if not to loathsome brutality.

Frances Wright (1827)

Another function of prostitution has been to accommodate sexual tastes that men are unwilling or unable to express within their marriages:

Keep a small book containing a series of birch scenes, written in a dramatic form, which when your visitor calls, you should put in his hands, and ask of him which of them he would most like to enact.

Anon. advice to Victorian brothel-keepers, quoted by Ian Gibson in *The English Vice* (1979)

A special facet of the Harlem night world, where Negroes catered to married white people's weird sexual tastes. Rich men, middle-aged men and beyond, men well past their prime...Harlem was their sin-den, their fleshpot. They stole off among taboo black people, and took off whatever antiseptic, important, dignified masks they wore in their white world.

Malcolm X *The Autobiography of Malcolm X* (1965)

Whether or not prostitution is justifiable – it exists:

Prostitution is hard, if not impossible, to eradicate. Everywhere men (and women) seek sexual gratification and are willing to pay for it. Accordingly, every society has to compromise, to find a way to contain this 'necessary evil'.

P. U. Venema and J. Visser *Safer Prostitution: a New Approach in Holland* (1990)

Those men who find a need for this 'necessary evil' have opinions too, which can sometimes be quite eloquent:

A man has missed something if he has never woken up in an anonymous bed beside a face he'll never see again, and if he has never left a brothel at dawn, feeling like jumping off a bridge into the river out of sheer physical disgust with life.

Gustave Flaubert, quoted by Baldrick in *Dinner at Magny's*

But, in rank itchy lust, desire and love
The nakedness and bareness to enjoy
Of thy plump muddy whore or prostitute boy.

John Donne *Satires* (1593–98)

Make-up is the badge of a harlot; rotten posts are painted, and gilded nutmegs are usually the worst.

Thomas Hall *The Loathsomnesse of Long Haire...* (1654)

Germaine was different...Sauntering along the boulevard I had noticed her verging toward me with that curious trot-about air of a whore and the run-down heels and cheap jewelry and the pasty look of their kind which the rouge only accentuates. It was not difficult to come to terms with her...In a few minutes we were in a five franc room on the Rue Amelot, the curtains drawn and the covers thrown back. She didn't rush things, Germaine. She sat on the bidet *soaping herself and talked to me pleasantly about this and that...As she stood up to dry herself, still talking to me pleasantly, suddenly she dropped the towel and, advancing toward me leisurely, she commenced rubbing her pussy affectionately, stroking it with her two hands, caressing it, patting it, patting it. There was something about her eloquence at that moment and the way she thrust that rosebush under my nose which remains unforgettable...it was no longer just her private organ, but a treasure, a magic, potent treasure, a God-given thing – and none the less so because she traded it day in and day out for a few pieces of silver.*

Henry Miller *Tropic of Cancer* (1934)

'Now,' he says, 'I'm going to pay you as usual,' and taking a bill out of his pocket he crumbles it and then shoves it up her quim.

Henry Miller *Black Spring* (1936)

How haughtily he cries: "Page, fetch a whore;
Damn her, she's ugly; rascal, fetch me more;
Bring in that black-ey'd wench; woman, come near;
Rot you, you draggled bitch, what is't you fear?"
Trembling she comes, and with as little flame,
As he for the dear part from whence he came.
But by the help of an assisting thumb
Squeezes his chitterling into her bum;
And if it prove a straight, well-sphincter'd arse,
Perhaps it rears a little his feeble tarse.

Charles Sackville, Sixth Earl of Dorset *A Faithful Catalogue of the Most Eminent Ninnies* (mid-17th century)

She's lousy, she's frowsy,
She works on the street,
Whenever you meet her she's always on heat,
You can frig her for fourpence no less and no more,
Charlotte the harlot, the cowpuncher's whore.

Rugger song (20th century)

Some men frankly admit to enjoying the services of prostitutes:

My dear little Lillie Costello
I met you and crammed you today
And I would I might be your best fellow
So I with you more often would play.
Today for the first time I met you
And played with your pussy so cute
And Lillie if e'er I forget you
Then I am a crank and a galoot.
But Lillie you treated me kindly
Your price I paid freely & more
I'll say that I will not blindly
Forget me & call you a 'whore'.

Frederick Ryman *Diary* (Feb. 1885)

I'm not surprised that our Lord Christ
liked to live with harlots and sinners,
that's just how it is with me too.

J. W. von Goethe *Venetian Epigrams* (c. 1786)

Just as some women are more blatant than others:

Oh, my name is Diamond Lily,
I'm a whore in Piccadilly
And my father runs a brothel in the Strand
My brother sells his arsehole
To the Guards at Windsor Castle.
We're the finest fucking family in the land.

Anon. 'Diamond Lily'

Prostitution did not earn its epithet 'the oldest profession' for nothing:

> *The Actor and the Streetwalker...the two oldest professions in the world – ruined by amateurs.*
>
> Alexander Woollcott *Shouts and Murmurs* (1922)

Its history is, indeed, long. The earliest records of prostitution come from the ancient Middle East, around 3000 BC, and are associated with the worship of the Great Goddess, Ishtar:

> *...wherever she was worshipped, sacred prostitution was a focal point of the holy ritual. With Ishtar herself identified as a prostitute, and with prostitute-priestesses staffing the temples that were still at the centre of religion, political and economic power in Mesopotamia, the status of whores was high...*
>
> *It is here that the true story of prostitution begins; with the temple priestesses who were both sacred women and prostitutes, the first whores in history.*
>
> Nickie Roberts *Whores in History* (1992)

> *The Babylonians have one most shameful custom. Every woman born in the country must once in her life go and sit down in the precinct of Aphrodite, and there have intercourse with a stranger...A woman who has once taken her seat is not allowed to return home until* [a stranger] *throws a silver coin into her lap, and takes her with him beyond the holy ground. When he throws the coin he says these words: 'I summon you in the name of the goddess Mylitta.'...The woman goes with the first man who throws her money, and rejects no one. When she has had intercourse with him, and so satisfied the goddess, she returns home, and from that time on no gift however great will prevail with her.*
>
> *In the land of the Lydians all the daughters go whoring so as to procure a dowry, and they do this until they are regularly married.*
>
> Herodotus *History of the Persian Wars* (5th century BC)

Indeed, the tradition of sacred prostitution has persisted in some parts of our world until modern times. In northern India:

> *They feed the idol every day, for they say that he eats; and when he eats, women dance before him who belong to the pagoda, and they give him food, and all that is necessary, and all the girls born of these women belong to the temple. These women are of loose character, and live in the best streets that are in the city...any respectable man may go to their houses without any blame attaching thereto.*
>
> Domingo Paes (16th century)

> *And when they approached with it, all the harlots came out of the church, pagóga and sirke or temple harlots, to dance before the gods, and with them their master, who is called baldor. He hires them out every day for money, both to the soldiers and bachelors in the town, and this money is put into the treasure-house of the temple and is used for its upkeep, but the harlots get their keep out of the revenues of the temple, paid to them by its warders.*
>
> Jón Ólaffsson, describing the arrival of the Hindu festal car at a temple in Tanjore (1623)

> *And these lewd women, who make a public traffic of their charms, are consecrated in a special manner to the worship of the divinities of India. Every temple of any importance has in its service a band of eight, twelve or more.*
>
> Abbé J. A. Dubois *Hindu Manners, Customs and Ceremonies* (1816)

> *...as soon as a girl reaches maturity, her virginity, if not debauched by the pagoda brahmins, is sold to outsiders in proportion to the wealth of the party seeking the honour, if such it may be termed, after which she leads a continuous course of prostitution – prostituting her person at random, to all but outcasts, for any trifling sum.*
>
> Dr John Shorrt 'The Bayadere: or Dancing Girls of Southern India', paper read to the Anthropological Society (1868)

and in Africa:

The chief business of the female kosi [young girl dedicated to the god] *is prostitution, and in every town there is at least one institution in which the best looking girls are received. Here they remain for three years, learning the chants and dances peculiar to the worship of the gods, and prostituting themselves to the priests and inmates of the male seminaries; and at the termination of their novitiate they become public prostitutes. This condition, however, is not regarded as one for reproach; they are considered to be married to the god...*

A. B. Ellis *The Ewe-speaking Peoples of the Slave Coast of West Africa* (1887)

The secularization of sacred prostitution in the ancient world was a gradual and insidious affair:

As male rulers and priests consolidated their power, many of the temple women were ousted from the temples and formed troupes of professional singer-dancer-prostitutes travelling the rounds of the religious and social festivals in order to provide the entertainment and ritual sex that always formed part of the celebration.

Nickie Roberts *Whores in History* (1992)

In ancient Greece and Rome, some prostitutes could command high prices – perhaps reflecting the high esteem in which their sacred predecessors were held:

A foreigner visiting Athens
a satrap, very old about ninety,
saw Gnaithainon at the festival of Kranos going
with Gnaithaina out of a temple of Aphrodite.
And after he'd perused her figure and her movements,
he'd asked her how much she'd charge
for the night. Gnaithaina, glancing at his purple gown
and spearmen, put the price at a thousand drachmas.

Machon (250 BC)

Here she graciously received all comers, asking from each his fee: and when at length the keeper dismissed the rest, she remained to the very last before closing her cell, and with passion still raging hot within her went sorrowfully away.

Juvenal *Satire VI* (2nd century)

However, when its sacred origins were forgotten, prostitution became just another amenity:

A common harlot shall not veil herself as other women do; her head shall be uncovered. Anyone who sees a common harlot veiled shall arrest her. They shall beat her with 50 strokes with rods, and they shall pour pitch on her head.

Assyrian law (c. 2000 BC), quoted by H. W. F. Saggs in *Everyday Life in Babylonia and Assyria* (1965)

One [ancient Greek] *streetwalker's sandal has survived the centuries. Studded in reverse on the sole is a message that would print itself on the roadway for the next passerby to read. The message, of course, is 'follow me'.*

Reay Tannahill *Sex in History* (1990)

HIC HABITAT FELICITAS
Here dwells happiness.

Anon. inscription in a pastry cook's shop where whores were kept for the customers (79 AD)

Once, just as Cato was pausing by a brothel, a young man, very embarrassed at the sight of him, came out and did his best to sneak secretly round the corner. But Cato called to him and said, that there was nothing to blame in what he was doing. When then he afterwards saw the young man frequently coming out of the same brothel, he stopped him and said, "I praised you then, since I assumed that you came here now and then, not that you lived here".

Cato, quoted in the commentary to Horace (2nd century)

He's been the round of the whores, and they've all cost money: then only the other day he got sick of them, I suppose, and announced his intention of marrying.

Terence *The Brothers* (160 BC)

We all know Galla's services as a whore
Cost two gold bits; throw in a couple more
And you get the fancy extras too. Why, then,
Does your bill, Aeschylus, amount to ten?
She sucks off for far less than that. What is it
You pay her for? Silence after your visit.

Martial *Epigrams* (1st century AD)

When Antisthenes once saw an adulterer running away, he said "You ass, you could have had that without any risk for an obol!" [about 1½p]

Diogenes Laertius (3rd century)

In ancient Greece prostitution was mainly confined to slaves and other non-citizens. Any male citizen who prostituted himself lost the privileges of his status:

It is to be feared that anyone who sells his own body for money will also lightly sacrifice the common interests of the state.

Any Athenian citizen who prostitutes himself shall be excluded from exercising any public function or even expressing his opinion in the Assembly of the Council. He will be charged with hetairesis [lack of principle] *an offence punishable with the utmost rigour of the law.*

Aeschines *Contra Timarchum* (4th century BC)

Biblical attitudes to prostitution are uncompromising:

One who keeps company with harlots squanders his substance.

Proverbs 29:3

Know ye not that your bodies are the members of Christ? shall I then take the members of Christ, and make them *the members of an harlot? God forbid. What? know ye not that he which is joined to an harlot is one body? for two, saith he, shall be one flesh.*

I Corinthians 6:15–16

However, centuries of Christian denunciation did nothing to stem the practice:

There is scarcely a town in Italy, or in France, or in Gaul, where English prostitutes are not found.

St Boniface (8th century)

The Second Council of Aachen in 836 complained that certain convents were little better than brothels, a complaint repeated a century later in a letter from the Bishop of Würzburg to Rabanus Maurus.

James A. Brundage *Law, Sex and Christian Society in Medieval Europe* (1987)

By the later Middle Ages attempts were made to control and regularize prostitution with the establishment of well-run brothels. Their inhabitants were not necessarily regarded as beyond hope of redemption:

...prostitutes should be counted among wage earners. In effect they hire out their bodies and provide labour. If they repent they may keep the profits from prostitution for charitable purposes. But if they prostitute themselves for pleasure and hire out their bodies so that they may gain enjoyment, then this is not work and the wage is as shameful as the act.

Thomas of Chobham (13th century)

Since we came here we have effected great improvements. When we came, we found out three or four brothels. We leave behind us but one. We must add, however, that it extends without interruption from the eastern to the western gate.

Cardinal Hugo, on leaving Lyons in 1250 after 8-years in exile there with Pope Innocent IV, quoted by H. C. Lea in *A History of Sacerdotal Celibacy in the Christian Church* (1907)

In Venice

...in 1358 the Grand Council declared prostitution 'absolutely indispensable to the world' (thus echoing the teaching of the canonists and theologians) and authorized an official house of prostitu-

tion to cater for the large numbers of men visiting the city [opened in 1360].

Jeffrey Richards *Sex, Dissidence and Damnation* (1990)

In 13th-century France, however, mere proximity to prostitutes was regarded as a serious health hazard:

We prohibit public prostitutes (frequent cohabitation with whom is more effective than the plague in bringing harm) from being permitted to live in the city or bourg but rather should be set apart as is the custom with lepers.

Council of Paris, decree (1213)

Although by the 15th century

...prostitution was not merely tolerated or hidden away, but that even in quite small places there were prostibula publica belonging to the community, or under seignorial control in towns with no communal governing body. Sometimes, as in Avignon or Paris, instead of the grande maison, there would be one or several precincts officially reserved for public prostitution.

Jacques Rossiaud 'Prostitution, Sex and Society in French Towns in the Fifteenth Century', quoted in Philippe Ariès and André Béjin *Western Society* (1985)

In 1816, French prostitutes were obliged to register themselves, to carry a card, and to comply with certain conditions:

They are forbidden to practise their profession by day...They must be simple and decently dressed...They may not go about bare-headed. They are expressly forbidden to address men who are in the company of women or children. They must never, at any hour, show themselves at their windows but must keep these shut and curtained at all times.

De la Prostitution dans la Ville de Paris (1857)

In the UK, even now, the legal position of prostitutes is confused:

Prostitution itself is not a crime, but various activities related to it are...attempting to obtain prospective clients in a street or public place [soliciting] *is punishable by a fine of up to £100 on a first conviction and up to £400 on a subsequent conviction.*

Elizabeth Martin *A Concise Dictionary of Law* (1990 ed.)

Although this seems rather pointless:

The most obvious problem is the fact that when a woman is fined for prostitution, she has to work harder to raise the money to pay the fines.

Lyn Matthews *Outreach Work with Female Prostitutes in Liverpool* (1990)

Inspector Dick Powell...knows that roughly half an hour elapses between the arrest of a prostitute and her return to the street. He also knows that she is likely to be fined an insignificant sum which she will earn by repeating the offence. Measured by results, it is an exercise in futility...Teresa has given up paying fines, she said. "I just go to jail two or three times a year. I rest up and eat and use the gym. It's like a health cure. Holloway's my second home."

Independent on Sunday (13 Sept. 1992)

Campaigners for prostitutes' rights maintain that, far from protecting women, the offence of 'living off immoral earnings' (pimping) effectively prevents a prostitute from having a steady boyfriend:

Prostitutes have a right to a private life.

P. U. Venema and J. Visser *Safer Prostitution: a New Approach in Holland* (1990)

I may be a prostitute, but I'm not promiscuous.

Barbra Streisand in *The Owl and the Pussycat* (1970)

Some feminists go further, arguing that the effective criminalization of prostitution is a threat to all women:

Punishing the prostitute promotes the rape of all women. When prostitution is a crime, the message conveyed is that women who are sexual are 'bad' and therefore legitimate victims of sexual as-

sault. Sex becomes a weapon to be used by men.

Margo St James,, US prostitute quoted in *San Francisco Examiner* (29 Apr. 1979)

British police have traditionally tolerated prostitutes – even to the extent of being quite paternal towards them:

It must be clearly understood that it is the duty of the police in dealing with prostitutes more to prevent loitering and importuning than to detect it. Of course, considerable forbearance should be shown by constables in dealing with these unfortunate women, many of whom are greatly to be pitied.

Report of the Street Offences Committee (1928)

Police should carefully avoid gossiping with prostitutes, for unfounded charges and suspicions may easily arise therefrom. At the same time they should avoid bullying or harassing these unfortunate persons if their conduct is orderly.

Howard Vincent *Police Code and General Manual of the Criminal Law* (1934)

The constable on the beat may sometimes be crudely jocular at the expense of toms and tarts, but he will usually defend prostitution as a natural relationship, a thing on quite a different plane from male homosexuality, about which in common with so many men he expresses his disgust.

C. H. Rolph *Women of the Streets* (1955)

'Toms and tarts' – throughout their long history prostitutes have gone by many names: whore, harlot, strumpet, hooker, trollop, cocotte, hustler, streetwalker, sporting lady, call girl, and dollymop, are just a few of the commoner ones. However, to be politically correct, one now has to call them 'sex workers'.

Rape

A female definition of rape can be contained in a single sentence. If a woman chooses not to have intercourse with a specific man and the man chooses to proceed against her will, that is a criminal act of rape.

Susan Brownmiller *Against Our Will* (1976)

The law, however, has not and does not always take this simple view. Ancient Jewish teaching made little distinction between rape and illicit but consensual intercourse, while Roman law regarded rape as primarily an offence against property until well into the Christian era:

No cities had been destroyed by God's wrath because of [female] *rape. In fact, biblical injunctions against rape seem to have been rare at best.*

Guido Ruggiero *The Boundaries of Eros: Sex Crime in Renaissance Venice* (1989)

In Roman law, raptus was abduction and did not necessarily involve sex. The offence was a property offence – stealing a female from her family or guardian. It was a private matter rather than a public crime. The early penitentials took the same view of raptus, and rape as we understand it did not appear…[In the 4th century] *Gratian and his successors redefined the crime to bring it closer to what we now see as rape. They considered it a major crime not against property but against the person and defined it as having four constituent elements: abduction, violence, sexual intercourse, and the absence of consent. This strongly suggests that we should see the development of the offence of rape as a corollary of the Church's development of the idea of consent in marriage.*

Jeffrey Richards *Sex, Dissidence and Damnation* (1990)

Until a landmark judgment in 1991 altered the situation, UK law did not recognize forced sex within marriage as rape. In the words of the eminent but, in modern terms, chauvinist jurist Sir Matthew Hale:

The husband cannot be guilty of a rape committed by himself upon his lawful wife, for by their mutual matrimonial consent and contract the wife hath given up herself in this kind unto her husband, which she cannot retract.

Sir Matthew Hale, quoted by R.H. Small in *History of the Pleas of the Crown* (1736)

See also MARRIAGE

Such attitudes have roused the anger of women campaigners in many countries:

A mutual and satisfied sexual act is of great benefit to the average woman, the magnetism of it is health giving. When it is not desired on the part of the woman and she has no response, it should not take place. *This is an act of prostitution and is degrading to the woman's finer sensibility, all the marriage certificates on earth to the contrary notwithstanding.*

Margaret Sanger *Family Limitations* (1917)

To gain a conviction in the English Courts it is not enough to establish that sex took place without the woman's consent:

If an accused man believed the woman had consented, whether or not that belief was based on reasonable grounds, he could not be found guilty of rape.

House of Lords ruling (1975)

Recently feminist attention has focused on the issue of 'date rape' – the greyish area between rape and seduction, in which women are pressurized into sex against their better judgment (see SEDUCTION). The law recognizes no such grey areas:

It is not rape if she consents even if her will is weakened, unless fraud or threats are used to that end. Seduction is not rape.

M. D. A. Freeman *The Law and Sexual Deviation* (1964)

'Fraud' encompasses those cases (presumably very rare) in which a man obtains a woman's consent by impersonating her husband or lover. In addition many countries have an offence of 'statutory rape', meaning:

...a man's taking sexual advantage of a child, a mental defective, or other person presumed to lack comprehension of the physical and other consequences of sexual intercourse. Consent is not relevant. The definition of this lack of comprehension, however, is often overreaching, for...a child may be designated as someone as old as 18 years. The term statutory rape may also refer to those laws, as in France, against taking sexual advantage of a person in a subservient position, such as an employee or ward.

Encyclopaedia Britannica

Who are rapists? Most informed opinion agrees that

Rapes are rarely committed by isolated maniacs; they are more often brutal acts carried out by ordinary perfectly 'normal' people.

Stern and Stern *Sex in the Soviet Union* (1981)

Contrary to the stereotype image of the stranger who strikes in a dark alleyway or churchyard, you are more likely to be raped by someone you know or have seen before the assault.

Jane Dowdeswell *Women on Rape* (1986)

It is also accepted that rapists are rarely, if ever, motivated by a simple desire for sex:

A primary goal of the sexual aggressor is the conquest and degradation of his victim...Sexual assaults are expressions of anger and aggression prompted by the same basic frustrations...summarised as an inability to achieve masculine identification and pride through avenues other than sex.

A. J. Davis *The Sexual Scene* (1970)

Rather than sexual satisfaction as a motive for rape, which has been the social understanding, women who had been raped presented sexual humiliation as the more obvious desire of the rapists.

Cathy Roberts *Women and Rape* (1989)

Apparently sexually well-adjusted youths have in one night committed a series of burglaries and, in the course of one of them, committed rape – apparently just as another act of plunder.

Dr Manfred Guttmacher *Sex Offenses* (1951)

It should be kept in mind that the rapist's motives involve feelings of domination, regardless of whether the 'victim' is a man or woman. Rape is a power trip – an act of aggression and an act of contempt – and in most cases is only secondarily sexual.

J. and H. Schwendinger *Rape Myths* (1974)

Male attitudes to rape have often been ambivalent. There is sometimes a tendency to sympathize with the perpetrator:

In one study, an account of forced sex was read to a group of male students (the word 'rape' was not used), and 53 per cent said there was some likelihood that they would behave in the same fashion as the man in the story if they could be sure of getting away with it.

The Times (23 Jan. 1992)

Rapists are victims of a disease from which many of them suffer more than their victims.

Benjamin Karpman *The Sexual Offender and His Offenses* (1954)

or to blame the victim:

A woman carrying a purse is not generally considered to be asking to be mugged, but a woman in a short skirt is often accused of asking to be raped.

Jane Dowdeswell *Women on Rape* (1986)

The notion that if a woman did not exactly consent to sexual intercourse, she by her conduct in some way 'asked for it', deep down, really wanted it, is popular among men, though seldom among women. Way back in Viking days, rape was a capital offence – but only if the woman screamed as soon as she was touched.

Fenton Bresler *Sex and the Law* (1988)

or to suggest that it is, or can be, an enjoyable experience:

It is in female psychology to wish, to some extent, to be overcome by a superior male.

Reginald Paget MP, in a speech on the Attempted Rape Bill, 1948, *Parliamentary Debates*

Women are terrified of being raped, but somewhere in the back of every womb there is one rebellious nerve end that tingles with curiosity whenever the word is mentioned...Raped women have been divorced by their husbands – who couldn't bear to live with the awful knowledge, the visions, the possibility that it wasn't really rape.

Hunter S. Thompson *Hell's Angels* (1967)

Such attitudes are often at their most shocking in the statements of the judiciary:

Women who say no do not always mean no. It is not just a question of saying no, it is a question of how she says it, how she shows and makes it clear. If she doesn't want it she only has to keep her legs shut and she would not get it without force and there will be marks of force being used.

Judge David Wild, summing up to Cambridgeshire Crown Court jury (1982)

When it was said that a victim had suffered severe internal injuries when a guardsman wearing chunky rings forced his hand inside her vagina, Lord Justice Roskill commented that her injuries would not have been so severe if she had submitted to the rape!

Fenton Bresler *Sex and the Law* (1988)

Rape trials are often conducted by remote and unsympathetic judges in a manner that creates further trauma for the victim:

Where rape is concerned the traditional methods of criminological analysis, criminal motivation and criminal behaviour are superseded by a preoccupation with the victim, her motivation, her proclivity for sexual experience and her moral behaviour. And yet it is not the sexual experience of the complainant that is on trial, but a man who it is alleged has had intercourse with her by force.

Susan Edwards *Female Sexuality and the Law* (1981)

The law recognizes only one issue in rape cases other than the fact of intercourse: whether there was consent at the moment of intercourse. The jury does not limit itself to this one issue; it goes on to weigh the woman's conduct in the prior history of the affair.

Harry Kalven and Hans Zeisel *The American Jury* (1966)

Although it seems improbable that any one would lightly choose to undergo such an ordeal, a suspicion persists that women are prone to making false accusations for frivolous reasons:

There are many adult females of loose morals who, although consenting parties to sexual connection at the time, later become conscience-stricken, and to alter the complexion of their act after it has been committed, lay a charge of rape against the partner of their illicit intercourse.

J. Glaister *Legal Medicine* (1925)

As Alfred Kinsey often said, the difference between a 'good time' and a 'rape' may hinge on whether the girl's parents were awake when she finally arrived home.

Paul Gebhard, John H. Gagnon, W. B. Pomeroy, and Cornelia V. Christenson *Sex Offenders: An Analysis of Types* (1965)

I am sure that everyone agrees that men and youths must be protected from wild accusations which can be made very easily by a woman seeking to get herself out of trouble with her husband, boyfriend or parents, out of spite or, simple fantasy.

L. M. Blair, female police surgeon, *The Problem of Rape* (1977)

History, sacred and profane, and the common experience of mankind teaches that women are prone for selfish reasons to make false accusations both of rape and of insult upon the slightest provocation , or even without provocation, for ulterior motives...this tendence shows they are predisposed to make false accusations upon any occasion whereby their selfish ends may be gained.

Judge James E. Horton 'Opinion of Judge James E. Horton of the Alabama Circuit Court' (1934)

The prevalence of such attitudes has led to the extreme feminist view that rape is part of a systematic conspiracy of men against women, in which all heterosexual males are implicated:

Man's discovery that his genitalia could serve as a weapon to generate fear must rank as one of the most important discoveries of prehistoric times, along with the use of fire...Female fear of an open season of rape, and not a natural inclination toward monogamy, motherhood, or love, was probably the single causative factor in the original subjugation of woman by man...

Rather than society's aberrants or 'spoilers of purity', men who commit rape have served in effect as front-line masculine shock troops, terrorist guerrillas in the longest sustained battle the world has ever known.

Susan Brownmiller *Against Our Will* (1975)

Whatever they may be in public life, whatever their relations with men, in their relations with women, all men are rapists, and that's all they are. They rape us with their eyes, their laws, and their codes.

Marilyn French *The Women's Room* (1977)

In our culture, heterosexual love finds an erotic expression through male dominence and female submission...if the professional rapist is to be separated from the average dominant heterosexual, it may be mainly a quantitative difference.

Susan Griffin *Rape: the All American Crime* (1971)

However, not all recent commentators accept the view that rape is a product of socialization:

Rape is a mode of natural aggression that can be controlled only by the social contract. Modern feminism's most naive formulation is its assertion that rape is a crime of violence but not of sex, that it is merely power masquerading as sex. But sex is power, and all power is inherently aggressive. Rape is male power fighting female power. It is no more to be excused than murder is or any other assault on another's civil rights. Society is woman's protection against rape, not, as some feminists absurdly maintain, the cause of rape...the rapist is a man with too little socialization rather than too much. Worldwide evidence is overwhelming that whenever social controls are weakened, as in war or mob rule, even civilized men behave in uncivilized ways, among which is the barbarity of rape.

Camille Paglia *Sexual Personae* (1990)

Rape has been an almost inevitable accompaniment of war and conquest from ancient times to the present day:

Rape is an integral part of human history. In the development of mankind, rape has been used as a weapon both in mass conflicts and everyday battles. For womankind, women's bodies have been used, not only to inflict pain on, but as the weapon with which to defeat and humiliate the opposing males – the presumed real owners of those female bodies.

Cathy Roberts *Women and Rape* (1989)

After they had destroyed the town of Carbina in Apulia, they dragged all the boys, girls, and young women into the temples and exposed them naked to the gaze of visitors. Anyone who liked might rush upon this unfortunate herd, and satisfy his lust upon the naked beauty of those exposed to view, before the eyes of all, and certainly those of the gods, which they least suspected. But the gods punished this crime, for soon after, all these debauchees were struck by lightning.

Clearchus of Soli (2nd century BC)

I then told him that, in spite of my most diligent efforts, there would unquestionably be some raping, and that I should like to have the details as early as possible so that the offenders could be properly hanged.

George S. Patton Jr *War As I Knew It* (1947)

What do soldiers talk about in barracks? Women and sex. Put a gun in their hands and tell them to go out and frighten the wits out of a population and what will be the first thing that leaps to their mind? Remember, some of our Bengali women are very beautiful.

Unidentified Bengali politician, quoted by Aubrey Menen in 'The Rape of Bangladesh' *New York Times* (23 July 1972)

In 1993 the world was shocked by reports that Serbs had carried out mass rapes of Bosnian Muslim women as a policy of war:

It is clear that at least some of the rapes are being committed in particularly sadistic ways so as to inflict maximum humiliation on the victims. Rape had, therefore, become an instrument and not a by-product of war.

David Andrews *Independent* (6 Jan. 1993)

This [the raping of Muslim women] *was done systematically. It is a plan. Firstly, the rapes are to keep the women out of their villages, to prevent them ever going back. These are Muslim women and the rapists were trying to kill their personality by forcing them to have children. It is not just a physical crime against a woman. It is also a psychological crime.*

Senad Saric, doctor treating Bosnian rape victims, *Independent* (8 Feb. 1993)

In peacetime, too, rape can sometimes be an expression of racial hatred. For the militant Black activist Eldridge Cleaver

Rape was an insurrectory act. It delighted me that I was defying and trampling upon the white man's law, upon his system of values, and that I was defiling his women – and this point, I believe, was the most satisfying to me because I was very resentful over the historical fact of how the white man had used the black woman. I felt I was getting revenge.

Eldridge Cleaver *Soul on Ice* (1968)

A Black US sociologist has written:

I am well aware that, like murder, rape has many motives. But when the motive for rape, however psychotic, is basically racial, that is a different matter. I think now that, at one time or another, in every Negro who grows up in the South, there is a rapist, no matter how hidden. And that rapist has been conceived in the Negro by a system of morals based on guilt, hatred, and human denial.

Calvin C. Hernton *Sex and Racism in America* (1966)

Similarly, the fear of rape has often been used to exacerbate racial fears. In the Southern US:

The charge of 'rape' was consciously forged as a matter of state policy…It has since consistently been used to terrorize militant Negroes with the ever-present menace of death by lynching or by 'legal

murder' through police, incited mobs, and venal courts. Examples of how the cry of 'rape' is used, invariably on the basis of race, abound. The genocidal, murderous quality of the charge of 'rape' is apparent.

Petition of the Civil Rights Congress to the UN *We Charge Genocide* (1951)

There is now growing recognition of the reality of male rape, for long obscured by taboo and disbelief. Even so:

Male rape is perhaps the easiest crime to get away with in this country... If you and I decided, as two men, that we were going to go out tonight and rape a boy or a man, we could almost guarantee – 99.9 per cent certain – that we're going to get away with it. The reason we're going to get away with it is because we know the victim is not going to report the crime. His sexual identity is going to be brought into question. He's going to be made to look a fool in front of his family and friends. He'll be asked 'How on earth *could you let that happen to you?'*

Richie J. McMullen, male rape victim, in a BBC interview; quoted in the *Independent on Sunday* (6 Dec. 1992)

Male rape has always been common in enclosed single-sex institutions such as prisons:

Virtually every slightly built young man committed by the courts is sexually approached within a day or two after his admission to prison. Many of these young men are repeatedly raped by gangs of inmates.

A. J. Davis *The Sexual Scene* (1970)

Findings suggest that the majority of male rapes are carried out by heterosexuals – further evidence that the crime has more to do with the urge to violate and degrade than with the desire for sexual gratification. Cases in which women have compelled unwilling men to engage in sexual acts are rare but not unheard of:

The most extraordinary cases of rape are undoubtedly those committed by women upon men. This occurs in situations where the women are sexually starved. In the Kuril Islands this kind of thing is common. Fishing boat captains dare not let sailors go ashore, for there are thousands of women working in the canneries who have no man for years on end, and the sailors genuinely run the risk of death.

Stern and Stern *Sex in the Soviet Union* (1981)

At present, British law does not recognize that a man can be 'raped' by an attacker of either sex; the offences of indecent assault and 'non-consensual buggery' both carry lesser penalties. (A private member's bill to alter this situation passed its first reading in 1992.)

Personal accounts given by survivors of rape suggest that the burden of suffering is much the same for both men and women. For long after the attack, victims experience feelings of defilement, depression, and unreality so acute as to make normal life impossible.

It's like living through your own murder.

Rape victim, quoted in Fenton Bresler *Sex and the Law* (1988)

The process of recovery is painful and long-drawn-out, calling on great resources of courage and determination:

The question you ask is, will the rapist win, or will you win? Every step is a fight, literally pushing myself.... Because unless you can gather together every single piece of your life that he smashed against the wall, seize back every single one, and make your life whole again, then the rapist has won.

Male rape victim, quoted in the *Independent on Sunday* (6 Dec. 1992)

I no longer feel tainted by my victimisation. It's an honour to be a survivor, and although it's not the sort of thing I can put on my résumé, it's the accomplishment of which I'm most proud.

Susan Brisan, rape victim, *Guardian* (10 Apr. 1993)

Reproduction

Amoebas at the start
Were not complex;
They tore themselves apart
And started sex.

Arthur Guiterman *Sex* (20th century)

In most adult human beings the sexual imperative retains an element of blind biological instinct:

Let's fuck, dear heart, let's have it in and out,
For we're obliged to fuck for being born,
And as I crave for cunt, you ache for horn,
Because the world would not make sense without.

Pietro Aretino 'Let's Fuck, Dear Heart' (16th century)

A sense of the power of the sexual instinct and of the fertility of nature underlay most ancient religions:

The goat, being so strongly sexually inclined, it was considered that his genital organ, the instrument of generation, should be worshipped; as it is through this comes the birth of living things. But not only by many other nations is the male sex-organ worshipped as the principal object of generation.

Herodotus (5th century BC)

Love moves the pure Heaven to wed the Earth; and Love takes hold on Earth to join in marriage. And the rain, dropping from the husband Heaven impregnates Earth, and she brings forth for men pasture for flocks, and corn, the life of men.

Aeschylus *Danaids* (5th century BC)

Most primitive cultures saw human fertility as a sign of divine approbation – and infertility as a curse or stigma. The ability to bear children was a woman's chief marketable asset:

To know a woman who will bear from a woman who will not bear: water-melon, pounded and bottled with the milk of a woman who has borne a male child; make it into a dose. To be swallowed by the woman. If she vomits, she will bear. If she belches, she will never bear.

Mesopotamian papyrus (c. 2000 BC)

In the Jewish scriptures human reproduction is generally seen as an awesome mystery, only to be understood in terms of God's power and goodness:

I do not know how you appeared in my womb; it was not I who endowed you with breath and life, I had not the shaping of your every part.
It is the creator of the world, ordaining the process of man's birth and presiding over the origin of all things.

II Maccabees 7:22–23

For many early Christian thinkers, however, human reproduction was tainted with disgust for the body in general and the sexual act in particular:

Inter faeces et urinam nascimur.
Between shit and urine we are born.

St Augustine *Confessions* (4th century)

We are conceived somewhere between pissing and shitting, and as long as these excretory functions are regarded as intrinsically disgusting, the other one, ejaculation, will be so regarded.

Germaine Greer *The Female Eunuch* (1970)

Some Christians have gone so far as to express their regret that reproduction cannot be achieved by other, non-sexual, means:

The reproduction of mankind is a great marvel and mystery. Had God consulted me in the matter, I should have advised him to continue the generation of the species by fashioning them of clay.

Martin Luther (16th century)

The physician Sir Thomas Browne was of a similar opinion:

Who would not be curious to see the lineaments of a man who, having himself been twice married, wished that mankind were propagated like trees.

Charles Lamb on Sir Thomas Browne, *New Monthly Magazine* (Jan. 1826)

The taboos surrounding sex, reproduction, and childbirth have been particularly hard for women:

Certain other taboos seem to us to spring from the general horror of violence; for instance, the taboos associated with menstruation and the loss of blood at childbirth. These discharges are thought of as manifestations of internal violence... The menstrual discharge is further associated with sexual activity and the accompanying suggestion of degradation... Childbearing cannot be dissociated from this complex of feelings. Is it not itself a vending process, something excessive and outside the orderly course of permitted activity? Does it not imply the denial of the established order...?

Georges Bataille *Eroticism* (1987)

The female reproductive system has often been cited as evidence for the physical, mental, and moral inferiority of women: some of the arguments employed are distinctly odd:

Nature placed the female testicles internally... Woman is a most arrogant and extremely intractable animal; and she would be worse if she came to realize that she is no less perfect and no less fit to wear breeches than man... I believe that is why nature, while endowing her with what is necessary for our procreation, did so in such a way as to keep her from perceiving and ascertaining her sufficient perfection.

P. Borgarucci *Della contemplatione anatomica sopra tutte le parti del corpo umano* (1564)

Even in the 19th century

The assumption that women were dominated by their reproductive systems (women belonged to nature, while men belonged to culture) was implicit in all medical attitudes.

Jeffrey Weeks *Sex, Politics, and Society* (1987)

Prescientific accounts of conception often tended to minimize or denigrate the role of the female:

The male provides the 'form' and the 'principle of the movement', the female provides the body, in other words the material.

Aristotle *History of Animals* (347-335 BC)

Or to see the conception of female offspring as some kind of mishap:

Men produce female as well as male seed. So do women. Male seed is stronger than female seed... This is what happens: if the stronger seed comes from both sides, the product is male; if the weaker, then the product is female.

Hippocrates (4th century BC)

Woman is defective and accidental... a male gone awry... the result of some weakness in the father's generative power.

St Thomas Aquinas (13th century)

See also FEMINISM

Traditional Catholic teaching has always maintained that sexuality is only sanctioned by the need to reproduce and continue the species. Such an assumption also influenced many Protestant pronouncements on the subject until quite recently. This failure to honour the non-procreative aspects of sex has drawn indignant protests:

The failure to see sexual relationship in any other light but the functional ones of reproduction has resulted in the limitation of sex to the purely physical with no concept at all of the depth of significant interpersonal trust, empathy, and love of which sexual intercourse, at best, is the expression...the pall of centuries of sin-obsessed taboos and misanthropic caricatures of human nature still blankets our culture and informs our mores.

Rev. Robert L. Treese *Homosexuality: A Contemporary View of the Biblical Perspective* (1972)

Sex is not the same as reproduction: the relation between the two is especially tenuous for human beings, who may copulate when they will, not only when they are driven thereto by heat or an instinctual urge.

Germaine Greer *The Female Eunuch* (1970)
See also MORALITY

The Catholic Church's continuing ban on artificial contraception has provoked much anger and ridicule:

Every sperm is sacred,
Every sperm is great,
If a sperm is wasted,
God gets quite irate.

Monty Python *The Meaning of Life* (1982)
See also CONTRACEPTION

Traditional views of fertility as a religious and social duty clearly need to be revised in the light of world population trends:

The command 'Be fruitful and multiply' was promulgated according to our authorities, when the population of the world consisted of two people.

Dean Inge *More Lay Thoughts of a Dean* (1931)

India's government, headed by a Prime Minister who has fathered eight children, introduced a bill yesterday seeking to bar people with more than two babies from becoming MPs, in an attempt to promote small families.

Independent (23 Dec. 1992)

Governments have also been urged to prevent women and girls from becoming pregnant at too young an age:

Recognising that pregnancy occurring in adolescent girls, whether married or unmarried, has adverse effects on the morbidity and mortality of both mother and child, Governments are urged to develop policies to encourage delay in the commencement of childbearing.

Report of UN Secretary General to World Conference to Review and Appraise the Achievements of the UN Decade for Women (1985)

Before the advent of safe and effective contraception, the threat of unwanted pregnancy hung over most casual heterosexual encounters:

Then he'll take me by the hand
And lay me down upon the land
And make my buttocks feel like sand
Upon this high holiday.

Spindle, bobbin, and spool, away,
For joy that it's a holiday!

In he'll push and out he'll go,
With me beneath him lying low:
'By God's death you do me woe
Upon this high holiday!

Spindle, bobbin, and spool, away,
For joy that it's a holiday!

Soon my belly began to swell
As round and great as any bell;
And to my dame I dared not tell
What happened to me that holiday.

Spindle, bobbin, and spool, away,
For joy that it's a holiday!

Anon. 'The Servant Girl's Holiday' (c. 14th century)

Whilst they did embrace unspied,
The conscious willow seemed to smile,
That them with privacy supplied,
Holding the door, as 'twere o'er,
The willows, to oblige them more,
Bowing, did seem to say, as they withdrew,
'We can supply you with a cradle too.'

William D'Avenant 'Under the Willow-Shades' (17th century)

Familiarity breeds contempt – and children.

Mark Twain *Notebooks* (19th century)

There are no illegitimate children – only illegitimate parents.

Léon R. Yankwich, quoting columnist O. O. McIntyre. Decision, State District Court, Southern District of California (June 1928)

He said it was artificial respiration but now I find I'm to have his child.

Anthony Burgess *Inside Mr. Enderby* (1963)

Various methods of minimizing the risk of conception were, of course, employed. Few were as ingenious as this Roman matron, who contrived to conduct liaisons only when she knew herself to be already pregnant by her husband:

A grave wise man that had a great rich lady,
Such as perhaps in these days found there may be,
Did she think she played him false and more than think,
Save that in wisdom he thereat did wink.
Howbeit one time disposed to sport and play
Thus to his wife he pleasantly did say,
"Since strangers lodge their arrows in thy quiver,
Dear Dame, I pray you yet the cause deliver,
If you can tell the cause and not dissemble,
How all our children me so much resemble?"
The lady blushed but yet this answer made
"Though I have used some traffic in my trade,
And must confess, as you have touched before,
My bark was sometimes steered with foreign oar,
Yet stowed I no man's stuff but first persuaded
The bottom with your ballast full was laded."

Sir John Harington 'Of an Heroical Answer of a Great Roman Lady to her Husband' (16th century)

Even when a child is much wanted, the parents are often ill-prepared for its arrival:

Who of us is mature enough for offspring before the offspring themselves arrive? The value of marriage is not that adults produce children but that children produce adults.

Peter De Vries *Tunnel of Love* (1954)

In the late 20th century a variety of medical techniques have been devised to help couples who have found difficulty in conceiving. Where the husband is fertile but unable to perform sexually, the woman may be impregnated with his sperm using artificial insemination (AIH); where he is infertile, the sperm of an anonymous donor may be used (AID). Certain kinds of female infertility can now be overcome using in vitro fertilization (IVF), in which a woman's egg is fertilized outside her body and then introduced to the womb. These techniques – and such related developments as surrogate motherhood and embryo storage – have raised a host of ethical and legal dilemmas.

Los Angeles: *A judge ruled that a man could not will his sperm to his girlfriend and ordered that it be destroyed. The will of William Kane, a millionaire lawyer who committed suicide, is being contested by his children. The girlfriend, Deborah Hecht, wept and said: 'I really want his baby.'*

The Times (11 Dec. 1992)

Because of these developments, it is now possible for a woman to bear children without ever having sexual intercourse with a man. Some women have taken the opportunity to claim that men are no longer necessary:

> *The world cannot do without women, which is why there's resentment from men. They realize the future lies with us.*
>
> Joan Collins *Independent* (13 Apr. 1991)

> *It is now technically possible to reproduce without the aid of males, and to produce only females. We must begin immediately to do so.*
>
> Valerie Solanas *SCUM* (Society for Cutting Up Men) *Manifesto* (1967)

In reality, of course, neither sex can do without the other. Mark Twain is supposed to have replied to the question 'In a world without women what would men become?' thus:

> *Scarce, sir. Mighty scarce.*

Sadism and Masochism

I ache for the touch of your lips dear
But much more for the touch of your whips dear.
You can raise welts
Like nobody else
As we dance to the Masochism Tango.

Tom Lehrer *Masochism Tango* (1959)

What are sadism and masochism (S & M)?

Dear God, what have we here? A Prodigy? That pleasure should come from pain, sweet from bitter, lust from bloody wounds? Does the same road lead to torment and to delight?

Giovanni Sinibaldi *Genean Thropeiae* (1642)

We comprehend this form of sex as sexual pleasure roused, or exclusively finding satisfaction in, tortures of one kind or another. We speak of an active *form,* sadism, *after the Marquis de Sade, who wrote books on the subject, and a* passive *form,* masochism, *after Sacher-Masoch, who described this form.*

J. Fabricius-Møller *Sexual Life* (1944)

Both terms were coined by the 19th-century German sexologist Richard von Krafft-Ebing:

Masochism is the opposite of sadism. While the latter is the desire to cause pain and use force, the former is the wish to suffer pain and be subjected to force.

I feel justified in calling this sexual anomaly 'masochism' because the author Sacher-Masoch frequently made this perversion, which up to his time was quite unknown to the scientific world as such, the substratum of his writings.

Psychopathia Sexualis (1886)

Krafft-Ebing realized that the sadomasochist was fascinated by something deeper and more complex than the physical aspects of beating and being beaten (see FLAGELLATION):

In coining the term masochism, Krafft-Ebing was giving Masoch credit for having redefined a clinical entity, not merely in terms of the link between pain and sexual pleasure, but in terms of something more fundamental connected with bondage and humiliation.

Gilles Deleuze *Masochism: Coldness and Cruelty* (1989)

Domination versus submission; freedom versus slavery; absolute power versus absolute helplessness – these are the opposites which constitute the basis of sadomasochism, and to which any preoccupation with pain is secondary.

Dr Anthony Storr *Sexual Deviation* (1964)

S & M's more articulate advocates view it as a challenge to the accepted social concepts of personal identity, gender role, consent and dissent, as well as to the nature of sexual pleasure:

S & M is deliberate, premeditated, erotic blasphemy. It is a form of sexual extremism and sexual dissent.

Pat Califia *Guardian* (28 Nov. 1992)

What I really like about S & M, in its funny little ant-sized way, is how it stands down there at the base of the mighty colossus of social authority and shakes it as hard as it can.

Anon. quoted by Robert J. Stoller in *Pain & Pleasure: a Psychiatrist Explores the World of S & M* (1989)

For many advocates of SM from within the sexual subcultures of the West, it provides unique insights into the nature of sexual power, therapeutic and cathartic sex revealing the nature of sex as ritual and play. Such claims...pose very dramatically the question of the relationship between context and choice, subjectivity and consent in thinking about sexuality. Should people have the right to consent to activities which are conventionally regarded as painful and potentially harmful? What are the conditions that make such choices valid? Is there the same possibility of free choice between say a man and a woman as there is between people of 'the same caste' (gay, two women)? The activities of the 'sexual fringe'...may remain marginal to the mainstream of most people's sexual lives, but...what are the limits of normality, what are the boundaries of valid sexual activity, and what are the extremes to which we should go in the pursuit of pleasure?

Jeffrey Weeks *Sexuality* (1986)

Attempts to explain the deeper significance of sadomasochism often become rather esoteric:

The male masochist magnifies the losses and divisions upon which cultural identity is based, refusing to be sutured or recompensed. In short, he radiates a negativity inimical to the social order.

Kaja Silverman 'Masochism and Male Subjectivity' *Camera Obscura* (1988)

Masochism is a search for recognition of the self by another who alone is powerful enough to bestow this recognition.

Jessica Benjamin *Master and Slave: the Fantasy of Erotic Domination* (1983)

A master is superior to God because he exists in the flesh.

Anon. quoted by Dr Anthony Storr in *Sexual Deviation* (1964)

...erotic masochism or submission expresses the same need for transcendence of self – the same flight from separation and discontinuity – formerly satisfied and expressed by religion.

Jessica Benjamin *Master and Slave* (1983)

The aim of sadism is to transform a man into a thing, something animate into something inanimate, since by complete and absolute control the living loses one essential quality of life – freedom.

Erich Fromm *The Heart of Man* (1964)

It is interesting that binding one's lover up, and so rendering him or her helpless, can itself provide a sexual stimulus. In some cases bondage is an end in itself, in others it is a prelude to more painful stimuli:

I don't know what got into him. It started out as a game. I trusted him and thought that he was playing. He wanted to tie me down to the bed during sex – I thought it might be kinda fun so I agreed. I had no idea what could happen. He seemed content at first but after a while he started talking mean to me and slapping me on the face and breasts. I was getting scared and begged him to untie me. He went to the dresser and got a hairbrush and shoved it up my vagina over and over again. I screamed and thought he was going to kill me. I nearly passed out from the pain.

Anon. quoted in C. D. Tollison and H. E. Adams *Sexual Disorders* (1979)

A handkerchief was thrust into my mouth, I was made to clasp the tree in a tight embrace and was bound at the shoulders and legs, which left my body free of the ropes so that I should have no protection from the beating which I was about to receive. The Marquis, marvellously excited, seized a thong. Before striking me, he was cruel enough to wish to observe my face, and it was as though he was feasting his eyes not only on my tears but also on the expressions of pain and fear with which my countenance was suffused. He then placed himself behind me at a distance of about three feet and I immediately felt, from the middle of my back to the top of my legs, the stroke of the lash which he applied with all the strength he could muster. My tormentor paused for a moment and ran his hands roughly over the areas which he had just beaten black and blue.

Marquis de Sade *Justine, or the Misfortunes of Virtue* (1791)

Sometimes the bondage can be self-inflicted:

He sat naked in his rocking chair of undressed teak, guaranteed not to crack, warp, shrink, corrode or creak at night. It was his own, it never left him. The corner in which he sat was curtained off from the sun, the poor old sun in the Virgin for the billionth time. Seven scarves held him in position. Two fastened his shins to the rockers, one his thighs to the seat, two his breast and belly to the back, one his wrists to the strut behind. Only the most local movements were possible. Sweat poured off him, tightening the thongs...He sat in his chair in this way because it gave him pleasure!

Samuel Beckett *Murphy* (1938)

Sometimes these inclinations can begin very early in life; this letter from a six-year-old boy in 1984 to Jimmy Savile for his BBC programme 'Jim'll Fix It' is an example:

Dear Jim,
Can you please fix it for me to meet the girls on page 39 of the 'Mothercare' catalogue. I would like them to chase me through the woods and tie me to a tree.

and another example, from the founder of the Corrective Party:

I loved the Guides, that was where I learned to tie knots.

Lindi St Clair *Independent* (1 July 1992)

One of the numerous paradoxes of sadomasochism is that, in practice, the masochist is usually the dominant partner:

It should be recognized that the masochist gives himself a sense of control of what transpires. He is the master of operations, determining – often to the finest degree – in what he will suffer in the role of the victim.

Mervin Glasser *Role of Aggression in the Perversions* (1964)

The fact is, S&M is controlled and responsible sexual activity. We have a very highly developed sense of ethics. We have a golden rule that when the bottom [masochist] *says enough, the activity stops. The bottom will often use a special word when he or she does not want to go further.*

Anon. *Guardian* (28 Nov. 1992)

There is the bottom who is so controlling in the scene that the tops [sadists] *begin to suspect they are dealing with a top in bottom drag. Some tops like the adversarial quality of these encounters, but most tops seem to come away from them feeling topped by the bottom.*

Anon. quoted by Robert J. Stoller in *Pain & Pleasure: a Psychiatrist Explores the World of S & M* (1989)

The masochist is a revolutionist of self-surrender. The lambskin he wears hides a wolf. His yielding includes defiance, his submissiveness opposition. Beneath his softness there is hardness; beneath his obsequiousness rebellion is concealed.

Theodor Reik *Masochism in Modern Man* (1957)

As creator of the performance, the masochist is never truly a victim, because he never really relinquishes control, and in that sense the whole scenario is known to portray only fraudulent suffering.

Robert J. Stoller *Perversion* (1976)

This being the case, it is legitimate to ask whether *true* masochism can be said to exist at all:

Masochists seek only certain specific and individually variable forms of suffering and humiliation. As soon as these reach greater intensity or take a different form, they are reacted to with the habitual fear and pain.

R. M. Loewenstein *A Contribution to the Psychoanalytic Theory of Masochism* (1956)

But is there such a thing as genuine masochism? Does anyone really seek pain for its own sake and enjoy pain? The truth is that no one really knows.

Paula J. Caplan *The Myth of Women's Masochism* (1984)

In the past, it has often been assumed that a degree of masochism is natural to women, and a degree of sadism to men:

There is not a man who doesn't want to be a despot when he's excited.

Marquis de Sade *Philosophy in the Bedroom* (1795)

While in men it is possible to trace a tendency to inflict pain, or the simulacrum of pain, on the women they love, it is still easier to trace in women a delight in experiencing physical pain when inflicted by a lover, and an eagerness to accept subjugation to his will. Such a tendency is certainly normal.

H. Havelock Ellis *The Psychology of Sex* (1897–1928)

Although Freud wrote about masochism in both sexes, he explicitly said many times that masochism is feminine. Even masochistic behaviour in a man was labeled feminine by Freud, so that masochism, which was not considered normal or typical in a man, was thought to be both in a woman.

Paula J. Caplan *The Myth of Women's Masochism* (1984)

The simplest and most elementary pattern of masochism is the enjoyable misery of a woman who wears beautiful, but too small shoes. There is a proverb, 'Vanity has to suffer'. It is often applied to women who have to undergo painful sensations in beauty-salons. The feminine character of masochism becomes transparent when you turn the sentence around. Suffering appears then as motivated or accompanied by satisfaction of vanity.

Theodor Reik *Sex in Man and Woman* (1960)

Any self-respecting John Wayne fan will tell you that all women really want to be slapped around occasionally.

Andrea Blanch *Cornell Journal of Social Relations* (1970)

These assumptions seem to proceed from women's traditionally subordinate role in relation to men and from the usual female role in lovemaking:

In coitus, the woman, in effect, is subjected to a sort of beating by the man's penis. She receives its blows and often, even, loves their violence.

Marie Bonaparte *Half the Human Experience: the Psychology of Women* (1980)

Heterosexual intercourse has been thought to give rise to masochism because it was assumed that for biological reasons intercourse has to take place with the woman underneath the man.

Paula J. Caplan *The Myth of Woman's Masochism* (1984)

Others deny that there is any essential connection between being a heterosexual woman and being a masochist:

Even most women who become aroused by fantasies of sexual masochism are immediately turned off by real masochism.

Robin Morgan *Against Sadomasochism: A Radical Feminist Analysis* (1982)

The suffering of pain, being beaten or tied up, disgrace and humiliations, do not belong to the sexual aims of the normal woman.

Theodor Reik *Masochism in Modern Man* (1957)

There is nothing essentially more masochistic about a housewife running herself ragged waiting on her husband hand and foot than there is about a businessman driving himself to a heart attack to further pad an already solid bank account. The only difference lies in the social value attributed to each activity.

Andrea Blanch *Cornell Journal of Social Relations* (1970)

The evidence suggests that male masochism is at least as common as female:

The beautiful woman bent on her adorer a strange look from her green eyes, icy and devouring, then she crossed the room, slowly donned a splendid loose coat of red satin, richly trimmed with princely ermine, and took from her dressing table a whip, a long thong with a short handle, with which she was wont to punish her great mastiff. 'You want it,' she said, 'then I will whip you.' Still on his knees, 'Whip me' implored her lover, 'I implore you'.

Ritter Leopold von Sacher-Masoch *Under the Whip* (1873)

As he was unbuttoned to me, and tried to provoke and rouse to action his unactive torpid machine, he blushingly own'd that no good was to be expected from it, unless I took it in hand to re-excite its languid loitering powers, by just refreshing the smart of the yet recent blood-drawn cuts.

John Cleland *Fanny Hill: Memoirs of a Woman of Pleasure* (1749)

There are Persons who are stimulated to VENERY by STROKES OF RODS, and WORKED UP INTO A FLAME OF LUST by BLOWS, and that the PART, which distinguishes us to be MEN, should be raised by the charm of invigorating LASHES.

Johann Heinrich Meibom *On the Use of Rods in Venereal Matters and in the Office of the Loins* (1718)

Male masochism often seems to involve a deliberate element of role reversal:

It cannot be doubted that the masochist considers himself in a passive feminine role towards his mistress. The pleasurable feeling, call it lust, resulting from this act differs per se in no wise from the feeling which women derive from the sexual act.

Richard von Krafft-Ebing *Psychopathia Sexualis* (1886)

Here James Joyce's Leopold Bloom fantasizes about being dominated and unmanned by the 'massive whore mistress' Bella Cohen:

Bow, bondslave, before the throne of your despot's glorious heels, so glistening in their proud erectness...I'm the tartar to settle your little lot and break you in! I'll bet Kentucky cocktails all round I shame it out of you, old son. Cheek me, I dare you. If you do tremble in anticipation of heel discipline to be inflicted in gym costume...I want a word with you, darling, just to administer correction. Just a little heart to heart talk, sweety. I only want to correct you for your own good on a soft safe spot...
What you longed for has come to pass. Henceforth you are unmanned and mine in earnest, a thing under the yoke. Now for your punishment frock. You will shed your male garments, you understand Ruby Cohen? and don the shot silk luxuriously rustling over head and shoulders and quickly too...Tape measurements will be taken next to your skin. You will be laced with cruel force into vicelike corsets of soft dove coutille...
By day you will souse and bat our smelling underclothes, also when we ladies are unwell, and swab out our latrines with dress pinned up and a dishclout tied to your tail. Won't that be nice?...You will make the beds, get my tub ready, empty the pisspots in the different rooms...Ay, and rinse the seven of them well, mind, or lap it up like champagne. Drink me piping hot. Hop! you will dance attendance or I'll lecture you on your misdeeds, Miss Ruby, and spank your bare bot right well, miss, with the hairbrush. You'll be taught the error of your ways.

James Joyce *Ulysses* (1922)

Not all women who adopt the role of dominatrix do so purely to gratify a masochistic partner: some evidently find a satisfaction of their own:

> *"I enjoy putting Gerry in his kennel." Sadie, a small, heavily made up woman in her late 30s, gestures outside the back door. "He has to wear his 'fifi' dog outfit, with his testicles chained to his ankles, and eat only dog food and pee like a dog. I've left him out there for up to a week sometimes."*
>
> *Guardian* (28 Nov. 1992)

> *History provides thousands of examples of female cruelty, and it is on account of their natural inclination to such behaviour that I should like women to make a habit of employing active flagellation...A few women do, I know, but not nearly as many as I should like.*
>
> Marquis de Sade *Philosophy in the Bedroom* (1795)

> *It is a well known fact that women are, and always have been, even more fond of wielding the rod than men, and that this passion pervades the higher, rather than the lower classes.*
>
> Pisanus Fraxi (pseud. of Henry Spencer Ashbee) *Index Librorum Prohibitorum* (1877)

So what is it about pain and humiliation that makes them such a turn-on for both some women and some men? Ritualized punishment can provide a means of coming to terms with guilt:

> *A sense of guilt is invariably the factor that transforms sadism into masochism.*
>
> Sigmund Freud *A Child is Being Beaten* (1919)

> *In masochistic perversions, there is a conflict between the hostile wish and the placatory expiation of guilt to preserve the loved object.*
>
> Ismond Rosen *The General Psychoanalytical Theory of Perversion* (1964)

Or a more general emotional catharsis:

> *The basic dynamic of S&M is the power dichotomy...Handcuffs, dog collars, kneeling, being bound, tit clamps, hot wax, enemas, penetration, and giving sexual service are all metaphors for the power imbalance...A good scene doesn't end with orgasm – it ends with catharsis.*
>
> Pat Califia *Guardian* (28 Nov. 1992)

> *One woman who had formerly been involved in sexual masochism said that when she suffered actual physical pain it was in an attempt to release a great deal of emotional pain, not to suffer for the sake of suffering.*
>
> Robin Morgan *Against Sadomasochism: A Radical Feminist Analysis* (1982)

Others find excitement in the sense of transgression and challenge to authority:

> *There's an enormous hard-on beneath the priest's robe, the cop's uniform, the president's business suit, the soldier's khakis. But that phallus is powerful only as long as it is concealed, elevated to the level of a symbol, never exposed or used in literal fucking. In an S & M context, the uniforms and roles and the dialogue become a parody of authority, a challenge to it, a recognition of its secret sexual nature.*
>
> Pat Califia *Guardian* (28 Nov. 1992)

As Freud noted:

> *The history of civilization shows beyond any doubt...an intimate connection between cruelty and the sexual instinct.*
>
> Sigmund Freud *Three Essays on the Theory of Sexuality* (1905)

More prosaically, masochism can be seen as an extreme case of the normal human tendency to increase pleasure by deferring it:

> *It is argued, justifiably, that the masochist is not a strange being who finds pleasure in pain, but that he is like everyone else, and finds pleasure where others do, the simple difference being that for him pain, punishment and humiliation are necessary pre-requisites to obtaining gratification.*
>
> Gilles Deleuze *Masochism: Coldness and Cruelty* (1989)

The masochist acts like a man who returns from a long journey home in a cold winter night. He already sees the lighted windows of his home and he needs only a little effort to arrive at home. But he falls into the next pub on the road.

Sigmund Freud, quoted in Theodor Reik *Sex in Man and Woman* (1960)

There are also physiological aspects to be considered alongside the psychological motives:

Discomfort, stress or actual pain can contribute to some women's sexual pleasure. First of all, these sensations increase tension, speed up breathing, and reproduce or intensify many of the physiological changes associated with arousal. This is also a way to express trust or devotion to a lover...Breaking through mental and physical barriers creates a feeling of elation.

Pat Califia *Sapphistry: The Book of Lesbian Sexuality* (1983)

An element of threat can facilitate orgasm. Research shows we are often turned on by a degree of dominance and power.

Dr Glenn Wilson *Guardian* (28 Nov. 1992)

Perhaps, the whole mysterious business of S&M is best summed up by one of the progenitors:

Whoever allows himself to be whipped, deserves to be whipped.

Ritter Leopold von Sacher-Masoch *Venus in Furs* (1870)

Seduction

Seduction operates somewhere between courtship and rape. At best, with its ritual techniques of persuasion it promises all the pleasures of courtship. At worst, it is a way of despoiling, only distinguishable from crime because it does not involve brute force. Seduction, unlike a marriage proposal, can never occur between equals. Its inherent imbalance explains why it is always exploitative in one way or another.

Jenny Norman 'Introduction' *The Faber Book of Seductions* (1988)

In many people's minds, the distinction between rape and seduction is largely one of pace. The word 'seduce' seems to imply effort of a persevering, thoughtful sort...

A seduction is the very opposite of the abrupt, which is, of course, rape.

Elizabeth Hardwick *Seduction and Betrayal* (1970)

Well, no. Legally, the distinction hinges entirely on the issue of informed consent. Seduction can be quick and brutal, but if the seducee is willing it can hardly qualify as rape:

Then with a violent movement Laurent stopped, took the young woman, and held her against his breast. He pushed her head back, crushing her lips beneath his own. She made one wild instinctive effort to resist and then yielded, slipping down on to the floor. Not a single word was exchanged. The act was silent and brutal.

Émile Zola *Thérèse Raquin* (1867–68)

The popular male belief that women are excited by a degree of rough treatment may not always be self-serving nonsense:

What they love to yield
They would often rather have stolen.
Rough seduction
Delights them, the boldness of near rape
Is a compliment.

Ovid *Ars Amatoria* (1st century BC)

Perhaps these two opinions from Fenton Bresler's *Sex and the Law* (1988) may help to clarify the distinction:

The difference between rape and seduction is salesmanship.

Lord Thomson of Fleet

Conquest by a 'con job', however reprehensible, is seduction, not rape. Every man is free to be a gentleman or a cad.

Judge Edward Greenfield

In law:

The seducer may resort to various devices in order to obtain the consent of his victim – soft lights, sweet music, flattery, and drink.

J. C. Smith 'The Heilbron Report' *Criminal Law Review* (1976)

More recently, some feminists have started to apply the term 'date rape' to situations in which the woman's consent is judged to have been obtained by 'unfair' means. Although the terminology is new, the phenomenon is ancient:

With wine and words of love and every vow
He lulled me into bed and closed my eyes,
A sleepy stupid innocent...So now

I dedicate the spoils of my surprise:
The silk that bound my breasts, my virgin zone,
The cherished purity I could not keep.
Goodness, remember we were all alone,
And he was strong – and I was half asleep.

Hedylos 'Seduced Girl'

The redefinition of such cases as 'rape' has not been universally accepted:

The date rape thing has become propaganda and hysteria. We cannot legislate what happens on a date. Sex is a dangerous sport.

Camille Paglia, CNN television (1991)

See also RAPE

Arguably, women often fall victim to their tendency to idealize an unsatisfactory situation:

The impulse to yield militates against the impulse to impose the right form on the circumstances, and most often a girl breathing out her soul on the lips of her callow lover seduces herself with an inflated notion of what is really happening...

The desire to have sex built up into an important occasion has a curious relationship with the alleged slowness of feminine response, for many women seek in sex not physical release but exaltation, physical worship as promised in the marriage service.

Germaine Greer *The Female Eunuch* (1970)

Seduction is perhaps best thought of as extending from the preliminary enticement, through the foreplay, to the moment at which consent is unambiguously granted. The seducer may be male or female and the seducee may be of the same or the opposite sex.

In literature, the seducer is often lyrical, stressing the transience of life, youth, and beauty:

Thy beauty shall no more be found,
Nor, in thy marble vault shall sound
My echoing song; then worms shall try
That long-preserved virginity,
And your quaint honour turn to dust,
And into ashes all my lust:
The grave's a fine and private place,
But none I think do there embrace.

Andrew Marvell 'To His Coy Mistress' (17th century)

Darling, each morning a blooded rose
Lures the sunlight in, and shows
Her soft, moist and secret part.
See now, before you go to bed,
Her skirts replaced, her deeper red –
A colour much like yours, dear heart.

Alas, her petals will blow away,
Her beauties in a single day
Vanish like ashes on the wind.
O savage Time! that what we prize
Should flutter down before our eyes –
Who also, late or soon, descend.

Then scatter, darling your caresses
While you may, and wear green dresses;
Gather roses, gather me –
Tomorrow, aching for your charms,
Death shall take you in his arms
And shatter your virginity.

Pierre de Ronsard 'Corinna in Vendome' (16th century)

Or given to moral sophistries:

I've oft been told by learned friars,
That wishing and the crime are one,
And Heaven punishes desires
As much as if the deed were done.

If wishing damns us, you and I
Are damned to all our heart's content;
Come then, at least we may enjoy
Some pleasure for our punishment!

Thomas Moore 'An Argument' (19th century)

Others are straightforwardly randy:

Please, my sweet Losithilta, my delightful girl, my charmer, order me to come to you this noon. And if you will have so ordered, add this also: do not let anyone bar your doorsill, and do not go outside, but stay at home and prepare nine consecutive acts of sexual intercourse for me. Truly, if you will do anything, give orders immediately, for as I lie on my back, hav-

ing lunched and full of food, I am poking through my tunic and my cloak.

Catullus (1st century BC)

Then straight before the wandering maid,
The tree of life I gently laid;
Observe sweet Sue, his drooping head,
How pale, how languid, and how dead;
Yet, let the sun of thy bright eyes,
Shine but a moment, it shall rise;
Let but the dew of thy soft hand
Refresh the stem, it straight shall stand;
Already, see, it swells, it grows,
Its head is redder than the rose,
Its shrivelled fruit, of dusky hue,
Now glows, a present fit for Sue:
The balm of life each artery fills,
And in o'erflowing drops distils.
Oh me! cried Sue, when is this?
What strange tumultuous throbs of bliss!
Sure, never mortal, till this hour,
Felt such emotion at a flower:
Oh, serpent, cunning to deceive,
Sure 'tis this tree that tempted Eve;
The crimson apples hang so fair,
Alas! what woman could forbear?
Well hast thou guessed, my love, I cried.
It is the tree by which she died;
The tree which could content her,
All nature, Susan, seeks the centre;
Yet, let us still, poor Eve forgive,
It's the tree by which we live;
For lonely woman still it grows,
And in the centre only blows.
But chief for thee, it spreads its charms,
For paradise is in thy arms –
I ceased for nature kindly here
Began to whisper in her ear:
And lovely Sue lay softly panting,
While the geranium tree was planting.
'Till in the heat of amorous strife,
She burst the mellow tree of life.

Richard Brinsley Sheridan 'The Geranium' (18th century)

In romantic fiction, seduction is pursued both by gentlemen, who are never randy, and by cads, who are never anything else:

For all their prudish insistence on blushing and the excision of any suggestion of less intense and less decorous human contact, [Barbara] *Cartland and* [Georgette] *Heyer are preparing the way for seducers – not lovers, seducers.*

Germaine Greer *The Female Eunuch* (1970)

The gentlemanly lover may proceed by appealing to the mercy of his beloved – as John Keats here does with Fanny Brawne (although they almost certainly never became lovers):

I cry your mercy – pity – love! – aye, love!
Merciful love that tantalizes not,
One-thoughted, never-wandering, guileless love,
Unmasked, and being seen – without a blot!
O! let me have thee whole, – all – all – be mine!
That shape, that fairness, that sweet minor zest
Of love, your kiss, – those hands, those eyes divine,
That warm, white, lucent, million-pleasured breast, –
Yourself – your soul – in pity give me all,
Withhold no atom's atom or I die,
Or living on perhaps, your wretched thrall,
Forget, in the midst of idle misery,
Life's purposes, – the palate of my mind
Losing its gust, and my ambition blind.

'I Cry Your Mercy' (1820)

The cad, on the other hand, takes a more cynical attitude to his desires:

When innocence, beauty, and wit do conspire
To betray, and engage, and inflame my desire,
Why should I decline what I cannot avoid,
And let pleasing hope by base fear be destroyed?

John Wilmot, Earl of Rochester 'The Submission' (1680)

For the truly compulsive seducer, sensual pleasure seems to be far less important than the sense of power that accompanies his successes:

Think of the Don Juan, that paradigm of promiscuity…his interests are in seduction, not love, and in recounting for friends how many women he has had and how they degraded themselves in the needfulness of the passion he induced.

Robert J. Stoller *Perversion* (1976)

See also PROMISCUITY

Of course, the seducer can equally well be a female:

When she raises her eyelids it's as if she were taking off all her clothes.

Colette *Claudine and Annie* (1903)

A lady is one who never shows her underwear unintentionally.

Lillian Day *Kiss and Tell* (1931)

It wouldn't be a good idea
To let him stay.
When they knew each other better –
Not today.
But she put on her new black knickers
Anyway.

Wendy Cope 'Prelude' (1980s)

She gave me a smile I could feel in my hip pocket.

Raymond Chandler *Farewell, My Lovely* (1940)

On a sofa upholstered in panther skin
Mona did researches in original sin.

William Plomer *Mews Flat Mona* (20th century)

In the narrowest of little side streets – one could hardly get through between the walls – I once found a girl sitting in my path, as I was walking through Venice. She was charming; a charming place, and I, the foreigner, let myself be seduced. Alas! my explorations took me into a wide canal. If only, Venice, you had girls like your canals, and cunts like your side-streets, you would be the world's finest town.

J. W. von Goethe *Venetian Epigrams* (c. 1786)

There was a little girl
Who had a little curl
Right in the middle of her forehead,
When she was good she was very very good
And when she was bad she was very very popular.

Max Miller *The Max Miller Blue Book* (20th century)

or as Mae West is supposed to have said:

When I'm good I'm very good, but when I'm bad I'm better.

Fanny Hill was just 15 when seduced by the experienced Phoebe:

…she now attempts the main-spot, and began to twitch, to insinuate, and at length to force an introduction of a finger into the quick itself, in such a manner, that had she not proceeded by insensible gradations, that enflamed me beyond the power of modesty to oppose its resistance to their progress, I should have jump'd out of bed, and cried out for help against such strange assaults.
Instead of which, her lascivious touches had lighted up a new fire that wanton'd through all my veins…

John Cleland *Fanny Hill: Memoirs of a Woman of Pleasure* (1748–49)

Men have often accused women of being the 'real seducers':

Reality shows us that the real seducers are the daughters of Eve who sashay their way through God's world with their miniskirts, low-cut and see-through blouses and tight-tight pants, for the sole purpose of exhibiting their curvaceous bodies to attract the attention and eyes of men.

Emerson Pereia (1975)

When Eve ate this particular apple, she became aware of her own womanhood, mentally. And mentally she began to experiment with it. She has been experimenting ever since. So has man. To the rage and horror of both of them.

D. H. Lawrence *Fantasia of the Unconscious* (1922)

Females are naturally libidinous, incite the males to copulation, and cry out during the act of coition.

Aristotle *History of Animals* (347–335 BC)

What is specific to women lies in the diffraction of the erogenous zones, in a decentered eroticism, the diffuse polyvalence of sexual pleasure and transfiguration of the entire body by desire.

Seduction is always more singular and sublime than sex, and it commands the higher price.

Jean Baudrillard *Seduction* (1979)

In some cases it is certainly more singular than in others:

Of course, Salvador Dali seduced many ladies, particularly American heiresses; but these seductions usually entailed stripping them naked in his apartment, frying a couple of eggs, putting them on the woman's shoulders, and without a word showing them the door.

Luis Buñuel *Conversations with Buñuel* (1985)

Sex in old age

The subject of geriatric sex has been taboo for far too long and, because of this, the elderly are discriminated against.

Roy Eskapa *Bizarre Sex* (1987)

There are probably several reasons for this silence, the most likely being the embarrassment many people feel at asking the elderly questions about sex – particularly in view of the widespread belief that they don't have any:

The sexuality of the elderly is no place for the evangelist. The recognition that continued physical intimacy benefits both the psychological and physical health of the individual must be tempered by a willingness to allow elderly people to make their own decisions unpressured by those who are younger. The embarrassment of the patients will be overcome only if the doctor can take the lead in introducing the topic — which is not easy for those of us who have been taught that elderly people don't do it.

J. Kellet 'Sex and the Elderly' *British Medical Journal* (Oct. 1989)

The discrepancy between earlier findings of low levels of sexual activity and interest among the elderly and recent findings to the contrary is that earlier studies were guided by the self-fulfilling prophesy – little sex was expected and consquently little was found. Researchers were even discouraged from pursuing the topic in the belief that older people would be resistant or unresponsive to sexual queries...or that their adult children would stop them from participating in such research...

One of the most powerful statements that Kinsey made about the status of sex and aging is the number of pages he devoted to the subject: four pages on older women and three pages on older men, out of 1,646 pages in his two volumes.

B. D. Starr *Sexuality and Aging* (1985)

Health-care professionals often seem to have difficulties in acknowledging the sexuality of the aged:

The literature suggests that health workers need to look at their own sexuality and also gain some understanding of the subject. Perhaps we can then cater for the client's needs. I think that this is particularly important for nurses. We claim to be concerned with the whole individual and yet we ignore an essential part of that individual's life...The elderly often get a rough deal; perhaps we can start improving the situation by acknowledging their sexuality.

D. Wright 'Sex and the Elderly' *Nursing Mirror* (1985)

There are two main reasons why sexuality in the elderly is difficult to discuss. First, nurses historically have not been trained to cope with sexuality. Their sexuality is 'suppressed and repressed,' with the aim of 'purity' and 'asexuality' and they suffer from sexism and stereotyping at work. But if nurses are not aware of their own attitudes, beliefs and values they will not be able to help others.

E. Griffiths 'No Sex Please, We're Over 60' *Nursing Times* (1988)

It's an old British custom that in the interests of military good order and discipline any institution, school, hospital, or home should be run like a good gaol – people in it should be clean, tidy, idle and not called on to make choices. Older people in Britain are spared the excesses of the American nursing-home racket; there fit people are kept in bed because the owners get higher subvention for the bedridden. Here they may be kept unnecessarily in bed because it's tidier like that...Sexuality is a particular bugbear of the British institution. It's only recently that homes (some of them) ceased to separate married couples, and any formation of new relationships may still cause acute administrative embarrassment.

Dr Alex Comfort *A Good Age* (1989)

Elderly people are often stereotyped as being decrepit, sexually impotent, or even asexual:

In old age, marriage is not to be recommended. Two decaying bodies in one bed can never be endured.

Philip of Novara *Of the Four Ages of Man's Life* (c. 1265)

While coition's long forgotten; should you try, varicocele and stunted nerve be limp,
And though they be caressed all night, limp them remain.

Juvenal *Satire X* (2nd century)

Tragically, yet understandably, tens of thousands of men have moved from effective sexual functioning to varying degrees of secondary impotence because they did not understand the natural restraints that physiological aging imposes on previously established patterns of sexual functioning. From a psychosexual point of view, the male over 50 has to contend with one of the great fallacies of the culture. Every man in this age group is arbitrarily defined by both public and professional alike as sexually impaired. When the aging male is faced by the unexplained but natural involutional sexual changes, and deflated by widespread psychosocial acceptance of the fallacy of sexual incompetence as a natural component of the aging process, is it any wonder that he carries a constantly increasing fear of sexual performance.

William Masters and Virginia Johnson *Human Sexual Inadequacy* (1970)

Let us look at the stereotype of the ideal aged person as past folklore presents it. He or she is white haired, inactive and unemployed, making no demands on anyone, least of all of the family, docile with putting up with the loneliness, cons of every kind and type of boredom, and able to live on a pittance. He or she, although not demented, which would be a nuisance to other people, is slightly deficient in intellect, and tiresome to talk to, because folklore says that old people are weak in the head, asexual, because old people are incapable of sexual activity, and it is unseemly if they are not.

Dr Alex Comfort *A Good Age* (1989)

In old age the sexual function gradually ceases, sexual difference turns again into indifference, and the change is revealed in the fact that the sexes come to resemble each other once again in appearance, and the condition of the body, as they did in childhood.

Encyclopädisches Wörterbuch (1828)

After sixty, the inclination to be alone grows into a kind of real, natural instinct; for at that age everything combines in favour of it. The strongest impulse – the love of women's society – has little or no effect; it is the sexless condition of old age which lays the foundation of a certain self-sufficiency, and that gradually absorbs all desire for other's company.

Arthur Schopenhauer *Counsels and Maxims* (1851)

For women these problems are compounded:

Nobody minds if your husband looks his age. Men are lucky. They needn't look young to be still attractive. They often get better looking with the years. Unfortu-

nately the same can't be said for us women. From the first moment a tiny line appears we need to take extra care of our skins with the special moisturizing treatment...

Catherine Itzen *The Double Jeopardy of Ageism and Sexism* (1984)

A soldier's discharged and he may be bald and toothless yet he'll find a pretty young thing to go to bed with. But a woman! Her beauty is gone with the first grey hair. She can spend her time consulting the oracles and fortune-tellers, but they'll never send her a husband.

Aristophanes *Lysistrata* (411 BC)

Now ther ye seye that I am foul and old,
Than drede you noght to been a cokewold;
For filthe and eelde, also moot I thee,
Been grete wardeyns upon chastitee.

Geoffrey Chaucer *The Canterbury Tales*, 'The Wife of Bath's Tale (late 14th century)

This is how beauty dies:
humped shoulders, barrenness
of mind; I've lost my hips,
vagina, and my lips.
My breasts? They're a retreat!
Short breath – how I repeat
my silly list! My thighs
are blotched like sausages.

François Villon 'The Old Lady's Lament for Her Youth' (15th century)

A man is as old as he's feeling,
A woman as old as she looks.

Mortimer Collins *The Unknown Quantity* (19th century)

Many respondents thought it was just as well that men prefer younger women because mentally, they said, men do not mature as fast as women. Although this is commonly said about adolescent boys and girls, it is surprising that this view is projected to the later years and mentioned so frequently by older women.

L. H. Croft *Sexuality in Later Life* (1982)

My dear, when you are my age you will realise that what you need is the maturer man.

Lady Diana Cooper, aged 86, on her name being linked with that of 99-year-old Sir Richard Mayer

Most of the taboos are taboos of the young. The elderly, themselves, have different views:

Relatively few of our respondents, it turned out, wanted to write about religion in the later years, or about transportation problems after age 50. What interested them most – and what they wrote about most eloquently and at greatest length – was, quite simply, love and sexuality.

E. M. Brecher *Love, Sex and Aging* (1984)

In early 1984, the Star *(Johannesburg) reported that a Danish sexologist suggested that 'male prostitutes be brought into Danish old age homes to help old ladies with their sexual needs.' The sexologist, Professor Sten Hegeler, said that women prostitutes were already servicing elderly males. In other words, he felt that there should be equality between the sexes so far as prostitution is concerned.*

Roy Eskapa *Bizarre Sex* (1987)

Because many of the bricks from which the edifice of self-esteem is built are lacking for the elderly, sexuality, perhaps, becomes increasingly important. Independence, social position, and professional or commercial success, may no longer be available to bolster the ego of the pensioner – the ability to express love physically may be:

When a man grows old wisdom will not help him, but emotion will preserve him. He should be careful to feed passion.

Mark Rutherford *Last Pages from a Journal* (1913)

For the older man, an active sex life appears to be crucial to his feelings of self-worth and his feeling that he is respected by his friends and secure socially. As with the younger man, dissatisfaction with sex-

ual activity is related to depression and feelings of worthlessness.

Stinson et al. *Sexuality and Self-Esteem among the Aged* (1981)

It is important to be aware that a satisfactory sexual relationship is important for most people's well-being at any age. In the elderly the increased need for love, self-esteem and for close human contact give sexuality an enhanced value...Professional staff need to be aware of compounding the problem through projecting their own taboos, by, for instance discouraging developing liaisons.

Robin Skinner 'Young at Heart' *Community Care* (11 Feb. 1988)

When the elderly are deprived of physical contact, they can quickly descend into depression:

Now King David was old and stricken with years; and they covered him with clothes, but he gat no heat. Wherefore his servants said unto him, Let there be sought for my lord the king a young virgin: and let her stand before the king, and let her cherish him, and let her lie in thy bosom, that my lord the king may get heat.

I Kings 1:1–2

I am rather prone to senile lechery just now – want to touch the right person in the right place, in order to shake off bodily loneliness.

E. M. Forster, letter to Joe Archerley (16 Oct. 1961)

In the past, it was often assumed that sexual function in men and women ceased punctually at certain specifiable ages:

Old age begins with the disappearance of the sexual function, as a rule at 60 years of age in men and 50 in women. A decline in nourishment and in the energy of all functions characterizes this section of life which in the normal way ends with death.

Hauslexicon der Gesundheitslehre (ed. H. Klencke et al.; 1872)

Until a man reaches forty he is usually full of vigorous passion. But as soon as he has reached his fortieth year he will suddenly notice that his potency is decreasing. Just at that time the countless diseases will descend on him like a swarm of bees. If this situation is allowed to continue for long, he will finally be beyond cure.

Sun-Szu-mo *Priceless Recipes* (7th century)

More recent research has suggested that sexual capacity does not disappear with age but undergoes a gradual decline:

Our 4,246 respondents constitute the largest geriatric sample ever assembled for a sexuality study – not only for the total period after the age of 50 but also for each decade from the fifties through the eighties. Our sample is the first one large enough to permit charting sexual changes between the fifties and the sixties and between the sixties and subsequent years – for women and for men separately.
Our two central findings can be stated with confidence: Male sexual function undergoes a gradual, steady decline from the fifties on.
Female sexual function also undergoes a decline from the fifties on.

E. M. Brecher *Love, Sex and Aging* (1984)

In both sexes the normal process of ageing brings about certain changes in sexual capacity and the emotional and sensory experience of sexuality. This is to be expected, for many of the body's functions change as we age. In our sixties we no longer expect to run as fast as we did in our twenties even if we are perfectly healthy, and in more subtle ways the body changes in its resistance to stress and disease.

H. B. Gibson *The Emotional and Sexual Lives of Older People* (1992)

The incidences of responding males, and the frequencies of response to the point of orgasm reach their peak within three to four years after the onset of adolescence.

On the other hand, the maximum incidence of sexual responding females are not approached until some time in the late twenties and in the thirties.
The frequencies of sexual response in the male begin to decline after the late teens or early twenties, and drop steadily into old age. On the other hand...among females the median frequencies of those sexual activities that are not dependent upon the male's initiation of socio-sexual contacts (e.g. masturbation) remain more or less constant from the late teens into the fifties and sixties.

Alfred Kinsey et al. *Sexual Behaviour in the Human Female* (1953)

Along with a gradual diminution of sexual capacity, subtle changes occur in the nature of sexuality itself:

We must all understand and accept that getting older produces changes in our patterns of sexual interest and responsiveness, and one crucial change is that we simply have to begin paying more attention to our conditions for being interested and responsive. This becomes progressively more important as we get older.

W. Williams *Man, Woman and Sexual Desire* (1986)

If sexual desire in the elderly manifestly cannot be denied, it has often been seen in wholly negative terms – as in the popular stereotypes of the dirty old man or desperate old maid:

The general decline in our physical powers has led to a false belief that sexuality, both in terms of performance, needs and interest, should normally fade out somewhere in the late fifties, and that, if it persists it takes pathological forms.

H. B. Gibson *The Emotional and Sexual Lives of Older People* (1992)

There is a frequent well marked tendency in women at the menopause to an eruption of sexual desire, the last flaring of a dying flame, which may easily take on a morbid form. Similarly in men, when the approach of age begins to be felt, the sexual impulse may become suddenly urgent. In this instinctive reaction it may tend to roam, normally or abnormally, beyond legitimate grounds. This late exacerbation of sexuality becomes still more dangerous if it takes the form of an attraction to girls who are no more than children, and to acts of indecent familiarity with children.

H. Havelock Ellis *Studies in the Psychology of Sex* (1933)

Until very recently, the question of homosexuality in old age had received particularly little attention:

Having completed this study I feel more disturbed than ever about the fact that almost every gerontological researcher and commentator has chosen to ignore older folk who happen to be homosexual. Can these researchers believe that homosexuals self-destruct at the age of forty? Or have they simply been unaware of the millions of older people who are homosexual?

R. Berger *Gay and Gray* (1980)

Gerontology, the social science of aging, began well before World War II, experienced rapid growth after the war, and has recently became a major field, as an ever larger proportion of the population reaches sixty. For many years, gerontological research assumed that all older people were heterosexual, even though upwards of three million North Americans over sixty are lesbian or gay. This scientific blindness was hardly accidental. The social science of 'deviant behavior' knew that older homosexuals existed, but it propagated the myth that 'old aunties' and 'aging dykes' lived lonely, miserable lives, shunned by a homosexual subculture obsessed with youth...Only in the late 1980s did gay gerontology become established as a field of research...There is certainly no evidence to persuade any homosexual, whether very open or very hidden, that the elder years must be less satisfactory merely because of sexual orientation.

John Allen Lee in *Encyclopaedia of Homosexuality* (ed. Wayne R. Dynes; 1990)

What finally appears to emerge is that sexuality among the aged, physical restrictions apart, is much like sexuality among any other age group – a matter of individual preference and choice:

Sexual boredom is very common among older married couples, who tend to fall into routine patterns in which they do the same old thing sexually, time after time, year after year.

R. M. Butler, and M. I. Lewis *Love and Sex After Sixty* (1988)

Age cannot wither her, nor custom stale
Her infinite variety.

William Shakespeare *Antony and Cleopatra* (c. 1607)

As an elderly man he [Augustus] *is said to have still harboured a passion for deflowering girls, who were collected for him from every quarter, even by his wife!*

Suetonius *Lives of the Twelve Caesars* (2nd century)

[Cato the Elder] *by his strong make and good habit of body, lasted long; so that even in old age, he frequently indulged his inclination for the sex, and at an unseasonable time of life married a young woman.*

Plutarch *Lives* (2nd century)

At the most positive, they said that their sexual feelings were "diminished", but still important to them; "It's not strong, but it's there"; "okay, not the be all and end all, no". [Some] *women clearly felt that sex had always been more a husband's privilege than a pleasure of their own, and had never been much interested themselves. "I think it's more for a man than a woman"; "no, not me particularly, but to a man it is right." As one wife put it, "I think if you want to keep your husband, if he's interested in sex, well, you've got to be as well – I don't see any difference in the age you are." One was glad this phase was past: "I think it's a thing that you serve your time at, when you're younger, and then when you get older it doesn't appeal to you so much."*

Paul Thompson, Catherine Itzen, and Michele Abendstern *I Don't Feel Old* (1990)

And finally, the lament of Oliver Wendell Holmes Jnr while watching a pretty girl in his 87th year:

Oh, to be seventy again!

Sexual Fantasies

Love in action is a harsh and dreadful thing, as compared with love in dreams.

Fyodor Dostoevsky

Surveys suggest that sexual fantasy is almost universal in adult human beings, who use it to meet a variety of different needs. Most obviously, and perhaps most frequently, it serves a purpose for those with no sexual partner available, who wish to excite themselves in order to masturbate. Sexual fantasy of this kind is particularly prevalent amongst such groups as adolescents –

On an outing of our family association, I once cored an apple, saw to my astonishment (and with the aid of my obsession) what it looked like, and ran off into the woods to fall upon the orifice of the fruit, pretending that the cool and mealy hole was actually between the legs of that mythical being who always called me Big Boy when she pleaded for what no girl in all recorded history had ever had. 'Oh shove it in me, Big Boy,' cried the cored apple that I banged silly on that picnic. 'Big Boy, Big Boy, oh give me all you've got,' begged the empty milk bottle that I kept hidden in our storage bin in the basement, to drive wild after school with my vaselined upright. 'Come, Big Boy, come,' screamed the maddened piece of liver, that, in my own insanity, I bought one afternoon at a butcher shop and, believe it or not, violated behind a billboard on the way to a bar mitzvah lesson.

Philip Roth *Portnoy's Complaint* (1969)

and prisoners. This example concerns two political prisoners in the Soviet Union; one, Rubashov, has just established contact with his neighbour by tapping in code on the cell wall between them:

WHEN DID YOU LAST SLEEP WITH A WOMAN?
...Rubashov thought it over for a bit, then tapped:
THREE WEEKS AGO.
The answer came at once:
TELL ME ALL ABOUT IT.
...Rubashov racked his brain...He sighed resignedly and tapped with his pince-nez:
SNOWY BREASTS FITTING INTO CHAMPAGNE GLASSES...THIGHS LIKE A WILD MARE...
MORE – PLEASE, PLEASE

Arthur Koestler *Darkness at Noon* (1940)

However, men and women with physically and emotionally fulfilling sex lives appear just as prone to fantasize as those who are sex-starved. In these cases fantasy is often used to add excitement and variety to love making:

We are all immature, and have anxieties and aggressions. Coital play, like dreaming, is probably man's programmed way of dealing acceptably with these, just as children express their fears and aggressions in games...Bed is the place to play all the games you have ever wanted to play...

Dr Alex Comfort *The Joy of Sex* (1972)

Far from being a simple substitute for physical sex, fantasies are often enjoyed by one or both partners during the act itself:

She accepted her conjugal duties merely as a matter of unavoidable necessity. Her

only condition was that she should be in the upper position. In this position she obtained a sort of gratification, for she imagined his body to be that of a beloved woman in the lower position...
Female charms never attracted him. Coitus was only possible when aided by the thought of a beloved man.

Richard von Krafft-Ebing *Psychopathia Sexualis* (1886)

Many sexual fantasies present merely an exaggerated or simplified version of 'normal' sexual activity:

With barnyard studs, imagined or not, it's all about the visible turn-on of the prick, the incredible size of it more than anything. Imagine something that *big – which you first reacted to with such fascination, at least the first time you saw it, even if you almost immediately glanced away with embarrassment – imagine that penetrating you! How can a woman look at a prick that big and not imagine it going into her?*

Nancy Friday *My Secret Garden: Women's Sexual Fantasies* (1973)

The nude, like the prostitute, is an erotic commodity; her nakedness is valuable not for its marked individuality and subjective expression, but for its ability to feed male fantasies that erase woman's desiring subjectivity.

Charles Bernheimer in *Seduction and Theory* (ed. Diane Hunter; 1989)

Others are of a kind that could not easily be acted out in real life because this would be illegal, too demeaning, or would inflict damage on others:

Yes, I admit I am a libertine and in that area I have imagined everything that can be imagined. But I have absolutely not acted out everything that I imagined nor do I intend to. I am a libertine, but I am not a criminal or a murderer.

Marquis de Sade, in a letter to his wife (20 Feb. 1781)

"Wicked ways!" her husband replied coolly. "But don't you see, my dear, that I am working for my salvation by sleeping with my cousin? For she is a nun!"

Marquis de Sade *Tales and Fabliaux of the Eighteenth Century*, 'The Law of Talion' (1787)

Sometimes I thought of my father...for a father is disturbing! – and the things imagined! His knee, at times coaxing; his trousers whose fly my finger wanted to open – oh! no! – To have the thick dark cock of my father, whose hairy hand rocked me!

Arthur Rimbaud *Memories of the Simple-Minded Old Man* (1943)

I never dared to reveal my strange taste, but at least I got some pleasure from situations which pandered to the thought of it. To fall on my knees before a Masterful Mistress, to obey her commands, to have to beg for her forgiveness, have been to me the most delicate of pleasures, and the more like a spellbound lover I looked.

Jean-Jacques Rousseau *Confessions* (1782)

We were always so afraid to go in a taxi with him, recalled one anonymous old lady who in the 1950s bumped into a friend of Gerhardie's in the tea-shop of the British Museum. She would have been even more alarmed had she known of his private fantasy of sex in a taxi, specifically between the Marble Arch and Paddington Station. The crescendo *of ecstasy has to be timed and superintended to the progress of the drive – streets have to be watched. The climax falls in with the moment when the taxi pulls up. A porter opens the door and staggers back, unspeakably shocked. X cries out cheerfully: 'No, thank you, don't want a porter!'*

Dido Davies *William Gerhardie: A Biography* (1990)

The relationship between sexual fantasies and sexual behaviour is obviously far from simple. Many people derive intense excitement from imagining situations that they would find ridiculous or repellent in real life. Amongst the most familiar examples of this are the fantasies of being raped or otherwise overpowered enjoyed by many perfectly normal women:

A rape fantasy has nothing to do with having a couple of teeth knocked out. It's when Robert Redford won't take no for an answer.

Molly Haskell 'Rape Fantasy' *Ms* (1976)

Elements of violence, compulsion, or humiliation occur in the fantasy life of many apparently well-adjusted people:

...his boss steps into the room and orders the daydreamer at the point of his gun to copulate with his, the boss's, wife...One could doubt whether sexual intercourse under such conditions would be very pleasurable. The presence of the husband in the bedroom with a gun in his hand would almost certainly impair the mood of the lover.

Theodor Reik *Masochism in Modern Man* (1957)

I'm on one of those stirrup tables that gynecologists have when they spread your legs and look deep into you. But the table is in the middle of the ring, in Madison Square Garden, and it's mounted on a revolving platform. Thousands of men have paid fifty or a hundred dollars each for tickets, and the ushers are selling binoculars so they can get a better view.

Nancy Friday *My Secret Garden: Women's Sexual Fantasies* (1979)

It is not very uncommon to find intensely masochistic women who desire to be subjugated, beaten, and ill-treated before they can be fully erotically aroused: but it is rare to find women who actually want to beat or ill-treat men in order to obtain erotic satisfaction. Women in top-boots cracking whips are generally either creatures of the masochistic male's imagination or else prostitutes obliging their clients by trying to fulfil their fantasies.

Dr Anthony Storr *Sexual Deviation* (1964)

Many people find their sexual fantasies disturbing and have preferred to suppress or disown them:

Under the influence of a puritan shame of sex, the true subjective origins of our sexual dreams or day-time fantasies cannot be admitted. Therefore, theories of witchcraft and obscenity were invented.

Theodore Schroeder 'A Psychological Challenge to Prudery' *Nudist* (Mar. 1937)

It might be embarrassing to admit squarely that these edifying tales about valiant knights fighting perverse dragons who pant after lovely virgins and tender lads are actually transfigurations of sexual fantasies which pious persons cannot admit into the range of consciousness. But it is just as annoying to deny it.

André Guindon *The Sexual Language* (1976)

However, even if banished from one's waking life such material will often reemerge involuntarily in dreams:

I have known intimately a very learned man, whose name I shall omit for honour's sake, who, whenever in a school or elsewhere he sees a boy punished, unbreeched and beaten, and hears his cries, at once ejaculates semen copiously without any tension or erection of the penis but with such mental confusion that he could almost swoon, and the same thing happens to him frequently in sleep when he dreams of this subject.

Johann Matthias Nesterus, in a letter to a friend (24 Feb. 1677)

Girlish fantasies relating to rape often remain unconscious but evince their content in dreams, sometimes in symptoms, and often accompanying masturbating actions.

H. Deutsch *The Psychology of Women* (1944)

From his shelves he picked out a book about dreams and thumbed through...The setting afternoon sun lit up the room. "An emission during a dream indicates the sexual nature of the whole dream, however obscure and unlikely the contents are. Dreams culminating in emis-

sion may reveal the object of the dreamer's desire as well as his inner conflicts. An orgasm can not lie."

Ian McEwan *In Between the Sheets* (1978)

This quotation, probably from Freud, expresses the psychiatric view that sexual fantasies are not simply an indication of what turns one on but are, like dreams, an expression of some fear or anxiety dating back to one's early childhood or even infancy:

If hysterical subjects trace back their symptoms to traumas that are fictitious, then the new fact which emerges is precisely that they create such scenes in fantasy, *and this psychical reality requires to be taken into account alongside practical reality. This reflection was soon followed by the discovery that these fantasies were intended to cover up the autocratic activity of the first years of childhood, to embellish it and raise it to a higher plane. And now, from behind the fantasies, the whole range of a child's sexual life came to light.*

Sigmund Freud *On the History of the Psychoanalytic Movement* (1914)

The wishful fantasies revealed by analysis in night-dreams often turn out to be repetitions or modified versions of scenes from infancy; thus in some cases the façade of the dream directly reveals the dream's actual nucleus, distorted by an admixture of other material.

Sigmund Freud *On Dreams* (1901)

The contents of the clearly conscious fantasies of perverts (which in favourable circumstances can be transformed into manifest behaviour), of the delusional fears of paranoiacs (which are projected in a hostile sense on to other people), and of the unconscious fantasies of hysterics (which psychoanalysis reveals behind their symptoms) – all these coincide with one another even down to their details.

Sigmund Freud *Three Essays on the Theory of Sexuality* (1905)

Psychiatrists have been able to offer explanations for even the most extreme fantasies:

Even the phantasy scene in which a man has a woman urinate into his mouth obtains a meaning through revocation of the reversal of the phantasy. We know that babies wet only people they love, as if the wetting with urine were a gift of love.

Theodor Reik *Masochism in Modern Man* (1957)

Others, however, remain incomprehensible:

Sex experts are puzzling over the strange case of 'George' who fell in love with an Austin Metro and developed a close erotic relationship with the machine...George, 20, came from a family who belonged to a strict religious sect. He was a shy student with little social life and no sexual involvement with women because this would have invoked disapproval from his parents. But his life changed when the family acquired an Austin Metro car...George, confused but happy, began to masturbate inside the car, or crouching down behind it next to the exhaust pipe. He was excited by the exhaust pipe especially if the engine was running and it was emitting fumes.

Independent (7 Dec. 1992)

Sexual fantasy has been celebrated as a creative and life-enhancing activity – and attacked as immoral and dangerous:

Imagination is pleasure's spur...It is only by enlarging the scope of one's tastes and one's fantasies, by sacrificing everything to pleasure, that that unfortunate individual called man, thrown despite himself into this sad world, can succeed in gathering a few roses among life's thorns.

Marquis de Sade *Philosophy in the Bedroom* (1795)

While we have sex in the mind, we truly have none in the body.

D. H. Lawrence 'Leave Sex Alone' (1929)

In neither case can it be considered insignificant:

> *I do not see how fantasy can be left out of one's calculations about human sexual behaviour; it is no secret that fantasy, in the form of daydreams, is present consciously in much of sexual activity…*
> *Just as every human group has its myth, perhaps for every person there is* the *sexual fantasy. In it is summarized one's sexual life history – the development of his or her erotism and of masculinity or femininity…*
> *On hearing of a person without sexual fantasy, we suspect that an inhibition is in force.*

Robert J. Stoller *Perversion* (1976)

> *How many times a day do men think, perhaps only momentarily, of the shape and attributes of human flesh? How many tiny interstices are thus filled? How often and how vehemently do we look forward to going to bed – but not to sleep?…I can only confess that, judging from my own experience and having no reason to think that others are different from me, the thought or memory of that activity of our bodies, which is only openly acknowledged between lovers…and which reaches its fulfilment in physical union and orgasm, does in fact occupy, in greater or lesser degree, very many of the interstices of our waking lives and thus colour and inform and perfect or, it may be, mar our doings.*

Eric Gill *Autobiography* (1940)

> *Facing our sexual fantasies honestly would tell us a lot about ourselves.*

André Guindon *The Sexual Language* (1976)

And finally, the ultimate in sexual fantasies:

> *If you are having trouble with your love life, do not despair. Help may be at hand. Scientists in the United States are working to replace sexual intercourse between human beings with 'inter-facing' between humans and computers. They call the new technology 'cybersex'…potentially it could be better than the real thing because it could become the realisation of our fantasies…*
> *Lisa Palac, the editor of a trendy new San Francisco-based quarterly called* Future Sex, *believes that computers are bound to impinge more and more on our sex lives.*

James Bone *The Times* (11 Feb. 1993)

Sexually Transmitted Diseases

Life is a sexually transmitted disease.

Graffito in London Underground, quoted by D. J. Enright in the *Faber Book of Fevers and Frets* (1984)

The Gate that gave life to you, can also be the Gate leading to your death.

Chin-p'ing Mei *Wang-Chieh* (c. 1640)

The famous phrase in Genesis used after the Fall – 'it shall bruise thy head and thou shalt bruise his heel' – seems to have a phallic meaning. 'Head' and 'heel' are euphemisms for the sexual organs, and the real curse of Eden was being smitten by the 'love-disease' – syphilis.

H. Cutner *A Short History of Sex Worship* (1940)

Sexually transmitted diseases (STDs) are clearly not new. If Mr Cutner is to be believed, the authors of Genesis were well aware of them. According to one popular theory, syphilis was brought to Europe by Columbus's sailors on their return from the New World.

The introduction of syphilis into Europe by the crew of Columbus's expeditions was perhaps the greatest godsend to the older conception of sexual morality which history could possibly have provided. Venereal disease had been known to the Greeks, but it had not constituted a risk severe enough to restrict the freedom of the Hellenistic sexual tradition. Now at a single blow, that freedom was destroyed. For the first time the hierarchical conception of the sinfulness of sexuality received a physical and inescapable sanction.

Alex Comfort *Sexual Behaviour in Society* (1950)

And when his men pulled out again
And reckoned all their score up,
They'd caught a pox from every box
That syphilised all Europe.

Anon. 'Christopher Columbo' (19th century)

More recent research suggests that in the Middle Ages many supposed cases of 'leprosy' were in fact tertiary syphilis. Here, for instance, a medieval Welsh poet describes the effects of having sex with a girl who turns out to be a 'leper':

When I sat up from off the girl with snow coloured features I had too sudden a shock, deformed genitals and a scorched chisel and a scrotum which was far from well.

Ieuan Gethin 'A Misadventure' (mid 15th century)

Whatever the case, descriptions of the unsavoury consequences of STDs became increasingly common in European literature from the late 15th century onwards:

White pustules and fissures and corruptions that are formed on the penis and next to the prepuce, for having lived carnally with a woman who is dirty or poisonous, retained and trapped between the prepuce and the skin of the penis, and when it cannot be expelled or exhaled it grows and multiplies in the place and when at the beginning one ignores it, it multiplies again and corrupts the skin and blackens it and corrodes it with the substance of the penis which is never afterwards cured. With such corruption there came fevers and a flux of blood and very frequently death.

Guillaume de Salicet *La Cirurgie de Maistre Guillaume de Salicet* (1492)

Worse part of me, and henceforth hated most,
Through all the town a common fucking post,
On whom each whore relieves her tingling cunt
As hogs on gates do rub themselves and grunt,
Mayst thou to ravenous chancres be a prey,
Or in consuming weepings waste away;
May strangury and stone thy days attend;
Mayst thou ne'er piss, who dids't refuse to spend
When all my joys did on false thee depend.

John Wilmot, Earl of Rochester 'The Imperfect Enjoyment' (1680)

My prick is excessively inflamed,
I'll be damned if its head is smaller than a pole!
My scrotum has been blighted
Unhappy tribulation, grievous deformation.
Because of wantonness there is in my trousers,
Yes, I've a testicle bigger than a goose's body.

Dafydd Llwyd of Mathafarn 'The Poet's Revenge' (16th century)

Scarce, three-days past, bewails the dear-bought Bliss,
For now, tormented save with scalding heat
Of Urine, dread forerunners of a Clap!
With eye repentent, he surveys his shirt
Diversify'd with Spots of yellow Hue,
Sad symptom of ten thousand Woes to come!

The Reverend Mr Kennet 'Armour' (1741)

The greatest Evil that attends this Vice [whoring], *or could befal Mankind, is the Propagation of that infectious Disease call'd the* French Pox, *which in two Centuries has made such incredible Havock all over* Europe*...Men give it to their Wives, Women to their Husbands, or perhaps their Children; they to their Nurses, and the Nurses again to other Children; so that no Age, Sex, or Condition, can be entirely free from the Infection.*

Anon., from *Satan's Harvest Home, or The Present State of Whorecraft, Adultery, Fornication, Procuring, Pimping, Sodomy, And the Game at Flatts, And other Satanic Works, daily propagated in this good Protestant Kingdom* (18th century)

It was, and still is, a particular menace to armies:

In the sixteenth century, virulent and progressive, it [syphilis] *spread through opposing forces and often brought military operations to a halt.*

C. F. Brockington MD *Short History of Public Health* (1966)

During the Boer War as many as half the British troops suffered from venereal disease and in the First World War the proportion reached 20% in some military troops. This risk associated with combatant troops was identified again during the Second World War and a 1973 study of 400 Australian soldiers serving in Vietnam showed an STD incidence of 27%.

R. G. Masterton and P. W. Strike *STDs in a British Military Force in Peacetime Europe* (1988)

A consignment of condoms is being sent to Cambodia for UN peacekeeping soldiers. There have been 1251 cases of sexually transmitted diseases among UN forces.

The Times (19 Nov. 1992)

Soldiers on active service, in considerable numbers, so far from avoiding infection, welcomed it. In giving evidence before the Special Committee on Venereal Disease, appointed by the Birth Rate Commission, Miss Etti A. Roat (Hon Secretary, New Zealand Volunteer Sisters) stated it to be a fact that prostitutes suffering from venereal disease could command a higher fee than those free from disease...In her evidence Miss Roat said: "Some men wanted to get diseased during the war. They would sell the discharge to other men and they would infect their genital organs with it."

George Ryley Scott *A History of Prostitution* (1936)

But it is not only the soldiers themselves who suffer, as a World War I general pointed out:

The gonococcus is a germ of terrible social malignancy, while the spirochete of syphilis, transcending the imagination of Ezekiel, visits upon the innocent mother and children the iniquity of the father.

Sir William Osler (1915)

This has, of course, always been the case:

If she catch a clap, she divides it so equally between the master and the serving-man, as if she had cut out the getting of it by a thread.

Sir Thomas Overbury *A Chamber-Maid* (early 17th century)

He, perhaps, gives the disease to his housekeeper; she stoops as low to the horse's heels, and transmits it to the groom; he conveys it from the stable to the laundry, and from thence it goes back with the clean linen to their master. So that the pox in his family, like the blood in his veins, is in perpetual circulation.

Robert Gould *The Rival Sisters, or The Violence of Love* (late 17th century)

'nlike many diseases, STDs can be avoided mpletely. Just as food poisoning only afflicts ose who eat, so, with very rare exceptions, TDs are only caught by those who are sexually tive. There are occasional cases of congenital philis, in which the disease passes from an fected mother to her unborn child. In spite of e well-known rhyme:

It's no use standing on the seat,
A spirochaete can jump five feet.

TDs cannot be contracted from lavatory seats:

Contrary to popular rumour [gonorrhoea] *cannot be acquired by contact with an object such as a contaminated towel or a toilet seat.*

Peter Saunders *Womanwise, Every Woman's Guide to Gynaecology* (1980)

If one is not willing to be totally abstinent, the chances of infection can be reduced by being very selective in one's choice of sexual partners and by taking simple precautions:

Swear solemn with drawn sword not to be with women sine condom nisi Swiss lass.

James Boswell *Diary* (1764)

Of Allied troops who visited Paris on leave, but without prophylaxis, in the summer of 1917, 20 per cent contracted venereal disease, but in the five months from November 1917, when prophylaxis kits were provided, this figure fell to 3 per cent.

Richard Davenport-Hines *Sex, Death and Punishment* (1990)

Thinking about STDs has always been bedevilled by issues of sexual morality:

Sexually transmitted diseases have been wrapped so long in moral reasoning that dispassionate analyses of truly effective means of control have often been pushed aside in the past...the control of sexually transmitted diseases has very often been confused with the control of sexuality itself, a conceptualization which overlooks more pragmatic means of prophylaxis, and has led to the unintentional increase of the problem.

Barry D. Adam *The Rise of a Gay and Lesbian Movement* (1987)

The British Medical Association produced a report on 'Venereal Disease and Young People' in 1964 which hysterically suggested a vast increase in promiscuity among the young, and throughout the 1960s and 1970s the venereal disease figures were treated as an index of immorality, or in the vivid phrase of a leading expert on the subject, were part of a syndrome of illegitimacy, violence, drug tak-

ing and homosexuality as evidence of 'social pathology'.

Jeffrey Weeks *Sex, Politics and Society* (1981)

Such attitudes have also influenced the treatment of sufferers:

In 1505 the French government passed a decree providing for the building of a hospital for persons attacked by the 'large pox' but through the opposition of the clergy it was not until some thirty years later that provision was actually made for the treatment, along with sufferers from other diseases, of those afflicted with syphilis...the treatment was of the crudest, and, because of the moral obloquy attached to the infection, every patient suffering from a venereal disease was soundly whipped both on entering and on leaving the establishment.

George Ryley Scott *A History of Prostitution* (1936)

Four hundred years later, on the other side of the Channel, the change from Christian indignation to secular parsimony meant only that the whipping was omitted:

Just before the First World War, the House of Commons voted that £50,000 be spent on laboratories to diagnose and treat venereal diseases, the Treasury intervened to stop this sum being spent, and a figure of £25,000 was substituted.

Richard Davenport-Hines *Sex, Death and Punishment* (1990)

By the end of the Second World War, the main bacterial STDs – gonorrhoea and syphilis – had largely succumbed to treatment (if caught early enough) by sulphonamides and antibiotics. Together with the advent of the Pill, this set the scene for the swinging sixties. By the end of the 1970s however, an age-old viral STD staged an unnerving comeback – genital herpes:

It was the disease on everybody's lips (and other parts of their anatomy). Billy Graham thought it God's judgment on an immoral society. Thousands of people hit by it shunned the opposite sex for fear of passing it on. Women were afraid it caused cancer and still-births. Today herpes is still with us but few are worried by it.

Jeremy Laurence *The Times* (10 June 1993)

As fears about cancer proved to be unfounded and the drug acyclovir almost always cures it, herpes is now regarded more as an inconvenience than a danger. Science had succeeded, it appeared, in removing one of the last obstacles to promiscuity (see PROMISCUITY). There are, however, no loopholes in either God's law or Sod's law (depending on your beliefs). In 1981 the Aids syndrome was identified amongst members of the gay community in Los Angeles:

The belief that was handed to me was that sex was liberating and more sex was more liberating.

Aids Patient *Newsweek* (8 Aug. 1983)

If AIDS is not an act of God with consequences just as frightful as fire and brimstone, then just what the hell is it?

Headline *New York Post* (24 May 1983)

AIDS is the price we pay for the 'benefits' of the permissive society which, helped by the pill, liberal legislation and more 'enlightened' attitudes, has demolished the last defences of sexual restraint and self-discipline, leading to a collapse of nature's self-defence against degeneracy.

Chief Rabbi Sir Immanuel Jakobovits *The Times* (27 Dec. 1986)

The tone for religious condemnation in relation to AIDS was set by an announcement issued in December 1986 by the former Nonconformist now Catholic convert, Chief Constable of Greater Manchester James Anderton. God, he informed us, had, as happened on a previous occasion with Moses, spoken privately to him. This time there was no burning bush, but otherwise the scenario was similar to that described in Exodus 3. God told the Chief Constable, as He had earlier told Moses, that He had seen the affliction of His people and heard their cry, and knew their sorrows. Nevertheless it had to be pointed out that they were, as the Chief Constable put it (acting as God's trumpet), swirling in a cesspit of their own making.

Francis Bennion *The Sex Code* (1991)

Insidiously, almost imperceptibly, the perverts have got the heterosexual majority with their backs against the wall...The woofters have had a dreadful plague visited upon them, which we call AIDS...Since the perverts offend the laws of God and nature, is it fanciful to suggest that one or both is striking back?

Ray Mills 'The Angry Voice' *The Star* (9 Sept. 1986)

The image of an enraged God striking down promiscuous homosexuals proved irresistible to many religious spokesmen – and even to some members of the gay community:

The psychological impact of AIDS on the gay community is tremendous...Some people are saying 'maybe we are wrong, maybe this is a punishment'.

Richard Failla *Newsweek* (18 Aug. 1983)

Amidst this torrent of condemnation one Christian voice expressed compassion in referring to Aids sufferers:

Each one of them is Jesus in a distressing disguise.

Mother Theresa (1980s)

The President of the USA, in a speech, called for calm:

America faces a disease that is fatal and spreading. This calls for urgency, not panic. This calls for compassion, not blame. This calls for understanding, not ignorance.

Ronald Reagan (June 1987)

The British junior health minister, in a speech, was more specific and more practical:

My message to the businessmen of this country when they go abroad on business is that there is one thing above all they can take with them to stop them catching AIDS, and that is the wife...

Good Christian people who would not dream of misbehaving will not catch AIDS.

Edwina Currie *Guardian* (13 Feb. 1987)

The General Medical Council made a statement:

It is unethical for a registered medical practitioner to refuse treatment or investigation for which there are appropriate facilities on the ground that the patient suffers or may suffer from a condition which could expose the doctor to personal risk. It is equally unethical for a doctor to withhold treatment from any patient on the basis of a moral judgment that the patient's activities or lifestyle might have contributed to the condition for which treatment was sought. Unethical behaviour of this kind may raise a question of serious professional misconduct.

(May 1987)

A British royal, in a speech, was unusually philosophical:

It could be said that the AIDS pandemic is a classic 'own goal' scored by the human race on itself, a self-inflicted wound that only serves to remind homo sapiens *of his fallibility.*

There is a saying, which was often quoted at me in my youth...which is that prevention is better than cure. When there is no cure, prevention is the only answer.

The Princess Royal, in a speech to the World Summit of Ministers of Health on Programmes for Aids Prevention (Jan. 1988)

The Pope, in several proclamations, called for restraint and reiterated the Church's ban on the use of contraceptives. These seem to be fair comments:

The AIDS pandemic has presented the Catholic Church with another moral problem. Here, once again, it is speared on the horns of a dilemma between the ideal and reality. Deep in the Catholic heart is the conviction that if the world had listened to it in the first place, AIDS would not exist. The best way to avoid getting the disease is to abstain from sexual intercourse, in the best Catholic fashion.

Kate Saunders and Peter Stanford *Catholics and Sex* (1992)

Around the globe the Church's ban on artificial contraception is a virulent force for ignorance, repression and suffering...By their efforts they are hampering attempts to control soaring population growth. By their opposition to condoms, they are contributing to the spread of AIDS.

Brenda Maddox *The Pope and Contraception* (1991)

Despite the rising tide of concern, there were some who pretended that nothing had changed:

The present herpes and AIDS crises has about as little to do with sex values and ethics as a spate of air crashes have to do with flying.

Raymond J. Lawrence Jr *The Poisoning of Eros* (1989)

A whole new generation is sick of hearing of the dangers of Aids and think they are exaggerated.

J. Money, professor of medical psychology and paediatrics

Few people have changed their behaviour because of Aids.

Dr June Reinisch, director of the Kinsey Institute, Indiana University.

Sex is on the up. All this hooplah about Aids is rubbish. People I know rarely wear condoms. If it was true that Aids was a threat, swingers would be dropping like flies. There has not been one case of Aids from swinging.

Robert McGinley *Sunday Times* (14 June 1992)

It affects homosexual men, drug users, Haitians and haemophiliacs. Thank goodness it hasn't spread to human beings yet.

Caption to cartoon about public reaction to AIDS (1984)

In spite of the head-in-the-sand brigade, European and US governments began to address the problems, spending serious money on advertising campaigns:

Don't die of ignorance.

Every time you sleep with a boy you sleep with all his old girlfriends.

UK government-sponsored AIDS advertisements (1987)

It was now becoming clear to all but the wilfully blind that Aids was not a problem exclusive to homosexuals:

One of the most striking features of the AIDS crisis is that, unlike most illnesses, from the first its chief victims were chiefly blamed for causing the disease, whether because of their social attitudes or sexual practices. And as most people suffering from the disease in Western countries were male homosexuals...the term "gay plague" became the common description of it in the more scabrous parts of the media. In fact it was clear from the beginning that other groups of people were prone to the disease.

Jeffrey Weeks *Sexuality* (1986)

A homosexual man practising safe sex is less likely to be exposed to the AIDS virus than a heterosexual man who is not practising safe sex. It is the nature of the sexual activity that is important, not the sexual orientation.

Trevor Pearcy, of the Terence Higgins Trust, in a letter to *The Times* (1986

We must conquer AIDS before it affects the heterosexual population...the general population. We have a very strong public interest in stopping AIDS before it spreads outside the risk groups, before it becomes an overwhelming problem.

Margaret Heckler, director of the Departmer of Health and Human Services (15 April 1985

To this end, massive campaigns were commis sioned to convert dangerous casual sex into sa casual sex. The instrument chosen to effect this conversion was the condom:

We hope people will learn to love condoms. In the past people like Casanova had lots of fun with their condoms.

David Cox, TV producer (March 1987)

The condom is the third most popular method of contraception (16 per cent) after sterilisation (25 per cent) and the Pill (23 per cent of women), and about two million British women used condoms as their main method of contraception in 1991.

Aids hasn't ruined sex; it has made us more responsible. I would have hated to have lots of one-night stands, and Aids gives girls the perfect excuse to say no. I would ask a new partner about his background, but how can you know if they have Aids? It is a risk you have to take. You can't worry too much, otherwise you would never have any fun...

I have had two Aids tests and I have my own gynaecologist. Most of my friends have regular Aids tests, it's almost like a dental check-up. We are into safe sex not less sex. I had a Scottish nanny who died of Aids – it does frighten me...

'Is This the Age of the Condom' *The Times* (27 Oct. 1992)

These are fantasies I have dreamed up. Like most human beings, when I let my mind go, I rarely think of condoms. My fantasies take place in a perfect world, a place without Aids. Unfortunately, the world is not perfect and I know that condoms are not only necessary but mandatory.

Madonna *Sex* (1992)

See also CONTRACEPTION

The epidemic has raised a number of new legal issues:

In different parts of the world it has become an offence for a person known to have the [AIDS] *virus to have unsafe sex with someone who hasn't.*

Richie J. McMullen *Male Rape* (1990)

An HIV-infected man [in Portland, Oregon, USA] *was convicted of attempted murder for having unprotected sex with a 17-year old girl, knowing he could transmit the virus.*

Independent (27 Nov. 1992)

Kenneth Clarke, the Home Secretary, yesterday ruled out legislation to make it a criminal offence to transmit knowingly the HIV virus.

Independent (16 Dec. 1992)

Not all suggestions for halting the spread of the disease have been considered acceptable:

Perhaps eventually, if we ever get serious about controlling AIDS before we are inundated, persons who test (and are confirmed) positive might even have 'AIDS' tattooed just above their pubis.

Dr Seth Haber *US Medical Journal* (Aug. 1987)

One small benefit of the disease has been the way in which it has compelled open public discussion of many previously taboo subjects:

The epidemic is accomplishing what one million teenage pregnancies couldn't...get us talking about sex. People who were tongue-tied realise that they must *address something that is lethal.*

Marian Wright Edelman *New York Times* (14 Mar. 1987)

With the onset of HIV disease and the worry about casual sex, more emphasis is being placed on thinking up ways of making masturbation more interesting as a regular form of sexual behaviour. Mutual masturbation, where two or more men masturbate each other, is obviously thought of as safer sex.

John Green and Alana McCreaner *Counselling in HIV Infection and AIDS* (1989)

Although it is recognised by gay men that oral sex, with ejaculation into the partner's mouth, is not as unsafe as anal counterpart, there is a fear that HIV or the hepatitis B virus might enter the body through cuts in the gums. Therefore, while sucking is still popular, most men would not allow their partners to come into their mouth.

John Green and Alana McCreaner *Counselling in HIV Infection and AIDS* (1989)

Once HIV had become established in the gay male community it was quickly recognized that prostitutes, both male and female, could be a vector for carrying it into the heterosexual majority, especially via bisexual men:

Sexually transmitted diseases are more frequently found among female prostitutes who are street-walkers than among other women who have unprotected coitus with large numbers of men.

J. E. Exner et al. *Some Psychological Characteristics of Prostitutes* (1977)

The clientele of male prostitutes may include a relatively high number of bisexual men who want to hide their homosexuality, and in this way male prostitution could be a bridge for the spread of STDs and HIV into the general population.

R. A. Coutinbo et al. *Role of Male Prostitutes in Spread of STDs and HIV* (1988)

Prostitutes are considered a reservoir for transmission of certain sexually transmitted diseases. However a variety of studies suggest that human immunodeficiency virus (HIV) infection in prostitutes follows a different pattern than that for STDs: HIV infection in non-drug using prostitutes tends to be low or absent, implying that sexual activity alone does not place them at high risk, while prostitutes who use intravenous drugs are far more likely to be infected with HIV.

M. J. Rosenberg and J. M. Weiner *Prostitutes and AIDS: a Health Department Priority* (1988)

Prostitution, because of its ubiquity and its scale, is a potential 'flash point' from which HIV infection could spread more generally than it appears *to have done so far.*

Martin A. Plant *AIDS, Drugs and Prostitution* (1990)

AIDS is unlikely to stop boy prostitution any more than syphilis did. Indeed...there will be an increased demand for younger, unspoilt boys.

Richie J. McMullen *Male Rape* (1990)

It is interesting and anomalous that prostitutes are not as widely affected as expected (see PROSTITUTION). This has led to research on the relationship between tissue type and HIV infection:

Dr Francis Plummer of Manitoba University told an Aids conference yesterday that some prostitutes in Nairobi never seemed to become HIV-positive in spite of working in a country where at least 10 per cent of their clients were infected. Some of the women he had studied had remained immune for eight years – "which is extremely unlikely, given what we know about HIV transmission".

The Times (9 June 1993)

It may be that eventually some better understanding of the way the disease works will emerge from these studies. In the meantime it is equally interesting and anomalous that Aids in the UK has not spread as rapidly among heterosexuals as at first expected:

We [in Britain] *have one of the lowest rates of heterosexually acquired Aids and of that among injecting drug users in the European Community...In each of the last two years the recorded number of HIV positive tests among homosexuals has fallen by about 10 per cent.*

The Times (30 Nov. 1992)

Elsewhere the story is different — in Africa and the Caribbean, for instance:

HIV transmission is predominantly heterosexual. Equal numbers of men and women are infected.

Roger Gaitley and Philip Seed *HIV and AIDS* (1989)

Of an estimated 27,000 HIV positive people in England and Wales (*The Times* 9 June 1993), about 15,000 are homosexual or bisexual males, 4500 are injecting drug users, 1500 have been infected by blood products, and 6300 people have been infected by heterosexual intercourse. None are lesbians:

If we accept the notion…that AIDS represents God's punishment to erring homosexuals, then it stands to reason that lesbians – virtually untouched by AIDS or sexually transmitted diseases – must be God's chosen people.

Letter, *Newsweek* (1980s)

Sexual Nonsense

Probably more demonstrable – and dangerous – nonsense has been written about sex than about any other subject. This is not really surprising. The atmosphere of secrecy and taboo that surrounded the subject until relatively recently provided a fertile breeding ground for every kind of superstition. Moreover, such are the fears and perplexities aroused by the subject even today that anyone who offers 'authoritative' guidance is guaranteed a hearing. There has never been a shortage of experts in this field – from the sages and wise women of ancient times to the sexologists of today. Experts are notorious for their occasional follies, medical people being no exception:

There are special conditions, both physical and moral, which dispose to insanity; in women, menstruation with its irregularities, childbirth, and the change of life are potent influences.

T. C. Allbutt *A System of Medicine* (1899)

Married people often appear to think that connection may be repeated just as regularly and almost as often as their meals. Till they are told of the danger, the idea never enters their heads that they may have been guilty of great and almost criminal excess.

Dr William Acton *The Functions and Disorders of the Re-productive Organs* (1857)

In the 20th century, the assertions of psychoanalysts have found a wide acceptance, despite their sometimes surreal quality:

Pressing out the contents of the blackhead is clearly to him a substitution for masturbation. The cavity which then appears owing to his fault is the female genital.

Sigmund Freud *The Unconscious* (1915)

Infantile fixation of the libido on the father – the typical choice of object; anal auto-eroticism. The position she has chosen can be broken down into its components, for it seems to have still other factors added to it. Which factors? It must be possible, by the symptoms and even by the character, to recognize anal excitation as a motivation. Such people often show typical combinations of character traits. They are extremely neat, stingy and obstinate, traits which are in a manner of speaking sublimations of anal eroticism.

Sigmund Freud, in a letter to Carl Jung about a female patient who was fascinated by her own faeces (17 Oct. 1906)

It has also been explained to me why a chimney sweep is regarded as a good omen: chimney sweeping is an action symbolic of coitus, something Breuer certainly never dreamed of. All watch charms – pig, ladder, shoe, chimney sweep, etc. – are sexual consolations.

Sigmund Freud, in a letter to Carl Jung (21 Nov. 1909)

The psychoanalytic interpretation of transvestism runs as follows: The homosexual man replaces his love for his mother by an identification with her: the fetishist refuses to acknowledge that a woman has no penis. The male transvestite assumes both attitudes simultaneously. He fantasies that the woman possesses a penis, and thus overcomes his castration anxiety, and identifies himself with this phallic woman.

Dr Anthony Storr *Sexual Deviation* (1964)

Not one single neurotic individual possesses orgiastic potency.

Wilhelm Reich *Function of the Orgasm* (1942)

In the case of modern sexologists, the element of nonsense may have less to do with what is said than with the impenetrable way in which it is expressed:

Understandably, the maximum physiologic intensity of orgasmic response subjectively reported or objectively recorded has been achieved by self-regulated mechanical or auto-manipulative techniques...the lowest intensity of target-organ response was achieved during coition.

William Masters and Virginia Johnson *Human Sexual Response* (1966)

If the author had said that 'wanking gives the best orgasms' he might have been a more successful communicator.

Other contemporary pundits have distinctly eccentric views:

I think that testosterone is a rare poison.

Germaine Greer, in a Clive Anderson TV interview (19 June 1992)

Lesbian is a label invented by the man to throw at any woman who dares to be his equal, who dares to challenge his prerogatives...who dares to assert the primacy of her own needs.

Radicalesbians (a political activist group) *The Woman-Identified Woman (1970s)*

People who have a low self-esteem...have a tendency to cling to their own sex because it is less frightening.

Clara Thompson 'Changing Concepts of Homosexuality in Psychoanalysis' in *A Study of Interpersonal Relations, New Contributions to Psychiatry* (1949)

Our understanding of sexism is premised on the idea that in a free society everyone will be gay.

Allen Young *Out of the Closets: Voices of Gay Liberation* (1972)

Sex without class-consciousness cannot give satisfaction even if it is repeated until infinity.

Aldo Brandirali, Secretary-General of the Italian Marxist-Leninist Party (1973)

Sex is one of the nine reasons for reincarnation...The other eight are unimportant.

Henry Miller *Big Sur and the Oranges of Hieronymus Bosch* (1958)

Her parthenogenic birth from Adam's body makes Eve his daughter, so that the Judeo-Christian tradition rests on a primal father-daughter incest motif.

Naomi Goodman *Eve, Child bride of Adam* (1974)

I would not allow one of my babies to be adopted by a couple who practice contraception. People who use contraceptives do not understand the meaning of love.

Mother Teresa, in a radio interview during a visit to England (1983)

Some find it surprising that those who worship Jesus Christ, for whom love was the essence of life, should take such a negative view of its physical expression:

To be carnally minded is death.

Bible: Romans 8:6

You can no more dwell on sexual thoughts during sleep without suffering moral damage than you can hold on to burning coals without charring your flesh.

St Caesarius of Arles (5th century)

Let him who puts semen in the mouth do penance for seven years, for this is the worst evil.

Theodore of Tarsus (7th century)

All witchcraft comes from carnal lust which in women is insatiable.

Johann Sprenger and Heinrich Kraemer *Malleus Maleficarum* (1489)

More often than not it is ignorance that has led mankind into absurdity. If a mechanism is not understood, there will always be an expert to provide a spurious explanation:

The ancients say that if a woman hangs about her neck the finger and the anus of a dead foetus, she will not conceive while they are there.

It is also said that if one cuts off the foot of the female weasel, leaving her still alive, and if one puts this foot about the neck of a woman, she will not conceive while she wears it; and that if she takes it off she will become pregnant. If one takes the two testicles of a weasel and wraps them up, binding them to the thigh of a woman who wears also a weasel bone on her person, she will no longer conceive.

The Admirable Secrets of Albert the Great (16th century)

If the forehead of the mother-to-be is heavily freckled, the child she is carrying is a boy.

Mesopotamian papyrus (c. 2000 BC)

Many pronouncements of the ancient Greek philosophers fall into this category:

A kinswoman of mine owned a very valuable danseuse, whom she employed as a prostitute. It was important that this girl should not become pregnant and thereby lose her value. Now this girl had heard...that when a woman is going to conceive, the seed remains inside her and does not fall out...One day she noticed that the seed had not come out...When I heard it, I told her to jump up and down, touching her buttocks with her heels at each leap. After she had done this no more than seven times, there was a noise, the seed fell out upon the ground...

Hippocrates *The Nature of the Child* (5th century BC)

If in the act of copulation, the woman earnestly looks on the man, and fixes her mind on him, the child will resemble the father. Nay, if the woman, even in unlawful copulation, fix her mind upon her husband, the child will resemble him though he did not beget it.

Aristotle *The Nicomachean Ethics* (4th century BC)

Similarly with the Romans:

If a woman's loins are rubbed with blood taken from the ticks on a wild black bull she would be inspired with aversion to sexual intercourse.

Pliny the Elder *Natural History* (77 AD)

The kidneys are exciters of sexual desire...for the veins which empty into the testicles...pass directly through the kidneys, deriving hence a certain pungency provocative of lust.

Galen *De Usu Partium* (2nd century)

The Chinese, too, have left us with their share of absurdities:

The Yellow Emperor learned the Art of the Bedchamber from the Dark Girl. It consists of suppressing emissions, absorbing the woman's fluid, and making the semen return to strengthen the brain, thereby to obtain longevity.

Dien Jang *Chang-hua-fu* (c. 200)

All debility of man must be attributed to faulty exercise of the sexual act.

Su-nü-ching *Secrets of the Bedchamber* (c. 600)

If a man can copulate with 93 women and still contain himself, he will attain immortality.

Sun-Szu-Mo *Priceless Recipes* (7th century)

The Chinese had some particularly imaginative ideas about aphrodisiacs:

In the pastures of the Tartars wild horses often copulate with dragons. Drops of the semen will fall down and enter the earth, and put forth shoots resembling bamboo sprouts, of pointed shape...much like a penis. Some people say that lewd country women insert these things into their vagina; as soon as they meet the yin-essence they will suddenly swell and grow longer. The local people then dig these things out, wash them, peel them, and cut them into slices. After these slices have been dried they make excellent aphrodisiacs.

T'ao Tsung-i *Cho-kêng-lu* (c. 1360

The Burmese Bell is said to contain the semen of the bird P'eng. This bird is of extreme lasciviousness...If it meets a Burmese woman, the bird will want to have intercourse. So the aborigines make a puppet of straw, clothe it in women's clothes, and stick hairneedles and flowers in its head. The bird will then copulate with the dummy, and leave its sperm on it. The people gather this sperm and enclose it in a double golden pellet of the size of a small pea. If a man inserts this pellet in his member and then has intercourse with a woman, he will find his potency greatly increased.

T'an Chien *Tsao-lin-tsa-tsu* (c. 1400)

This subject has inspired a rich vein of fantasy in other cultures, too:

If he ejaculates little semen, then eats coconut, then a man has a great amount of semen. The semen is there in the buttocks.

Tikopian elder, quoted by Raymond Firth in *We the Tikopia* (1936)

The Greeks believed that the liver was the source of all generative power, and a recognition of the aphrodisiac potency of animal liver has persisted to the present day in parts of Europe. The idea that eating the generative organs of the obviously more potent beasts such as the stag, bull or stallion as a means of transferring that animal's characteristics to the consumer has been practised in most societies since prehistory.

Peter V. Taberner *Aphrodisiacs: The Science and the Myth* (1985)

Girls have been known to go to a graveyard at night, exhume a corpse that had been nine days buried, and tear down a strip of the skin from head to foot; this they manage to tie round the leg or arm of the man they love while he sleeps, taking care to remove it before his awaking. And so long as the girl keeps this strip of skin in her possession, secretly hidden from all eyes, so long will she retain the man's love.

Lady Wilde *Ancient Cures, Charms, and Usages of Ireland* (1890)

See also APHRODISIACS

From every corner of the earth, from every period, pours this torrent of spurious information about fertility and other sexual matters:

Water which has been used for the washing of a dead person is secretly given to a woman in order to make her infertile.

Edward A. Westermarck *Ritual and Belief in Morocco* (1926)

In the town of Qua, near old Calabar, there used to grow a palm tree, which used to ensure conception to any barren woman who ate a nut from its branches.

Sir James Frazer *The Golden Bough* (1913)

Whosoever shall lie in sexual intercourse with a woman who has an issue of blood; either out of the ordinary course or at the usual period, does no better deed than if he should burn the corpse of his own son, born of his own body, and killed by a spear, and drop its fat into the fire.

Fargard, Zoroastrian text (c. 10th century)

The man who often penetrates from behind risks having born to him from these women sons who are effeminate or dainty, especially if the woman requests it.

Yahyâ ibn Māsawaih *Aphorisms of the Nestorian Doctor* (11th century)

They say that Teiresias saw two snakes mating on Cithaeron and that, when he killed the female, he was changed into a woman, and again, when he killed the male, took again his own nature. This same Teiresias was chosen by Zeus and Hera to decide the question whether the male or the female has most pleasure in intercourse. And he said: "Of ten parts a man enjoys one only; but a woman's sense enjoys all ten in full."

Hesiod *The Melampodia* (8th century BC)

A certain noble gentleman, having lost his virile member through some devilish arts, went to a witch to see if it was possible to restore it or have it replaced. She showed him a nest at the foot of a tree which contained several, and indicated that he could take his choice. When, however, he chose a large one, she said: "Don't take that, it is not for you, it belongs to a man of the people."

Johann Sprenger and Heinrich Kraemer
Malleus Maleficarum (1489)

Interestingly, to these old myths have been added some peculiarly modern superstitions such as that sun lamps arouse sexual passion, that girls with contact lenses cannot take oral contraceptive pills, and that the wedding ceremony confers immunity to venereal disease! America, in particular, has become the home of some of the strangest sex superstitions to be found anywhere. ...Among men it is said that sex during a woman's period can lead to baldness, even impotence. Girls, for their part, have an idea that a Coca Cola douche will prevent pregnancy.

Philippa Waring *A Dictionary of Omens and Superstitions* (1978)

Finally, two Anglo-Saxon 'nonsense' riddles:

A strange thing hangs by a man's thigh
Under its master's clothes. It is pierced in front,
Is stiff and hard, has a good fixed place.
When the man lifts his own garment
Up above the knee, he wishes to visit
With the head of this hanging tool the familiar hole
Which it, when of equal length, has often filled before.

Answer: a key

I am a wonderful creature, bringing joy to women,
And useful to those who dwell near me. I harm
No citizen except only my destroyer.
My site is lofty; I stand in a bed;
Beneath, somewhere, I am shaggy. Sometimes
The very beautiful daughter of a peasant,
A courageous woman, ventures to lay hold on me,
Assaults my red skin, despoils my head,
Clamps me in a fashion. She who thus confines me,
This curly haired woman, soon feels
My meeting with her – her eye becomes wet

Answer: an onion

The Exeter Book (c. 1060)

Sexual Techniques

The physical essentials of coitus can be quickly summarized – as in this instructional work for small children:

The man loves the woman. So he gives her a kiss. And she gives him a kiss. And they hug each other very tight. And after a while, the man's penis becomes stiff and hard and much bigger than it usually is. It gets bigger because it has lots of work to do. The man wants to get as close to the woman as he can, because he's feeling very loving to her. And to get really close the best thing he can do is lie on top of her and put his penis inside her, into her vagina. Making love is a very nice feeling for both the man and the woman. He likes being inside her, and she likes him being inside her.

Peter Mayle *Where Did I Come From?* (1973)

The basic act may appear constant and unchanging:

If you watch lizards and lions copulating, then you will see that in 200,000,000 years the male has not had a single new idea.

Robert Ardrey *The Hunting Hypothesis* (1976)

In fact, this statement is not altogether true:

All animals except man customarily copulate in a rear-entry position; exceptions are rare. By contrast, there is no known human society in which rear-entry is the usual pattern of intercourse. The universality of face-to-face intercourse in human beings reflects the anatomical fact that the vaginal opening of the human female is further forward than in other mammals. Face-to-face copulation affords a better opportunity for intense stimulation of the woman's sexual organs, particularly the clitoris, than does rear-entry, and is therefore more apt to bring her to orgasm.

Clellan Ford and Frank Beach *Patterns of Sexual Behaviour* (1951)

Face-to-face activity also allows, or should allow, a greater personal rapport between the participants. Sadly, much sexual activity over the centuries could be summed up in this description of middle-class 'love-making' in 17th- and 18th-century England:

Man on top, woman on bottom, little foreplay, rapid ejaculation, masculine unconcern for feminine orgasm.

M. E. Shorter *Capitalism, Culture, and Sexuality* (1972)

A combination of male insensitivity with female indifference can probably be blamed:

Most men in love are like apes trying to play a violin.

Honoré de Balzac (19th century)

I can never understand why most people have sex so quickly. You'd think they didn't enjoy it, the way they plunge in, thrash up and down, and then turn their backs on each other and go to sleep.

Graham Masterton *How to Drive Your Man Wild in Bed* (1975)

I had one of those splittings of a second where the senses fly out and there in that instant the itch reached into me and drew me out and I jammed up her ass and came as if I'd been flung across the room. She let out a cry of rage.

Norman Mailer *An American Dream* (1964)

The male sexual ideal of virility without languor or amorousness is profoundly desolating: when the release is expressed in mechanical terms it is sought mechanically. Sex becomes masturbation in the vagina.

Germaine Greer *The Female Eunuch* (1970)

In terms of sexual expertise, what really distinguishes the men from the boys is skill and sensitivity in foreplay. Here is one of the boys depriving Fanny Hill of her virginity:

First he put one of the pillows under me, to give the blank of his aim a more favourable elevation, and another under my head, in ease of it: then spreading my thighs and placing himself between them, made them rest upon his hips: applying then the point of his machine to the slit, into which he sought entrance; it was so small, he could scarce assure himself of its being rightly pointed. He looks, feels, and satisfies himself; then driving forward with fury, its prodigious stiffness thus impacted, wedge-like, breaks the union of those parts, and gain'd him just the insertion of the tip of it, lip-deep; which being sensible of, he improves his advantage, and following well his stroke, in a strait line, forcibly deepens his penetration.

John Cleland *Fanny Hill: Memoirs of a Woman of Pleasure* (1748–49)

This young man had clearly not studied the ancient Greeks:

Let there be lewd touching first and games before the work.

Anon. (5th century BC)

or Erasmus:

...a man must hug, and dandle, and kittle, and play a hundred little tricks with his bed-fellow when he is disposed to make that use of her that nature designed her for.

The Praise of Folly (1509)

or the English poets:

Licence my roving hands, and let them go
Before, behind, between, above, below.
O my America, my new found land,
My kingdom, safeliest when with one man manned,
My mine of precious stones, my empery,
How blessed am I in this discovering thee!
To enter in these bonds, is to be free;
Then where my hand is set, my seal shall be.

John Donne 'To His Mistress Going to Bed' (late 16th century)

Naked she lay, clasped in my longing arms,
I filled with love, and she all over charms;
Both equally inspired with eager fire,
Melting through kindness, flaming in desire.
With arms, legs, lips close clinging to embrace,
She clips me to her breast, and sucks me to her face.
Her nimble tongue, Love's lesser lightning, played
Within my mouth, and to my thoughts conveyed
Swift orders that I should prepare to throw
The all-dissolving thunderbolt below.

John Wilmot, Earl of Rochester 'The Imperfect Enjoyment' (1680)

In the 18th century Princess Maria Theresa, worried that she had failed to provide the future Hapsburg emperor with an heir, received the following respectful advice:

I think the vulva of Her Most Holy Majesty should be titillated before intercourse.

Quoted in V. C. Medvei *A History of Endocrinology* (1982)

Another piece of advice for married ladies:

Use the man that you wed like your fav'rite guitar.
Tho' music in both, they are both apt to jar
How tuneful and smooth from a delicate touch

Not handled too roughly, nor play'd on too much!

Anon. rhyme from *Sketches of the Fair Sex* (ed. John Adams; 1807)

In this century, we have been told often enough about the physical and psychological importance of foreplay:

The man who neglects love-play is guilty not only of coarseness but of positive brutality; and his omission can not only offend and disgust a woman, but also injure her purely on the physical plane.

Theodor Van de Velde *Ideal Marriage* (1928)

True sexual proficiency can only be acquired from experience and a willingness to both learn and teach:

A good sex life isn't something that you're born with, any more than you're born with the ability to cook, or crochet, or take shorthand.

Graham Masterton *How to Drive Your Man Wild in Bed* (1975)

No art can be learned at once. And lovemaking is a sublime art that needs practice if it's to be true and significant.

Charles Chaplin, quoted by Irving et al. in *Intimate Sex Lives of Famous People* (1981)

Sometimes it is the woman who needs guidance:

'Just kiss me'
She kissed him on the cheek.
'No.'
'Where do the noses go? I always wondered where the noses would go.'
'Look, turn thy head.' and then their mouths were tight together.

Ernest Hemingway *For Whom the Bell Tolls* (1940)

sometimes the man:

A woman who wants to be caressed in a certain way will, if her wish is not fulfilled for a long time, caress her lover in this manner: she will, for instance, kiss him behind the ear if this is an erogenous zone for her. This is an indication that, generally, she does to him what she wishes he would do for her.

Theodor Reik *Sex in Man and Woman* (1960)

while often it is a learning experience for both:

may i feel said he
(i'll squeal said she
just once said he)
it's fun said she
(may i touch said he
how much said she
a lot said he)
why not said she
(let's go said he
not too far said she
what's too far said he
where you are said she)

e. e. cummings 'may i feel said he' (1930s)

Much detailed advice on foreplay and other aspects of sexual technique has been proffered over the centuries:

Fire [male sexuality] *easily flares up, but is easily extinguished by water; water* [female sexuality] *takes a long time to heat over the fire, but cools down very slowly.*

I-Ching (12th century BC)

Use force. Women like forceful men. They often seem to surrender unwillingly when they're really anxious to give in.

When you find the spot where a woman loves to be touched, don't be too shy to touch it... You'll see her eyes sparkle... She'll moan and whisper sweet nothings and sigh contentedly... But be careful that you don't gallop ahead, leaving her behind. And make sure that she doesn't reach the finish before you do.

Ovid *Ars Amatoria* (1st century AD)

Every man who has obtained a beautiful crucible will naturally love her with all his heart. But every time he copulates with her he should force himself to think of her as ugly and hateful.

Su-nii-ching *Fang Nei Chi* (*Secrets of the Bedchamber*) (c. 600)

When a man and a woman have intercourse for the first time, the man should sit down at the woman's left side and the woman should sit on the man's right. Then the man crosses his legs and places the woman in his lap...

The man sucks the woman's lower lip, the woman sucks the man's upper lip. They kiss each other, feeding on each other's saliva. Or the man softly bites the woman's tongue or gnaws her lips a little, places her head in his hands and pinches her ears. Thus patting and kissing, a thousand charms will unfold and the hundred sorrows will be forgotten...

The Jade Stalk should hover lightly around the precious entrance of the Cinnabar Gate, while the owner kisses the woman lovingly, or allows his eyes to linger over her body or look down upon her Golden Cleft. He should stroke her stomach and breast, and caress her Jewel Terrace. As her desire increases, he should begin to move his Positive Peak more decisively, back and forward, bringing it now into direct contact with the Golden Cleft and the Jade Veins, playing from side to side of the Examination Hall, and finally bringing it to rest at the side of the Jewel Terrace. Then, when the Cinnabar Cleft was in flood, it was time for the Vigorous Peak to thrust inward.

Li Tung-Hsuan *The Art of Love* (7th century)

Most gentle reader, [the clitoris is]*...pre-eminently the seat of woman's delight. If you touch it, you will find it rendered a little harder and oblong to such a degree that it shows itself as a sort of male member. Since no-one has discerned these projections and their workings, if it is permissible to give names to things discovered by me, it should be called the 'love sweetness of Venus.'*

Renaldus Columbus *De re anatomica* (1559)

Let her expressions be common ones, as my dear, my own heart, my soul, I am dying, let us die together, and such like, which will show a feigned sentiment, if not a true one. Let her add panting and sighing, and other gallantries, which will give her out to be melting, to be swooning, to be totally consumed, whereas in fact she is not even moved, but more as if she is made of wood or marble than of flesh. She must give pleasure through her words, if not her deeds, authenticating her words by closing her eyes, by anandoning herself as if lifeless, and by then rising up again in full strength with a vehement sigh, as if she were panting in the oppression of extreme joy, though in fact she be reduced and languid.

Ferrante Pallavicino *La Retorica della Putane* (1642)

Most discussion of coitus itself has focused on the activity and equipment of the male:

The change of the penis from the limp, soft, friendly, retiring appendage into a decidedly larger, stiff, erect, bold, proud and imperious organ...is surely one of Nature's greatest miracles.

Robert Chartham *Sex Manners for Men* (1967)

Deep and shallow, slow and quick, straight and slanting thrusts, all these are by no means uniform, each has its own characteristics.
A slow thrust should resemble the movement of a carp caught on the hook; a quick thrust should resemble the flight of birds against the wind. Inserting and withdrawing, moving up and down and from left to right...

Li Tung-Hsuan *The Art of Love* (7th century)

Size has been a particular preoccupation:

Take every pain in infancy to enlarge the privy member of boys (by massage and the application of stimulants), since a well-grown specimen never comes amiss.

Gabriello Fallopio *Obseruationes anatomicae* (1561)

The bites of insects, particularly bees, have been solicited by males both masochistically to enjoy the painful sensations, and in order to cause the penis to swell and thus enlarge the organ, after which sexual intercourse was engaged in before the swelling had a chance to recede.

Robert E. L. Masters *The Hidden World of Erotica* (1973)

Although, it may be that one is better off not tampering with what one has:

I fail to see any special merit in penises of more than the usual size. What more can they achieve than the smaller ones? I have read history carefully, and I nowhere find it of record that the sizes of Washington, Bonaparte, Franklin, Julius Caesar, or any of the worthies whose names illuminate history, it is fair to assume that they carried regular sizes. In this, as in everything else, quality is more to be considered than quantity.

Mark Twain *The Mammoth Cod* (1902)

The role of the female genitalia has elicited less comment:

A woman's body is well-lubricated in the clinch, and her lips are tender and soft for kissing. Therefore she holds a man's body wholly and congenially sedged into her embraces, into her very flesh, and her partner is totally incompassed with pleasure.

Achilles Tatius *Leukippe and Kleitophon* (4th century AD)

If the pelvic floor muscles are slack and you do not know how to use them, you are missing out on one whole aspect of sexual experience.

Sheila Kitzinger *Woman's Experience of Sex* (1983)

The vagina walls are quite insensitive in the great majority of females... There is no evidence that the vagina is ever the sole source of arousal, or even the primary source of erotic arousal in any female.

Alfred Kinsey et al. *Sexual Behaviour in the Human Female* (1953)

Many women admit to finding greater satisfaction in foreplay than in penetrative sex:

She loved it when Brian blew into her ear, gently bit the base of her thumb, or stroked her breasts in circles... 'Oh love, love,' she murmured. 'Oh bliss.' If only he had been satisfied to stop there, he could feel her thinking. But no, he always had to bring out, or up, what she called 'that thing'. 'Don't put that thing in yet please, darling; I'm not ready.'

Alison Lurie *The War Between the Tates* (1974)

In Christian Europe non-penetrative sexual activity has often been stigmatized as perverted or immoral:

In a tortuously worded decree of 342 the emperors Constantius and Constans prohibited sexual relations between man and wife in any fashion that did not involve penetration of the vagina by the penis. The intent, clearly enough, was to outlaw anal and oral sex between married persons.

James A. Brundage *Law, Sex and Christian Society in Medieval Europe* (1987)

Other cultures have had similar inhibitions:

The [Chinese] *sexual handbooks gave great detail of the various positions that could be adopted in sexual intercourse. Cunnilingus was approved, especially in Taoist texts, since it procured Yin esence for the Man. But anal penetration and fellatio should only be used as preliminaries and if there was no complete male emission.*

Geoffrey Parrinder *Sex in the World's Religions* (1980)

By contrast, modern sexologists have stressed the importance of variety and innovation:

There are many routes ('positions', 'techniques') to orgasms, and, say the sexologists, we must be ready to use them all. To limit oneself to particular techniques, to use only certain positions is to lose the chance of all manner of interesting possibilities out of a craven fear of the unknown.

Philippe Ariès and André Bejin *Western Sexuality* (1982)

There is nothing that a husband and wife can do with each other sexually that is de-

praved or perverse so long as they both enjoy it.

Robert Chartham *Sex Manners for Men* (1967)

There is no norm in sex. Norm is the name of a guy who lives in Brooklyn.

Dr Alex Comfort *Medical World News* (Nov. 1974)

It doesn't matter what you do in the bedroom as long as you don't do it in the street and frighten the horses.

Mrs Patrick Campbell, quoted by Daphne Fielding in *The Duchess of Jermyn Street* (1977)

Or as Woody Allen famously answered the question 'Is sex dirty?'

Only if it's done right!

Everything You Always Wanted to Know About Sex (1972)

It has also been remarked that for human beings the most important erogenous zone is always the mind:

If the psyche is unwilling, no amount of technique can persuade it; and if the psyche is willing, no lack of technique can dissuade it.

Ann Aldrich *We Walk Alone* (1970)

Transvestism and Transsexualism

What is the distinction between transvestism and transsexualism?

The term transsexual is the most appropriate term for the most extreme group of transvestites who wish to change their sex. Transvestism is the desire of a certain group of men to dress as women or of women to dress as men. It can be powerful and overwhelming, even to the point of wanting to belong to the other sex and correct nature's 'anatomical error'.

Harry Benjamin *Transsexualism and Sex Reassignment* (1969)

The…transsexual wishes to wear women's clothes always, because he wants to be a female all his life; the transvestite wears women's clothes intermittently, usually only for a few minutes or hours but does not want to be a female.

Robert J. Stoller *The Gender Disorders* (1964)

Although the nature of transsexualism is now much better understood, its cause remains a mystery. It is, however, indisputable that many biologically normal men and women have an overwhelming conviction that they 'really' belong to the opposite sex. This conviction, which may emerge at any time from childhood to old age, becomes unshakeable and does not usually respond to therapy:

For the transsexual, the psychiatrist's consulting room is a battlefield and the therapy sessions a bitter war. Armed only with his conviction that his body is alien to his 'true' identity, the transsexual is at a considerable disadvantage.

Rebecca Gardiner 'Diary of a Sex Change' *Observer* (28 June 1992)

I was three or perhaps four years old when I realized that I had been born into the wrong body, and should really be a girl. I remember the moment well, and it is the earliest memory of my life… What triggered so bizarre a thought I have long forgotten, but the conviction was unfaltering from the start…

Trans-sexualism is…not a sexual mode or preference. It is not an act of sex at all. It is a passionate, lifelong, ineradicable conviction, and no true trans-sexual has ever been disabused of it.

Jan Morris *Conundrum* (1974)

For the genuine transsexual, the only hope of contentment lies in assuming the identity of a member of the opposite sex. In the appropriate cases this can now be achieved by a combination of surgery and hormone therapy:

Male-to-female transsexuals may have their male organs surgically removed and an artificial vagina constructed. This operation has been performed now for more than 40 years and is very successful. Female hormone enables them to grow breasts, but most have silicone implants as well… Surgically, female-to-males have their breasts removed – these are always the feature they hate the most – and a hysterectomy. Most do not have a constructed penis, as the operation to perform phalloplasty is still experimental and, usually, not cosmetically acceptable.

Independent (Jan. 1993)

Although transvestism can be a symptom of the more extreme transsexuality, most cross-dressers are heterosexuals with an otherwise normal sex life. It just so happens that wearing female clothes turns them on – either as a prelude to masturbation or in some cases simply as a means of achieving a feeling of psychological release. Often their wives or girlfriends are unaware of their transvestism:

An essential part of transvestism is a fetishistic preoccupation partly with the female wardrobe and partly with the woman as such.

Preben Hertoft *Psychosexual Problems* (1976)

Cross-dressing for psychosexual reasons is almost exclusively a male phenomenon:

Most transvestites are men, in part because the practice of women wearing men's clothes is not seen as deviant behaviour in Western society and indeed has been fashionable from time to time.

Encyclopaedia Britannica

Fetishistic cross-dressing is essentially unheard of in women. While women cross-dress, they do not do so because the clothes excite them erotically.

Robert J. Stoller *The Gender Disorders* (1964)

Although not generally regarded as sexually deviant, female cross-dressing has often incurred moral and social disapproval. In the past, women have assumed male dress in order to escape the restrictions of their sexual role:

For my part, I am content to be in his Attire: for wearing a Man's Disguise always fills me with a Sense of Freedom, e'en Wantonness. I chase him round the Bed again, delighting in the Novelty of this Change in Status.

Erica Jong *Fanny* (1970)

In American history we have Deborah Sampson, a Massachusetts girl who taught school for two terms to earn money enough to put herself into men's clothes and join the army. As Robert Shurtleff, she served three years of the American Revolution in a fighting regiment, her sex undiscovered in camps, on marches or in battles (although she was twice wounded), until a fever sent her to a hospital.

David Loth *The Erotic in Literature* (1962)

Through her transvestism, she [Joan of Arc] *abrogated the destiny of womankind. She could thereby transcend her sex; she could set herself apart and usurp the privileges of the male and his claims to superiority. At the same time, by never pretending to be other than a woman and a maid, she was not only usurping a man's function but shaking off the trammels of his sex altogether to occupy a different, third order, neither male nor female but unearthly, like the angels whose company she loved.*

Marina Warner *Joan of Arc: The Image of Female Heroism* (1981)

Attitudes to male transvestism have varied widely from one age and culture to another. Many societies have accepted it within certain defined limits and conventions. In Tahiti, for instance:

When they get older these men-women continue to be treated with amused tolerance. They are not particularly common. They dress and behave as women, and always do women's work such as washing, sewing and looking after babies. They are called mahou. The Tahitians made no extra fuss of an old man known as the Queen's mahou. He sported a white beard, wore a colourful frock and paid attention to his hair. The venerable old gentleman was a completely accepted character on Papeete, far more than he would be in so-called Western civilization.

A. Denis *Taboo* (1966)

In ancient Greece and Rome cross-dressing played a role in the mythology and ritual of the mystery religions:

Ritual transvestism was fairly common in Greek cult. The procession of the

Oschophoria was led by two boys dressed as girls. Performers of Dionysus' ritual dance, the Ithyphallos, appeared in the costume of the opposite sex. In the Hybristika and Hysteria, Aphrodite's festival at Argos, men wore women's veils and women wore male dress. In the festival of Hera on Samos, men wore women's robes and adorned themselves with bracelets, necklaces and golden hairnets. On wedding nights at Cos, the bridegroom wore women's robes. At Sparta, the bride, head shaved, wore men's garments and boots. At Argos, the bride donned a false beard.

Camille Paglia *Sexual Personae* (1990)

Rhea castrated Atys, who thereupon dressed himself in female clothes, and travelled all over the earth, initiating orgies and singing hymns in her honour.

Lucian *Erotes* (2nd century)

Self-castration was a one way road to ritual impersonation. In the mystery religions, which influenced Christianity, the devotee initiated and sought union with his god. The priest of the Great Mother changed his sex in order to become her. Transsexualism was the severe choice, transvestism less so.

Camille Paglia *Sexual Personae* (1990)

On the whole, however, Greek and Roman writers treat the subject of cross-dressing with ridicule:

DIONYSUS *While sane he'll not consent to put on a woman's clothes; once free from the curb of reason, he will put them on. I long to set Thebes laughing at him, as he walks in female garb through all the streets.*

Euripides *The Bacchae* (407 BC)

Yet what will not other men do when you, Creticus, dress yourself in garments of gauze...you Creticus, you the keen unbending champion of human liberty, to be clothed in a transparency.

Juvenal *Satire II* (2nd century)

Many cultures – notably the Chinese and Japanese – have a tradition of female impersonation in the theatre. In England, female characters were played by men until after the Restoration (1660). Shakespeare's heroines were all originally played by boys – adding a further layer of ambiguity to plots that often turned on the assumption of male disguise by women:

ROSALIND *I could find it in my heart to disgrace my man's apparel and to cry like a woman; but I must comfort the weaker vessel, as doublet and hose ought to show itself courageous to petticoat...*

William Shakespeare *As You Like It* (1599)

The practice of dressing boys as women provoked furious denunciation from Puritans:

Our apparel was given to us as a sign distinctive to discern betwixt sex and sex, and therefore for one to wear the apparel of another sex, is to participate with the same and to adulterate the verity of his own kind.

Philip Stubbes *Anatomy of Abuses* (1583)

There is also the established tradition of the female impersonator – a male performer who presents a parodic version of femininity to broad comic effect:

Female impersonators do not refer to themselves as transvestites. Sometimes in interviews one would reluctantly say 'Well, I guess I'm sort of a transvestite,' but would then quickly add, 'but I only do it for a living,' or, 'this is my job.' To female impersonators, the real transvestites are the lone wolves whose individual and private experiments are described as 'freakish'. To them the transvestite is one who dresses as a woman for some 'perverted' sexual purpose.

E. Newton *Mother Camp: Female Impersonators in America* (1972)

Outside these accepted channels, transvestism has been a strictly underground phenomenon until very recently. Private clubs for cross-dressers are recorded as early as the 18th century:

They adopt all the small vanities natural to the feminine sex to such an extent that they try to speak, walk, chatter, shriek and scold as women do, aping them as well in other respects.

Edward Ward *History of the London Club* (1709–11)

The men calling one another 'my dear' and hugging, kissing, and tickling each other as if they were a mixture of wanton males and females, and assuming effeminate voices and airs; some telling others that they ought to be whipped for not coming to school more frequently...Some were completely rigged in gowns, petticoats, headcloths, fine laced shoes, furbelowed scarves, and masks; some had riding hoods; some were dressed like milkmaids, others like shepherdesses with green hats, waistcoats, and petticoats; and others had their faces patched and painted and wore very extensive hoop petticoats, which had been very lately introduced.

Samuel Stevens *Select Trials* (1725)

Even today transvestites endure frequent verbal and physical abuse. Many heterosexual men, in particular, find the cross-dresser a threat to their own masculine identity:

The queen is the most dangerous of creatures. He is always on the verge of threatening a man's virility. This is not solely because the queen represents a man's antithesis, the extreme evil to be avoided at all costs (American education as a whole being devoted to making boys different from girls), but because the queen is so nearly a woman that even a hidebound heterosexual may make a mistake.

Georges-Michel Sarotte *Like a Brother, Like a Lover* (1978)

The transvestite's chosen way of life demands great self-assurance:

...what you get with coming out about being TV is the confidence to walk down the street in a skirt and high heels and to say to the person who comes up to you and asks 'Are you a bloke in a dress?', 'Yes, I am thank you very much.'

Eddie Izzard, interviewed in the *Independent* (18 Feb. 1993)

It also requires unusual dedication in other respects:

I'm fascinated by boys who spend their lives trying to be girls, because they have to work so hard – double-time – getting rid of all the tell-tale male signs and drawing in all the female signs. I'm not saying its the right thing to do, I'm not saying it's a good idea, I'm not saying it's not self-defeating and self-destructive and I'm not saying it's not possibly the single most absurd thing a man can do with his life. What I'm saying is, it is very hard work. You can't take that away from them. It's hard work to look like the complete opposite of what nature made you.

Andy Warhol *From A to B and Back Again* (1975)

Just occasionally, the transvestite asks himself if it is all worth while:

All my life I wanted to look like Liz Taylor. Now I find that Liz Taylor is beginning to look like me.

Divine, 20-stone transvestite actor (1981)

Virginity

She was aye a virgin at Seventeen
A very rare thing in Aberdeen.

Anon. epitaph on Scottish tombstone, discovered by Spike Milligan and quoted in the *Independent on Sunday* (21 June 1992)

Traditionally, the virginity of a woman or girl has been taken as an outward sign of her purity and integrity. Poets and moralists have emphasized the beauty of the virgin state, the constant care required in preserving it, and the irreparable nature of its loss:

Look, how a flower in some close garden grows
Hid from rude cattle, bruised by no plows,
Wind-stroked, sun-strengthened, nurtured by rain;
To pluck it many a youth and maid is fain!
But once 'tis culled, its beauty fades away,
No youth, no maid, desires it from that day:
So is a virgin loved, while she is chaste.
But if within a lover's arms embraced
She lets her body's flower be gathered, then
No longer is she dear to maids or men.
Hymen alone is our defence and shield
To Hymen Hymenaeus all must yield.

Catullus (1st century BC)

In many prescientific cultures, reverence for virginity was expressed in a variety of folk beliefs and superstitions:

Some say no evil thing that walks by night,
In fog or fire, by lake or moorish fen,
Blue meagre hag, or stubborn unlaid ghost,
That breaks his magic chains at curfew time,
No goblin, or swart faery of the mine,
Hath hurtful power o'er true virginity.

John Milton *Comus* (1637)

We hear of a certain poor and very devout virgin, one of whose friends had been grievously bewitched in his foot, so that it was clear to the physicians that he could be cured by no medicines. But it happened that the virgin went to visit the sick man, and he at once begged her to apply some benediction to his foot. She consented, and did no more than silently say the Lord's Prayer...at the same time making...the sign of the life-giving Cross. The sick man then felt himself at once cured.

Johann Sprenger and Heinrich Kraemer *Malleus Maleficarum* (c. 1486)

A virgin should touch the patient with her right thumb – a circumstance that has led to the belief that persons suffering from epilepsy should eat the flesh of animals in a virgin state.

Pliny the Elder *Natural History* (77 AD)

Tests of virginity have been many and varied over the ages, most of them firmly rooted in superstition...In Britain, for example, it was said that if a girl could look into the sun it was a sure sign she still possessed her virginity...In Germany and Austria, only a virgin could blow back into life a still glowing candle, while in Hungary the one sure proof that a girl still had her maidenhead was that she could walk through a swarm of bees without being stung. The bees, apparently, would not touch a pure woman...In the depths of Poland an extraordinary claim was once advanced that a virgin had the power to roll water up in balls, while it would perhaps be hard to find a nastier belief than that which claimed that sexual intercourse with a virgin would cure venereal disease.

Philippa Waring *A Dictionary of Omens and Superstitions* (1978)

Many societies have inflicted severe penalties on women who lose their virginity while still unmarried:

Our forefathers were so severe where their honour was affected, and valued the purity of their children's morals so highly, that one of the citizens, becoming aware that his daughter had been violated and that she had not preserved her maidenhood until her marriage, shut her up with a horse in a lonely house, so that she died of hunger.

Aeschines *Contra Timarchum* (4th century BC)

The Old Testament prescribes this treatment for the bride found not to be a virgin on her wedding night:

Then they shall bring out the damsel to the door of her father's house, and the men of her city shall stone her with stones that she die: because she hath wrought folly in Israel, to play the whore in her father's house: so shalt thou put evil away from among you.

Deuteronomy 22:21

In most European countries, the penalties have been social and economic rather than legal:

The endeavour to protect virginity or otherwise to control female sexuality is a feature of most societies ancient and modern, though the diverse efforts to achieve this particular end change form, depending on patterns of kinship, economic and power relationships.

Michel Foucault *The Archaeology of Knowledge* (1972)

In particular, loss of virginity has been held to disqualify a girl from the marriage market:

Unhappy as the event must be for Lydia, we may draw from it this useful lesson: that loss of virtue in a female is retrievable; that one false step involves her in endless ruin; that her reputation is no less brittle than it is beautiful; and that she cannot be too much guarded in her behaviour towards the undeserving of the other sex.

Jane Austen *Pride and Prejudice* (1813)

I discovered how girls were sent ignorant through life into marriage, and pleaded that they, like men, had a right to know themselves and what was the nature of the contract to which they were giving themselves for life – then I remember I was told by one, who herself had the care of daughters, that that ignorance formed too valuable an addition to the virginal charm of womanhood in the marriage market.

Laurence Housman *The Immoral Effects of Ignorance* (1911)

Are there still virgins? One is tempted to answer no. There are only girls who have not yet crossed the line, because they want to preserve their market value...Call them virgins if you wish, these travelers in transit.

Françoise Giroud *Coronet* (Nov. 1960)

My mother used to say, Delia, if S-E-X ever rears its ugly head, close your eyes before you see the rest of it.

Alan Ayckbourn *Bedroom Farce* (1978)

In the pre-contraceptive era, fear of unwanted pregnancy was the all-powerful deterrent:

When he and I got under sheet,
I let him have his way complete,
And now my girdle will not meet
Dear God, what shall I say of it?

Ah dear God, I am forsaken,
Now my maidenhead is taken!

Anon., late medieval carol

There was a young lady called Wylde,
Who kept herself quite undefiled
By thinking of Jesus
Contagious diseases,
And the bother of having a child.

Norman Douglas *Some Limericks by Norman Douglas* (1917)

Loss of virginity has rarely carried any equivalent risk or stigma for men. Indeed, it has often been assumed that there is something pitiable or embarrassing about a sexually inexperienced adult male:

With regard to sexual relations, we should note that in giving herself to intercourse, the girl renounces her honour. This is not, however, the case with men, for they have yet another sphere for their ethical activity beyond that of the family.

G.W.F. Hegel *The Philosophy of Right* (1821)

What for a woman is a crime entailing dire legal and social consequences, is regarded in the case of a man as being honourable or, at most, as a slight moral stain that one bears with pleasure.

Friedrich Engels *The Origin of the Family, Private Property and the State* (1884)

In the male, of course, loss of virginity has no physical signs: the case is quite different with girls:

Although it is true that the hymen is often relaxed in virgins, or broken and diminished by accidents independent of all coition, such accidents are very rare, and the absence of the hymen is assuredly a good ground of strong suspicion.

Dr T. Bell *Kalogynomia* (1821)

In many cultures, husbands have demanded physical proof of virginity from their brides:

At a Samoan wedding there was a public demand for the tokens of virginity. The marriage of a chief's daughter took place in the village square before the assembled people; her virginity was tested publicly by the chief who inserted two fingers into her vulva. The crowd eagerly awaited the trickling of the blood, which was greeted with prolonged cheers. If, however, the girl failed to pass the test, her father and brothers would rush upon her with clubs, and despatch her in an instant.

G. Turner *Samoa, A Hundred Years Ago and Long Before* (1884)

Consequently some strange and cruel practices have been devised to maintain the pretence of virginity. Even in 1980s Britain, there were reported cases of doctors performing private operations to 'restore' the virginity of wealthy Asian brides. In the past astringents, such as alum, were sometimes used to contract the vagina:

The already Cuckold getts a Maidenhead,
Which is a toyle, made of restringent aide.
Cunt wash't with Allom makes a Whore a maid.

Anon. *Sodom, by E of R, written for the Royall Company of Whoremasters* (17th century)

Such stratagems have also been employed in brothels, where maidenheads have traditionally fetched a high price:

Once this sermon was done, the newcomer was presented to her companions, she was shown to her chamber in the house and the very next day her virginity was put up for sale. Within the space of four months, the same merchandise was sold in turn to eighty persons who each paid as though for unused goods, and it was only at the expiry of her thorny novitiate that Juliette was granted entry to the sisterhood.

Marquis de Sade *Justine, or the Misfortunes of Virtue* (1791)

By the eighteenth century in England the years at which a girl was regarded as choice by some sex maniacs had dropped even lower, and part of the mania was delight in the child's pain. Children described as coming hardly above a man's waist were pregnant: even more horrible was the practice in some brothers of renting out a little girl to be deflowered three or four times, sewing her up after each operation to get her ready for the next.

David Loth *The Erotic in Literature* (1962)

For men, deflowering a virgin has often been seen as a sign or test of virility:

As yet I have not destroyed the fortress of her maidenhood, which is still kept intact by delay since I avoided a fight. Yet if the battle begins anew, I will verily destroy her walls of virginity, nor shall any battlements hold me back.

Agathias of Myrina (6th century)

The satisfaction derived from the act may be partly or wholly sadistic:

No sooner did I feel the head lodged aright that I drove and shoved in with the utmost fury; feeling the head pretty well in I thrust and drove on, but gained so little that I drew it out, and wetting it with spittle I again effected the lodgement just within the lips. At length by my fierce rending and tearing thrusts the first defences gave way. I now recommenced my eager shoves, my fierce lungings, and I felt myself gaining at every move, till with one tremendous and cunt-rending thrust I buried myself in her up to the hilt. So great was the pain of this last shock that Rose could not suppress a sharp shrill scream, but I heeded it not: it was the note of final victory.

Anon. *Rose d'Amour* (19th century)

Although most cultures have required prenuptial virginity of women, and many religions have found an honoured role for celibacy, Roman Catholicism is unique in the emphasis it has placed on lifelong virginity as the ideal for both sexes:

There is nothing our Lord delighteth more in than virgins, nor wherein angels more gladly abide, and play with, and talk with.

Lewis Vives *The Instruction of Christian Woman* (1541)

In a very positive way, he [Peter Damian, Bishop of Ostia] *was passionately devoted to virginity, both in women and in men; he fervently believed that both Mary and Joseph has avoided all sexual intercourse, and that Jesus has entered the world without breaking Mary's hymen – a bizarre doctrine which he combined with the view that virginity, even if broken, could be miraculously restored.*

Christopher Brooke *The Medieval Idea of Marriage* (1989)

What is this gate [the hymen] *but Mary, closed because she is a virgin? Mary is the gate through which Christ entered the world, when he was born by a virgin birth, without opening the genital seal. The barrier of modesty remained intact and the seals of integrity were preserved.*

St Ambrose *De Institutione Virginis* (4th century)

Unlike the matriarchal societies...where physical virginity represented power, or ancient Greece where virginal intactness did not exist as a concept, in Christianity bodily purity is demanded in a context where women are conceived of as tainted beings. A virgin becomes defined as virgo intacta, a woman who has never experienced sexual intercourse, and this purity of body is to be combined with a purity of mind for God. Although men, too, are supposed to retain physical integrity, they can be rewarded with the priesthood and thus the ultimate closeness to the Lord. Women must settle for lesser status, and their physical virginity is given much greater emphasis.

Esther Lastique and Helen Rodnite Lemay 'A Medieval Guide to Virginity' in *Sex in the Middle Ages* (1991)

Traditional Catholic teaching has always seen virginity as superior to marriage:

Virginity stands as far above marriage as the heavens above the earth.

St John Chrysostom *De Virginitate* (c. 390)

The error of Jovian consisted in holding virginity not to be preferable to marriage. This error is refuted above all by the example of Christ Who both chose a virgin for His mother and remained Himself a virgin.

St Thomas Aquinas *Summa Theologica* (13th century)

Virginity seeks the soul's good in a life of contemplation mindful of the things of God. Marriage seeks the body's good – the bodily multiplication of the human race – in an active life in which husband and wife are mindful of the things of this world. Without doubt then the state of virginity is preferable to that of even continent marriage.

St Thomas Aquinas *Summa Theologica* (13th century)

Nuptiae terram replent, virginitas paradisum.

Marriage fills the earth, virginity heaven.

St Jerome *Adversus Iovinianum* (4th century)

See also CHASTITY AND CELIBACY

This attitude was not seriously challenged until the rise of Protestantism, which gave a new dignity to marriage and family life:

Only one woman in thousands has been endowed with the God-given aptitude to live in chastity and virginity...God fashioned her body so that she should be with a man, to have and to rear children. No woman should be ashamed of that for which God made and intended her.

Martin Luther *Kritische Gesamtausgabe* (1524)

After the break with Rome, with its conservative attitude to sexual relations, now no longer was virginity held to be a highest good, but a chastity of marriage was glorified by the Protestants.

Ivy Pinchbeck and Margaret Hewitt *Children in English Society* (1969)

The obvious retort to any insistence on virginity as a universal ideal is that, put into practice, such idealism would abolish the human race. This argument is adopted by Chaucer's Wife of Bath:

Did God at any time insist upon virginity? Everyone knows that when St Paul spoke of it, he said there was no law governing it. A woman may be advised to be a virgin, but that is only advice. It has been left for us to decide. If God had insisted upon virginity, he would have forbidden marriage. If that had happened, and no-one was ever born, where would we then find virginity?

Geoffrey Chaucer *The Canterbury Tales*, 'The Wife of Bath's Prologue' (late 14th century)

and extended by Shakespeare:

It is not politic in the commonwealth of nature to preserve virginity. Loss of virginity is rational increase and there was never virgin got till virginity was first lost. That you were made of is metal to make virgins. Virginity by being once lost may be ten times found; by being ever kept, it is ever lost: 'tis too cold a companion; away with 't!...To speak on the part of virginity, is to accuse your mothers; which is most infallible disobedience. He that hangs himself is a virgin: virginity murders itself; and should be buried in highways out of all sanctified limit, as a desperate offendress against nature. Virginity breeds mites, much like a cheese; consumes itself to the very paring, and so dies with feeding his own stomach. Besides, virginity is peevish, proud, idle, made of self-love, which is the most inhibited sin in the canon. Keep it not; you cannot choose but lose by 't: out with 't!

All's Well that Ends Well (c. 1602)

Others have mocked the cult of virginity from a variety of perspectives:

You spare your virginity. What's the use? When you're gone among the shades you won't find a lover, child. The ecstasies of Kypris are for the living. Down in Acheron, girl, as bones and dust we shall repose.

Asclepiades (300 BC)

It is clear that a young girl does not do well by remaining a virgin, or a married person by renouncing marriage...how then can it be that some who practise the virgin state make so great a thing of it, and say that they are 'filled with the Holy Spirit', for all the world like she who gave birth to Jesus!

Porphyrius *De Abstinentia* (3rd century AD)

It is one of the superstitions of the human mind to have imagined that virginity could be a virtue.

Voltaire *Notebooks* (1778)

A virgin is member of the army of the unenjoyed.

Leonard Louis Levison (20th century)

Nature abhors a virgin – a frozen asset.

Clare Boothe Luce (20th century)

To some, virginity is a burden to be shed as soon as possible:

Alas! I care not, Sir, what force you'd use
So I my Maiden-head could quickly lose:
Oft do I wish one skill'd in Cupid's Arts,
Would quickly dive into my private parts:
For as I am, at Home all sorts of weather,
I skit – as Heaven and Earth would come together,
Twirling a Wheel, I sit at home, hum drum,
And spit away my Nature on my thumb.

James Read *The Fifteen Plagues of a Maidenhead* (1707)

This, hotter than the other ten to one,
Longs to be put into her mother's trade,
And loud proclaims she lives too long a maid,
Wishing for one t'untie her virgin zone.

She finds virginity a kind of ware,
That's very troublesome to bear,
And being gone, she thinks will ne'er be missed:
And yet withal, the girl has so much grace,
To call for help I know she wants the face,
Though asked, I know not how she would resist.

Charles Cotton 'Two Rural Sisters' (17th century)

I thought of losing my virginity as a career move.

Madonna (1984)

In the permissive society of the 1960s and 1970s it even became an embarrassment:

An isolated outbreak of virginity like Lucinda's is a rash on the face of society. It arouses only pity from the married, and embarrassment from the single.

Charlotte Bingham *Lucinda* (1966)

Barbara Cartland, always the champion of the view that 'nice girls say no', was sure that fashion would come full circle:

I'll wager you that in 10 years it will be fashionable again to be a virgin.

Observer 'Sayings of the Week' (20 June 1976)

Ten years on, with growing recognition of the threat posed by the AIDS epidemic, she was claiming vindication:

I said 10 years ago that in 10 years time it would be smart to be a virgin. Now everyone is back to virgins again.

Observer 'Sayings of the Week' (12 July 1987)

This view is hardly borne out by social research. Surveys carried out in the late 1980s confirmed the trend of the previous two decades towards earlier loss of virginity in both boys and girls (in one 1989 survey nearly half the 16 year olds interviewed claimed to be sexually experienced):

There are many things which a girl under sixteen needs to practice but sex is not one of them.

Lord Templeman Appeal Court Hearing (1984)

At the same time, other surveys reveal that a considerable number of modern men would still 'ideally' like to marry a virgin. The double standard is obviously not entirely dead:

The men you meet aren't naive enough to expect virgins but they certainly don't want to hear about the 'ghosts' of your past life. Yet I can't imagine a man sticking around much after two or three months if you hadn't slept together.

Sacha Cowlam quoted by Angela Holdsworth in *Out of the Doll's House* (1988)

Wedding Nights

Much of the literature about wedding nights is preoccupied with the sexual state of the bride, dwelling on her loss of – or occasionally lack of – innocence:

> BRIDE *Maidenhood, maidenhood, where have you gone.*
> MAIDENHOOD *I have gone forever, forever.*
>
> Sappho 'Bride's Lament' (7th century BC)

> *Fears, fond and flight*
> *As the coy bride's, when night*
> *First does the longing lover right.*
>
> *Tears, quickly fled,*
> *And vain, as those are shed*
> *For a dying maidenhead.*
>
> Richard Crashaw 'Wishes to his Supposed Mistress' (1646)

> *Joy to the bridgroom and the bride*
> *That lie by one another's side!*
> *O fie upon the virgin beds,*
> *No loss is gain but maidenheads.*
> *Love quickly send this time may be*
> *When I shall deal my rosemary!*
>
> *I long to simper at a feast,*
> *To dance, and kiss, and do the rest.*
> *When I shall wed, and bedded be*
> *O then the qualm comes over me,*
> *And tells the sweetness of a theme*
> *That I ne'er knew but in a dream.*
>
> Thomas Randolph 'The Milkmaid's Epithalamium' (17th century)

> *When am'rous John in glowing hopes draws near;*
> *If my fair front to his I shall incline*
> *He'll say I'm bold and turn his head aside,*
> *And think he's purchased a lascivious bride.*
> *But that I no apology may lack*
> *I'm e'en resolved to lie upon my back.*
>
> Anon. (19th century)

> *O wha's the bride that cairries the bunch*
> *O' thistles blinterin' white?*
> *Her cuckold bridegroom little dreids*
> *What he sall ken this nicht.*
>
> *For closer than gudeman can come*
> *And closer to'r than hersel',*
> *What didna need her maidenhead*
> *Has wrocht his purpose fell.*
>
> *O wha's been here afore me, lass,*
> *And hoo did he get in?*
> – A man that deed or was I born
> This evil thing has din.
>
> *And left, as it were on a corpse,*
> *Your maidenhead to me?*
> – Nae less, gudeman, sin' Time began
> 'S hed ony mair to gi'e.
>
> Hugh MacDiarmid *A Drunk Man Looks at the Thistle* (1926)

The presumption that the bride would be a virgin seems often to have been little more than a polite convention. In the early 19th century

> *Juries seem to have paid little attention to arguments for the defence that "a girl who will so far forget herself as to anticipate the connubial rites, deserves little redress at the hands of the jury". The latter*

must have been only too aware that almost half of all English brides were pregnant on the day of their marriage.

Lawrence Stone *The Road to Divorce* (1989)

Nevertheless, for many inexperienced newlyweds the wedding night appears to have been something of a shock and an ordeal:

One woman, whose wedding night had been a deep shock because she had thought sleeping with a husband would be like sleeping with her sister, now thought sex unimportant.

Paul Thompson, Catherine Itzen, and Michele Abendstern *I Don't Feel Old* (1990)

Until comparatively recently...all too many women went to their wedding night without any idea at all how the sex act was performed.

Robert Chartham *Sex Manners for Men* (1967)

For some, the thought of the wedding night was so traumatic that they chose to take extreme measures:

One Victorian bridegroom, with admirable sensitivity, is said to have left the nuptial chamber to allow his blushing new wife to get ready for bed. After a suitable interval he returned. His heart leaped for joy, for there she lay, stretched out on the silken sheets, the object of all his desires. Unable to restrain himself any longer, he flung himself eagerly on the four-poster. But the bride did not stir. In fact she was out cold, drugged to the tip of her toes. Pinned to the pillow was this note, 'Mummy says you should do what you wish.'

Simon Welfare *Great Honeymoon Disasters* (1986)

Men were often advised to restrain their passions out of consideration for their brides:

Try to prevent your son-in-law from brutalizing your daughter on their wedding night, for many physical weaknesses and painful childbirths among delicate women stem from this cause alone. Men do not sufficiently understand that their pleasure is our martyrdom. So tell him to restrain his pleasure and to wait until he has little by little brought his wife to understanding and response. Nothing is more horrible than the terror, the sufferings, and the revulsion of a poor girl, ignorant of the facts of life, who finds herself raped by a brute. As far as possible we bring them up as saints, and then we hand them over as if they were fillies. If your son-in-law is an intelligent man, and if he truly loves your daughter, he will understand what must be done, and he will not resent your talking it over with him the day before.

George Sand, letter to her half-brother, Hippolyte Chatiron (19th century)

Although for some men the thought of inflicting this kind of a shock seems to have made the whole proceedings more exciting:

The Evening Star appears above Idalium
And brings Love's blessing to the nuptial bed,
New bride is overcome by modesty
And girlish teardrops mark the crimson veil.
But do not cease, young man, your close attack,
With love, subdue, opposing fingernail:
None can enjoy spring's perfumes or the honey
Of Hybla if he fears the scratch of a thorn.
Thorns arm the rose and bees defend their sweets,
And difficulties but increase the joy...
The kiss is sweeter stolen through tears.

Claudian 'Thorns Arm the Rose' (c. 400)

Women must often have discovered that men marry for many reasons, not all of them romantic:

Other elite couples were inspired to marry by more carnal ambitions. Few spelt it out more frankly than Frederick Mullins in 1747, when he complained that the trustees of his marriage settlement were unnecessarily delaying 'my taking possession of the charming Phoebe', adding by *way of explanation that they were 'not so eager for a f**k as I am.'*

A. P. W. Malcolmson *The Pursuit of the Heiress: Aristocratic Marriage in Ireland. 1750–1820*, quoted by Lawrence Stone in *The Road to Divorce* (1989)

Give me a Girl (if one I needs must meet)
Or in her Nuptial, or her winding sheet;
I know but two good Hours that women have,
One in the Bed, another in the Grave,
Thus of the whole Sex all I would desire,
Is to enjoy their Ashes, or their Fire.

William Cartwright 'Women' (17th century)

For men, too, the first night has often been a disturbing or disappointing experience. The case of John Ruskin, the Victorian art critic, is notorious:

He may have been impotent – as Effie later claimed when seeking an annulment – though Ruskin privately denied this. He himself hinted darkly that there were 'certain circumstances in her person' which 'completely checked' sexual passion. Whatever these may have been, they certainly did not discourage Effie's second husband, the Pre-Raphaelite painter John Everett Millais, by whom she had a number of children. For a long time it has been believed that Ruskin was indeed rendered impotent by the discovery that his wife's body differed from a statue of a classical goddess in having pubic hair. A more recent theory is that she was menstruating on their wedding night and that this disgusted him. But these explanations strike me as superficial. It is clear from Ruskin's writings that at this stage in his life he deeply distrusted all forms of sensuality.

David Barrie, Introduction to *Modern Painters* by John Ruskin (1987 abridged ed.)

Effie herself later complained in a letter to her father:

I had never been told the duties of married persons to each other and knew little or nothing about their relations in the closest union on earth.

Effie Ruskin, letter (Mar. 1854), quoted by Joan Abse in *John Ruskin: The Passionate Moralist* (1984)

That other great Victorian, Thomas Carlyle, similarly failed to consummate his marriage. In his (not too reliable) memoirs Frank Harris recounts Mrs Carlyle's alleged version of events:

"A little later he came up, undressed and got into bed beside me. I expected him to take me in his arms and kiss and caress me."
"Nothing of the sort, he lay there, jiggling like," ("I guessed what she meant," said Quain, "the poor devil in a blue funk was frigging himself to get a cock-stand.") "I thought for some time," Mrs Carlyle went on, "one moment I wanted to kiss and caress him; the next moment I felt indignant. Suddenly it occurred to me that in all my hopes and imaginings of a first night, I had never got near the reality: silent, the man lay there jiggling, jiggling. Suddenly I burst out laughing: it was all too wretched! too absurd!"
"At once he got out of bed with the one scornful word 'Woman!' and went into the next room: he never came back to my bed."

Frank Harris *My Life and Loves* (1923–27)

Whether through ignorance, anxiety, or more specialized psychosexual problems, men have often found difficulties in performing as expected:

On his marriage night he remained cold until, from necessity, he brought to his aid the memory-picture of an ugly woman's head with a nightcap. Coitus was immediately successful.

Richard von Krafft-Ebing *Psychopathia Sexualis* (1886)

One problem may be overindulgence at the wedding festivities:

Modesty forbids me to reveal the Secrets of the Marriage Bed, but nothing could have happen'd more suitable to my Circumstances than that, as above, *my Hus-*

band was so Fuddled when he came to Bed, that he could not remember in the Morning, whether he had had any Conversation with me or no, and I was oblig'd to tell him he had, *tho' in reality* he had not, *that I might be sure he could make no enquiry about any thing else.*

Daniel Defoe *Moll Flanders* (1722)

Why, happy bridegroom, why
Ere yet, the stars are kindled in the sky,
Ere twilight shades, or evening dews are shed,
Why dost thou steal so soon away to bed?...
Has Somnus brushed thy eyelids with his rod,
Or do thy legs refuse to bear thy load,
With flowing bowls of a more generous god?
If gentle slumber on thy temples creep,
(But naughty man, thou dost not mean to sleep)
Sleep by thyself and leave thy bride alone:
Go leave her with her maiden mates to play
At sports more harmless till the break of day.

Theocritus 'Song of the Sleepy Bridegroom' (3rd century BC)

At last came the moment when Abu Hasan was summoned to the bridal chamber. Slowly and solemnly he rose from his divan; but horror of horrors, being bloated with meat and drink, he let go a long and resounding fart. The embarrassed guests, whose attentions had been fixed upon the bridegroom, turned to one another speaking with raised voices and pretending to have heard nothing at all. Abu Hasan was so mortified with shame that he wished the ground would open up and swallow him. He mumbled a feeble excuse, and, instead of going to the bridal chamber, went straight to the courtyard, saddled his horse, and rode off into the night, weeping bitterly.

Tales from the Thousand and One Nights 'The Historic Fart'

Owing to embarrassment, inexperience, or exaggerated expectations, disappointment has been a common experience for both parties:

The embarrassments of our wedding night (Nancy and I being both virgins) were somewhat eased by an air raid: Zeppelin bombs dropping not far off set the hotel in an uproar.

Robert Graves *Goodbye to All That* (1929)

The First Time she was grave, as well she might,
For Women will be damn'd sullen the first Night;
But faith, they'll quickly mend, so be n't uneasie:
To Night she's brisk, and trys New Tricks to please ye.

Mary Griffith Pix *The Spanish Wives* (1696)

After Camille's murder, new desires seized them, but they had kept them under control, waiting for their wedding night, promising themselves frantic enjoyment when they could have it with impunity. And now at last their wedding night had come, and here they were, face to face, overcome with sudden uneasiness. They only had to stretch out their arms and crush each other in a passionate embrace, and lo! their arms seemed flabby as if they were already worn out with love-making. The oppression of the day weighed more and more heavily upon them, and they looked at each other with no desire but only timid awkwardness, irked at staying silent and cold. Their fevered dreams were turning into weird reality; the mere fact that they had succeeded in killing Camille and marrying, that Laurent's lips had touched Thérèse's shoulder, was enough to cool their lust to the point of nausea and horror.

Émile Zola *Thérèse Raquin* (1867–68)

Such disappointment is not, however, universal. Many writers have chosen to celebrate the sexual freedom that follows marriage:

Ma'aruf cast off all his clothes and, climbing into bed, threw himself upon the Prin-

cess as she lay on her back. He clasped her tight, and she pressed close to him, so that tongue met tongue in that hour when men forget their mothers. He slipped his hands under her armpits and strained her to his breast, squeezing all the honey and setting the dainties face to face. Then, threading the needle, he kindled the match, put it to the priming, and fired the shot. Thus the citadel was breached and the victory won.

Tales from One Thousand and One Nights
'The Tale of Ma'aruf the Cobbler'

"Ther nys no werkman, whatsoevere he be,
That may bothe werke wel and hastily;
This wol be doon at leyser parfitly.
It is no fors how longe that we pleye;
In trewe wedlok coupled be we tweye;
And blessed be the yok that we been inne,
For in oure actes we mowe do no synne.
A man may do no synne with his wyf,
Ne hurte hymselven with his owene knyf;
For we han leve to pleye us by the lawe."
Thus laboureth he til that the day gan dawe.

Geoffrey Chaucer *The Canterbury Tales*,
'The Merchant's Tale' (late 14th century)

*When in he came (*Dick*) there she lay*
Like new-faln snow melting away,
('Twas time I trow to part)
Kisses were now the onely stay,
Which soon she gave, as who would say,
Good Boy! *with all my heart.*

But just as heav'ns would have to crosse it,
In came the Bridesmaids with the Posset:
The Bridegroom eat in spight;
For had he left the Women to't
It would have cost two hours to do't,
Which were too much that night.

At length the candles out and out,
All that they had not done, they do't;
What that is, who can tell?
But I beleeve it was no more
Than thou and I have done before
With Bridget *and with* Nell.

Sir John Suckling 'A Ballade Upon a Wedding' (1646)

These snow-white breasts, which before you durst scarce touch with your little finger, you may now, without asking leave, grope by whole handfuls. Now you may practice delicious things to please your appetites.

Aphra Behn *The Curious Husband* (1671)

Other writers have emphasized a quieter kind of intimacy:

On my wedding night
I arrange the red candlesticks

Waiting for the morning
to wait on my in-laws

After my toilette
I whisper to my husband

Have I pencilled my eyebrows
sharply enough.

Chu Ching-yü 'The Toilette' (9th century)

It was my bridal night I remember,
An old man of seventy-three
I lay with my young bride in my arms,
A girl with t.b.
It was wartime, and overhead
The Germans were making a particularly heavy raid on Hampstead.
Harry, do they ever collide?
I do not think it has ever happened,
Oh my bride, my bride.

Stevie Smith 'I Remember' (20th century)

Many cultures have evolved distinct rituals and practices associated with the wedding night. To Westerners, some of these seem very strange:

Among the Dayaks of Dutch Borneo it is a rule that the bride and bridegroom must not sleep together on the wedding night, but their conduct before marriage is unrestricted…

Among the Swahili it is the rule that marriage must not be completely consum-

mated on the wedding night; the bridegroom has only partial connection with his wife, and completes the act with a girl who is at hand for the the purpose.

Robert Briffault *The Mothers: a Study of the Origins of Sentiments and Institutions* (1927)

The new-married couple are always disturbed toward morning by the women, who assemble to inspect the nuptial sheet, and dance around it. This ceremony is thought indispensably necessary nor is the marriage considered valid without it.

Mungo Park *Travels in the Interior Districts of Africa* (1799)

In the West, there is the tradition of wedding night advice and encouragement – such as Charles II's supposed remark to William of Orange as he led him and Mary to the bridal bed:

Now, nephew, to your work! Hey, St George for England!

and the advice of an anonymous 17th-century don to one of his undergraduates upon the occasion of his honeymoon:

Pleasures are augmented through their intermission, and the sweetness of a kiss will relish better after the cracking of a syllogism.

Quoted in *The Verney Family in the 17th Century* (ed. M. Slater)

Index

A

B

C

G

H

I

J

K

L

N

O

P

Q

R

S

T

U

V

W

Z